Essentials of
ORAL CANCER

Essentials of
ORAL CANCER

Editors

AK Dewan
MS MCh (Surgical Oncology)
Director
Department of Surgical Oncology
Rajiv Gandhi Cancer Institute
and Research Centre
New Delhi, India

Rajan Arora
MBBS MCh (Plastic Surgery)
Senior Reconstructive and
Microvascular Surgeon
Department of Surgical Oncology
Rajiv Gandhi Cancer Institute
and Research Centre
New Delhi, India

Swarupa Mitra
MBBS MD (Radiation Oncology)
Senior Consultant
Department of Radiation Oncology
Rajiv Gandhi Cancer Institute
and Research Centre
New Delhi, India

Ullas Batra
MBBS DM (Medical Oncology) ECMO FAGE
Senior Consultant and Co-Director
Department of Medical Oncology
Rajiv Gandhi Cancer Institute
and Research Centre
New Delhi, India

Foreword
Visweswar Bhattacharya

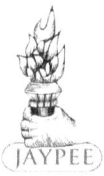

JAYPEE BROTHERS MEDICAL PUBLISHERS
The Health Sciences Publisher
New Delhi | London

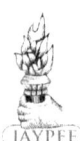
Jaypee Brothers Medical Publishers (P) Ltd

Headquarters
Jaypee Brothers Medical Publishers (P) Ltd
EMCA House, 23/23-B
Ansari Road, Daryaganj
New Delhi 110 002, India
Landline: +91-11-23272143, +91-11-23272703
+91-11-23282021, +91-11-23245672
Email: jaypee@jaypeebrothers.com

Corporate Office
Jaypee Brothers Medical Publishers (P) Ltd
4838/24, Ansari Road, Daryaganj
New Delhi 110 002, India
Phone: +91-11-43574357
Fax: +91-11-43574314
Email: jaypee@jaypeebrothers.com

Overseas Office
JP Medical Ltd
83 Victoria Street, London
SW1H 0HW (UK)
Phone: +44 20 3170 8910
Fax: +44 (0)20 3008 6180
Email: info@jpmedpub.com

Website: www.jaypeebrothers.com
Website: www.jaypeedigital.com

© 2022, Jaypee Brothers Medical Publishers

The views and opinions expressed in this book are solely those of the original contributor(s)/author(s) and do not necessarily represent those of editor(s) of the book.

All rights reserved. No part of this publication may be reproduced, stored or transmitted in any form or by any means, electronic, mechanical, photocopying, recording or otherwise, without the prior permission in writing of the publishers.

All brand names and product names used in this book are trade names, service marks, trademarks or registered trademarks of their respective owners. The publisher is not associated with any product or vendor mentioned in this book.

Medical knowledge and practice change constantly. This book is designed to provide accurate, authoritative information about the subject matter in question. However, readers are advised to check the most current information available on procedures included and check information from the manufacturer of each product to be administered, to verify the recommended dose, formula, method and duration of administration, adverse effects and contraindications. It is the responsibility of the practitioner to take all appropriate safety precautions. Neither the publisher nor the author(s)/editor(s) assume any liability for any injury and/or damage to persons or property arising from or related to use of material in this book.

This book is sold on the understanding that the publisher is not engaged in providing professional medical services. If such advice or services are required, the services of a competent medical professional should be sought.

Every effort has been made where necessary to contact holders of copyright to obtain permission to reproduce copyright material. If any have been inadvertently overlooked, the publisher will be pleased to make the necessary arrangements at the first opportunity. The **CD/DVD-ROM** (if any) provided in the sealed envelope with this book is complimentary and free of cost. **Not meant for sale.**

Inquiries for bulk sales may be solicited at: jaypee@jaypeebrothers.com

Essentials of Oral Cancer

First Edition: **2022**

ISBN: 978-93-5465-081-9

Dedicated to
My Parents

Contributors

Abhinav Dewan
MBBS DNB (Radiation Oncology)
Consultant
Department of Radiation Oncology
Rajiv Gandhi Cancer Institute and Research Centre
New Delhi, India

Abhishek Bansal
MBBS DNB (Radiodiagnosis)
Consultant
Department of Radiology
Rajiv Gandhi Cancer Institute and Research Centre
New Delhi, India

Abhishek Singh
BDS MDS (Oral and Maxillofacial Surgery)
Senior Resident
Department of Surgical Oncology
Rajiv Gandhi Cancer Institute and Research Centre
New Delhi, India

AK Dewan
MS MCh (Surgical Oncology)
Director
Department of Surgical Oncology
Rajiv Gandhi Cancer Institute and Research Centre
New Delhi, India

Ankita Jain
MBBS DNB (Surgical Oncology)
Attending Consultant
Department of Surgical Oncology
Rajiv Gandhi Cancer Institute and Research Centre
New Delhi, India

Bablesh Mahawar
MBBS DNB (Anesthesia)
FIPM and Palliative Care Physician
Fellowship in Pain Management
Consultant
MICU and Pain Physician
Department of Pain and Palliative Care
Rajiv Gandhi Cancer Institute and Research Centre
New Delhi, India

Ghanashyam Mandal
MBBS DLO DNB (ENT) Fellowship in Head and Neck Oncology
Consultant
Department of Surgical Oncology
Rajiv Gandhi Cancer Institute and Research Centre
New Delhi, India

Hemant T Bhoye
MBBS MS MCh (Plastic Surgery)
Consultant
Department of Plastic Surgery
Rajiv Gandhi Cancer Institute and Research Centre
New Delhi, India

Kinshuki Jain
MBBS DM (Oncoanesthesia)
Consultant
Department of Pain Management and Palliative Care
Rajiv Gandhi Cancer Institute and Research Centre
New Delhi, India

Kiran Joshi MS DNB (ENT)
Attending Consultant
Department of Surgical Oncology
Rajiv Gandhi Cancer Institute and Research Centre
New Delhi, India

Kripa Shankar Mishra
MBBS MS (General Surgery) MCh (Plastic Surgery) Fellow (Cancer Reconstructive Surgery)
Consultant
Department of Plastic Surgery
Rajiv Gandhi Cancer Institute and Research Centre
New Delhi, India

Meenakshi Kamboj
MBBS DNB Pathology
Fellowship in Oncopathology
Consultant Pathology
Rajiv Gandhi Cancer Institute and Research Centre
New Delhi, India

Mudit Agarwal
MS (Surgery) MRCS (Edinburg) MCh (Surgical Oncology)
Senior Consultant
Department of Surgical Oncology
Rajiv Gandhi Cancer Institute and Research Centre
New Delhi, India

Munish Gairola
MBBS MD DNB (Radiation Oncology)
Director
Department of Radiation Oncology
Rajiv Gandhi Cancer Institute and Research Centre
New Delhi, India

Contributors

Navneet Singh
BPT MPT
Senior Physiotherapist
Rajiv Gandhi Cancer Institute and Research Centre
New Delhi, India

Parveen Ahlawat
MBBS DMRT DNB (Radiation Oncology)
Consultant
Department of Radiation Oncology
Rajiv Gandhi Cancer Institute and Research Centre
New Delhi, India

Rajan Arora
MBBS MCh (Plastic Surgery)
Senior Reconstructive and Microvascular Surgeon
Department of Surgical Oncology
Rajiv Gandhi Cancer Institute and Research Centre
New Delhi, India

Rajeev Kumar
MS MCh (Surgical Oncology)
Senior Consultant
Department of Surgical Oncology
Rajiv Gandhi Cancer Institute and Research Centre
New Delhi, India

Ravi K Singh
MBBS FICS MCh DNB (Plastic Surgery) Fellowship in Plastic Surgery
Consultant
Department of Surgical Oncology
Rajiv Gandhi Cancer Institute and Research Centre
New Delhi, India

Sarthak Tandon
MBBS DNB (Radiation Oncology)
Attending Consultant
Department of Radiation Oncology
Rajiv Gandhi Cancer Institute and Research Centre
New Delhi, India

Shagun Bhatia Shah
MBBS DA DNB (Anesthesia)
Consultant
Department of Anesthesiology and Critical Care
Rajiv Gandhi Cancer Institute and Research Centre
New Delhi, India

Sheetal Bhalla BDS MIDA
Consultant
Rajiv Gandhi Cancer Institute and Research Centre
New Delhi, India

Sumit Goyal
MBBS DM (Medical Oncology) ECMO
Senior Consultant
Department of Medical Oncology
Rajiv Gandhi Cancer Institute and Research Centre
New Delhi, India

Sunil Pasricha
MD (Pathology) Fellowship in Oncopathology
Senior Consultant
Department of Pathology
Rajiv Gandhi Cancer Institute and Research Centre
New Delhi, India

Swarupa Mitra
MBBS MD (Radiation Oncology)
Senior Consultant
Department of Radiation Oncology
Rajiv Gandhi Cancer Institute and Research Centre
New Delhi, India

Ullas Batra
MBBS DM (Medical Oncology) ECMO FAGE
Senior Consultant and Co-Director
Department of Medical Oncology
Rajiv Gandhi Cancer Institute and Research Centre
New Delhi, India

Venkata Pradeep Babu Koyyala
MBBS DNB (Medical Oncology)
Assistant Professor
Department of Medical Oncology
Homi Bhabha Cancer Hospital and Research Centre
(A Unit of Tata Memorial Hospital), Visakhapatnam, Andhra Pradesh, India

Vikas Arora
MBBS MS (ENT) Fellowship in Head and Neck Oncology
Consultant
Department of Surgical Oncology
Rajiv Gandhi Cancer Institute and Research Centre
New Delhi, India

Vishal Yadav
MBBS MS (ENT) Fellowship in Head and Neck Oncology
Consultant
Department of Surgical Oncology
Rajiv Gandhi Cancer Institute and Research Centre
New Delhi, India

Vivek Mahawar
MBBS DNB DMRD DMRE (Radiology)
Consultant
Department of Radiology
Rajiv Gandhi Cancer Institute and Research Centre
New Delhi, India

Foreword

Cancer is a terrible disease, but I do not accept that the surgeon's scalpel can be more destructive than the disease itself. The war against the cancer (larynx) must stop, since its removal is unnecessary and ineffective in many cases. To take away the disease without excising a healthy glottis to make an effort to preserve the function of the organ to strive not to return a disabled person to the society: that is my motto.

–Alonso, 1951

The last two decades have seen an expanded interest in multimodality therapy combining surgery and radiotherapy or chemotherapy, and radiation with surgery reserved for salvage. This evolution in approach has evolved from surgeons becoming increasingly involved in clinical trials and the interest of surgeons in developing an evidentiary basis for the treatments they offer. The most important surgical innovations of the past 30 years have, however, been in the development of reconstructive approaches to ablative defects of the head and neck.

In the 1970s, the deltopectoral flap became the workhorse of reconstruction and things further improved with the advent of the pectoralis myocutaneous flap. We turned a blind eye to its incommodious bulk because of its unfailing reliability. Larger defects were closed with the latissimus dorsi flap, but we still had not solved the problem of replacing the mandible. We used free bone grafts carved to shape and wired into place, although many free bone grafts to the jaw failed and the mechanism by which those who did survive remained uncertain. All that was to end with the advent of the free flap. A surgeon could not only do better cancer surgery but also close any hole with tissue that was thin, that survived, and that functioned. The introduction of this new technology did wonders for the surgical civil war that had raged over the "ownership" of head and neck surgery for the previous 50 years. The only surgeons who could perform the whole repertoire on their own became those who could join blood vessels together—the rest had to call on help or do the fashionable thing and "work in teams." There is, of course, nothing to be criticized about team working; in fact, it is the tenet of modern surgery.

The original civil war had been between the General and ENT Surgeons in the United States and between Plastic Surgery and ENT in the United Kingdom. In both countries, the initial "winners" were the ENT Surgeons who went on to change the name of their specialty to Otolaryngology—Head and Neck Surgery.

Dr Conley had said, "If your treatment is worse than the disease, then you become the disease."

So what can readers of this book learn?
- Follow the Oslerian principle of not creating harm.
- In the local situation, work with your colleagues and do not compete, because the only loser will be the patient.

- Audit and believe the results.
- And, finally, be holistic and ask whether what you plan for a particular patient would be what you would do to a relative.

If you do these things, you will not make the mistake of not learning from the past and you will be a good head and neck "Doctor."

Visweswar Bhattacharya
MCh (Plastic Surgery) PhD FAMS FICS
Former Head
Department of Plastic Surgery
Institute of Medical Sciences
Banaras Hindu University
Varanasi, Uttar Pradesh, India

Preface

"Because the newer methods of treatment are good, it does not follow that the old ones were bad: for if our honourable and worshipful ancestors had not recovered from their ailments, you and I would not be here today."

–**Confucius, 551–478 BC**

The knowledge about head and neck cancers has undergone exponential growth over the last three decades. Although oral cancer is the leading cancer amongst all head and neck cancers, still clinicians keep struggling to collect information which will help them in decision-making in oral cancer management. We have selected key materials based on the combined wisdom and surgical expertise of an impressively well-informed institutional team. I regard it as a great pleasure and privilege to have been associated with such a wonderful team.

No one who reads this book believes in their heart that cancer is a surgical disease, but until the "magic bullet" is discovered, the head and neck surgeon has a role. In practicing this subspecialty, we are unlike other cancer surgeons. They are usually able to leave the patient with only a scar that can be hidden by clothes, even though they may have a catheter and a bag, a cough and a weak voice, or an ostomy bag near their trouser pocket into which their bowels empty. We, on the other hand, interfere with very visible anatomy and affect the physiology of speech, swallowing, chewing, and breathing in such a way that it is impossible to disguise and may attract unwanted attention from onlookers. Since I started to practice head and neck surgery, things have improved enormously because of the cascade of reconstructive procedures. In the past, survival figures were published, or rather claimed, in order to enhance the reputation of the surgeon, those were the days of eminence-based rather than evidence-based surgery.

We hope that in its current form, this book will continue to be a major resource not only for the trainees but also for established practitioners in otolaryngology, maxillofacial surgery, plastic surgery, and clinical oncology whose specific work includes a major head and neck practice.

In the next few years, further refinements will occur in the selection and application of the myriad of treatment options for oral malignancy. Increased characterization of genomic and proteomic profiles of tumors will allow us to better select patients for these therapies, providing a more individualized approach to oral cancer treatment. In the reconstructive arena, the major innovations are clearly in tissue engineering and transplantation. Tissue engineering may offer the potential to create composite tissue constructs that will replace the current approaches, including free tissue transfer and the associated donor site morbidity.

Essentials of Oral Cancer is in the form of tips and tricks for all oral cancer clinicians, not giving any details or trials or studies or references. This book is a joy to own, a pleasure to read and, above all, a powerful force to advance treatment standards in the huge variety of oral conditions. I would like to extend special thanks to my assistant, Mr Ranjeet, who has compiled and collated the manuscript, and helped me in bringing out the book in this shape.

I am indebted to Dr Shagun Bhatia Shah, Consultant, Department of Anesthesiology and Critical Care, who has edited the book and given important feedbacks. I am grateful to all the contributors in this book for their time, effort, and expertise in making it such a wonderful source of information for all oral cancer clinicians.

AK Dewan

Acknowledgments

Writing a book is not only satisfying but also rewarding. Today, it gives me immense pleasure as the book on Oral Cancer is ready to be published. I am grateful to everyone with whom I have had the pleasure to work during this entire journey. Every author has provided extensive personal and professional contribution. I would especially like to thank Dr Shagun Bhatia Shah and Dr Swarupa Mitra for their untiring effort in editing this book.

I am grateful to my co-editors who have stayed with me all along, lending me all the support that was required during this enormous task.

I would fail in my duty if I do not express my gratitude to my colleagues and assistants who have rendered their help from time to time for both academic and nonacademic issues.

This work has been made possible with the support of Ranjeet who has been constantly coordinating between authors and the other team members, and has taken care of the mundane technical work.

Nobody has been more important to me in the pursuit of this project than the members of my family. I would like to thank my wife, Rupali whose guidance and support are more than I can give credit for. Most importantly, I wish to thank my loving and supportive family especially my granddaughter, Kayra who provided an unending inspiration.

I am extremely thankful to Shri Jitendar P Vij (Group Chairman), Mr Ankit Vij (Managing Director), Mr MS Mani (Group President), Ms Chetna Malhotra Vohra (Associate Director—Content Strategy), and Ms Pooja Bhandari (Production Head) of M/s Jaypee Brothers Medical Publishers (P) Ltd, New Delhi, India, for giving the go-ahead at the very beginning and helping us in every way possible to bring out this book.

Not to forget, I owe in plenty to my patients and their family, who have been the reason behind writing this book.

AK Dewan

Contents

1. **Surgical Anatomy of Oral Cavity** 1
   AK Dewan

2. **Epidemiology and Etiology of Oral Cancer** 12
   Abhishek Singh, Mudit Agarwal

3. **Prevention and Chemoprevention** 23
   Kiran Joshi

4. **Histopathology and Molecular Pathology of Squamous Cell Carcinoma of Oral Cavity** 29
   Sunil Pasricha, Meenakshi Kamboj

5. **Evaluation and Staging of Oral Cancer** 40
   Vikas Arora

6. **Imaging in Carcinoma of Oral Cavity** 50
   Vivek Mahawar

7. **Principles of Oral Cancer Treatment** 58
   Vishal Yadav

8. **Management of Oral Premalignant Lesions** 66
   Vishal Yadav

9. **Trismus in Head and Neck Cancers** 73
   Ghanashyam Mandal

10. **Jaw Tumors** 79
    Vishal Yadav

11. **Nutrition in Oral Cancer** 101
    Ghanashyam Mandal

12. **Anesthesia in Oral Cancer Surgery** 108
    Shagun Bhatia Shah

13. **Preoperative, Peroperative, and Postoperative Nursing Care** 119
    Rajan Arora, Ghanashyam Mandal

14. **The Lip** 127
    Hemant T Bhoye

15. **Management of Buccal Mucosa and Retromolar Trigone Cancer** 140
    Vishal Yadav

16. **Carcinoma of Lower Alveolus** 150
    Rajeev Kumar

17. **Upper Alveolus and Palate** 153
    Vikas Arora

18. **Management of Tongue and Floor of Mouth Cancer** 163
    Ankita Jain, AK Dewan

19. **Management of Neck in Oral Cancer** 176
    Rajeev Kumar

20. **Neck Dissections in Oral Cancer** 183
    Kiran Joshi, Mudit Agarwal

21. **Complications of Surgery and Reconstructive Procedures** 193
    Kripa Shankar Mishra, Rajan Arora, AK Dewan

22. **Principles of Surgical Reconstruction in Oral Cancers** 200
    Rajan Arora, Ravi K Singh

23. **Reconstructions of Oral Mucosal Defects** 213
    Rajan Arora

24. **Reconstruction of Soft Tissues and Bony Defects of Oral Cavity** 222
    Rajan Arora

25. **Adjuvant Treatment in Oral Cavity Cancer** 230
    Abhinav Dewan, Swarupa Mitra

26. **Radiotherapy in Oral Cancer** 239
    Munish Gairola, Parveen Ahlawat, Sarthak Tandon

27. **Chemotherapy in Oral Cavity Cancer** 251
    Sumit Goyal

28. **Management of Recurrent Head and Neck Carcinoma** 255
    Sumit Goyal, Venkata Pradeep Babu Koyyala

29. **Role of Interventional Radiology in the Management of Oral Cancers** 260
    Abhishek Bansal

30. **Dental Management in Oral Cancer Patients** 264
    Sheetal Bhalla

31. **Swallowing and Speech Therapy in Oral Cancer** 273
    Navneet Singh

32. **Pain and Palliative Care in Oral Cavity Cancers** 283
    Bablesh Mahawar

33. **Quality of Life of Oral Cancer Patients** 290
    Kinshuki Jain

34. **Case Presentation for Postgraduate Students** 295
    Vikas Arora

35. **Cancer of the Oral Cavity (NCCN Guidelines)** 303
    Swarupa Mitra, Abhinav Dewan

36. **Oral Cancer–2021** 314
    Ullas Batra

Index *325*

CHAPTER 1

Surgical Anatomy of Oral Cavity

AK Dewan

EMBRYOLOGY

The oral cavity is a unique structure in that it forms from both ectodermal and endodermal structures. The tongue's embryological component derives from several different pharyngeal arches, each contributing toward the development of different regions of the tongue. In the 5th week of development, swellings, known as "lingual swellings," develop on the right and left sides of the first pharyngeal arch. These grow and develop to become the anterior two thirds of the tongue. The posterior one third of the tongue forms by the copula, a swelling that forms from the, the second and third pharyngeal arches, and a small portion of the fourth pharyngeal arch. The boundary between the anterior and posterior portions of the tongue is a V-shaped groove known as the terminal sulcus. The palate consists of primary and secondary embryological origins and forms between the 6th and 12th week. The primary palate arises from the embryonic frontonasal prominences. The secondary palate forms from the paired maxillary prominences fusion and contains the rest of the hard and soft palates. The upper lip forms during early embryogenesis from the maxillary, lateral nasal, and medial nasal facial prominences. These facial prominences develop from anteriorly migrating neural crest cells in combination with mesoderm and the head ectoderm. The mandibular processes fuse to form the lower lip.

BOUNDARIES OF ORAL CAVITY (FIG. 1)

The anterior limit of the oral cavity is the vermilion border of the upper and lower lips. The posterior limit of the oral cavity is the circumvallate papillae on the tongue, anterior tonsillar pillars, and the junction of the soft and hard palates. The hard palate separates the oral and nasal cavities. The contents of the oral cavity extending dorsally from the lips are the buccal mucosa, the upper and lower alveoli, the floor of mouth (FOM), the hard palate, the anterior two thirds of tongue, and retromolar trigone (RMT). The oral cavity forms the *entrance* of the passage for ingestion of food and liquids. The lips are a doorway to the oral cavity that aid in the intake of food and liquid.

Lips

- The lips are fleshy folds lined externally by skin and internally by mucous membrane. The mucocutaneous junction lines the "edge" of the lip; part of the mucosal surface is normally seen.
- Each lip is composed of: (1) skin, (2) superficial fascia, (3) the orbicularis oris muscle, (4) the submucosa containing mucous labial glands and blood vessels, and (5) mucous membrane.
- The lips bound the oral fissure. They meet laterally at the angle of the mouth. The inner surface of each lip is supported by

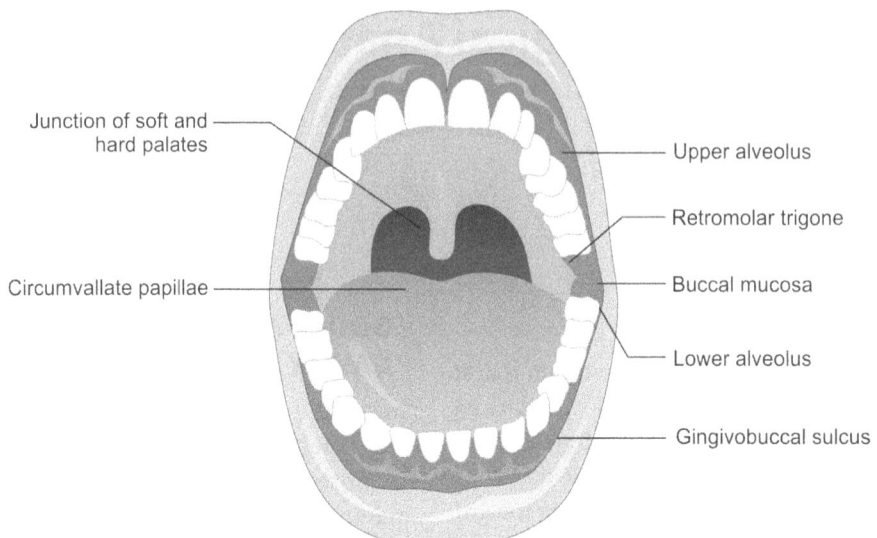

Fig. 1: Boundaries of oral cavity.

a frenulum which ties it to the gum. The outer surface of the upper lip presents a median vertical groove, the philtrum.
- Lymphatics of the central part of the lower lip drain to the submental nodes; the lymphatics from the rest of the lower lip pass to the submandibular nodes.
- The vascular supply of the lips are the labial arteries that come off from the facial artery.

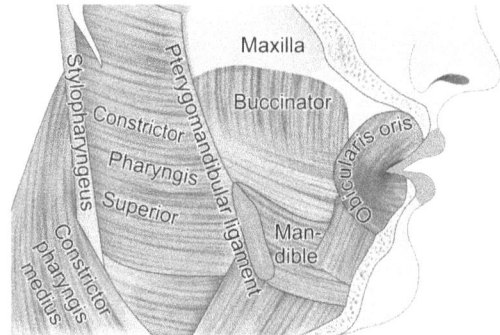

Fig. 2: Muscles of face.

Gingivobuccal Complex

The *cheek mucosa* covers the inside of the cheek, and is continuous with the upper and lower gingival mucosa. It would be thus appropriate to call this as gingivobuccal complex. The Stensen's duct from the parotid opens into the cheek mucosa opposite the upper second molar. The cheek mucosa has a thin layer of fat and buccinator muscle separating it from the skin of the cheek. Immediately lateral to the buccinator muscle is the facial artery, the buccal artery, and the vascular plexus that the buccinator myomucosal flap is based on. Lateral to the buccinator muscle is the buccal space that also contains fat which is traversed by the terminal branches of the facial nerve, and further posteriorly, the buccal fat pad, the zygomaticus major, the subcutaneous tissue and the skin. Stensen's duct opens in the buccal mucosa adjacent to the second upper molar tooth after crossing the masseter muscle and passing through the buccinator muscle (**Fig. 2**).

Gingival Mucosa

It overlies the alveolus from the point of abutment of the gingivobuccal sulcus to the FOM. The alveolus is the tooth-bearing area of the mandible and maxilla. It has an outer cortex and has inner trabeculae (medullary bone). The cortical lining of the dental socket is the *lamina dura*.

Retromolar Trigone

Retromolar trigone is a triangular area of mucosa overlying the ascending ramus of mandible. It extends from behind the third molar up to the maxillary tuberosity. Posteriorly the buccal mucosa is closely related to the medial pterygoid and masseter muscles, i.e., the masticator space and the infratemporal fossa (ITF). Tumors, particularly from the RMT, spread to these spaces. Posterior to the RMT is the pterygomandibular raphe; it extends between the pterygoid hamulus and the posterior end of the mylohyoid ridge of the mandible. The pterygomandibular space is enclosed by this raphe anteriorly and the medial pterygoid and ascending ramus of mandible on either side. It contains the lingual and alveolar nerves. Posteriorly it is related to the parapharyngeal space.

Arterial supply: The buccal mucosa is supplied by the facial and buccal arteries; the buccal artery originates from the pterygoid branch of the maxillary artery. The inferior alveolar artery is a branch of the mandibular branch of the maxillary artery and enters the mandibular canal to supply the inferior alveolus. The superior alveolus is supplied by the posterior superior alveolar artery, a branch of the pterygopalatine segment of the maxillary artery **(Fig. 3)**.

Venous drainage: The pterygoid plexus drains into the facial vein which eventually drains into the internal jugular vein.

Lymphatic drainage: The buccal mucosa drains into the deep cervical nodes. Level IB (submandibular node) is the first echelon of lymphatic spread of tumor.

Innervation: Sensory supply is via the maxillary and mandibular divisions of the trigeminal nerve. Motor supply to the muscles of mastication is by the mandibular nerve but the buccinator muscle is innervated by the buccal branch of the facial nerve **(Fig. 4)**.

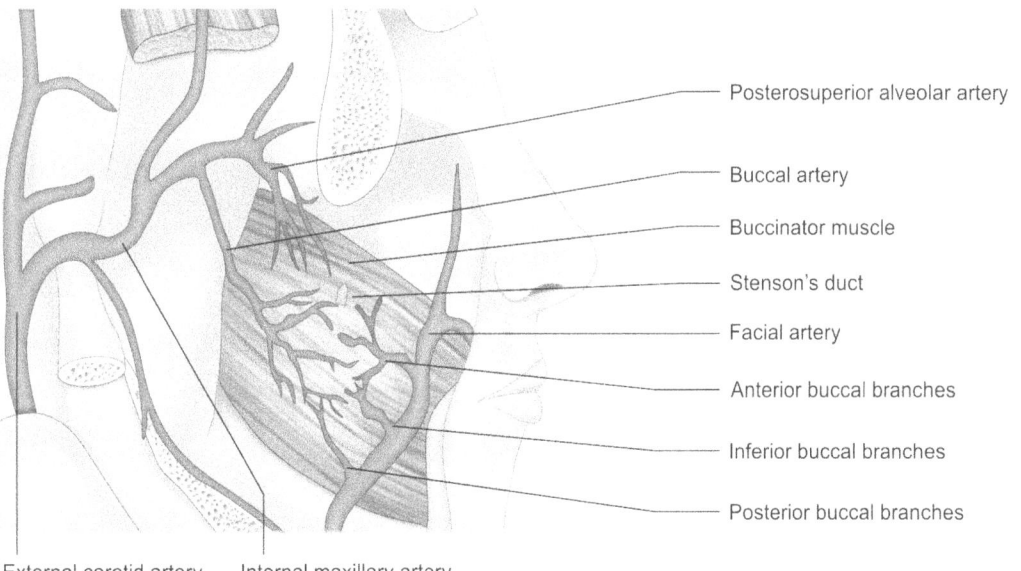

Fig. 3: Arterial supply of buccal mucosa.

4 Surgical Anatomy of Oral Cavity

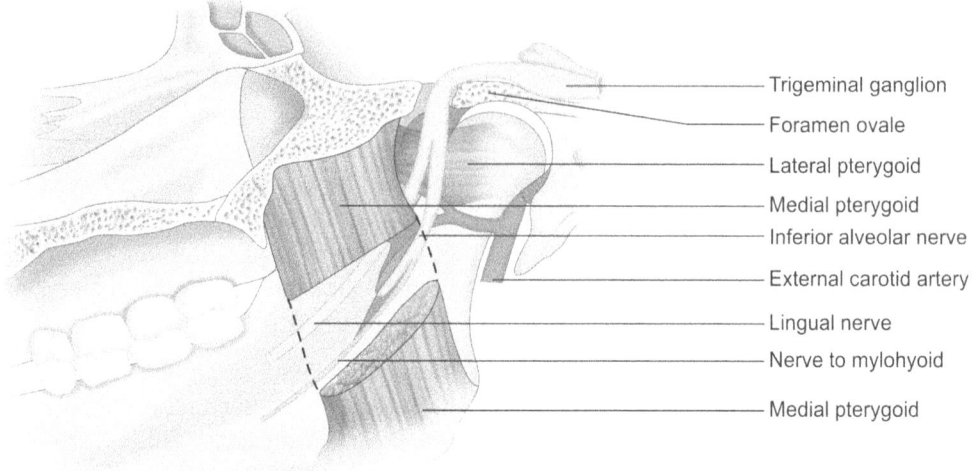

Fig. 4: Muscles and innervation of buccal mucosa.

Salient Surgical Anatomy

Masticator Space (Fig. 5)

Enclosed within superficial layer of deep cervical fascia covering muscles of mastication.

Inferior boundary: Lower border of mandible.

Superior boundary: Parietal calvarium.

Medial boundary: Fascia medial to medial pterygoid muscle.

Lateral boundary: Fascia overlying masseter and temporalis muscles.

Contents: Muscles of mastication, internal maxillary artery, mandibular nerve.

Clinical relevance: Involvement of masticator space is considered to be locally advanced disease, i.e., T4b stage.

Infratemporal Fossa

Medial boundary: Lateral pterygoid plate of sphenoid bone.

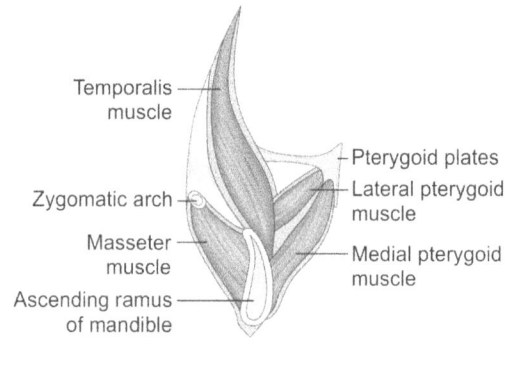

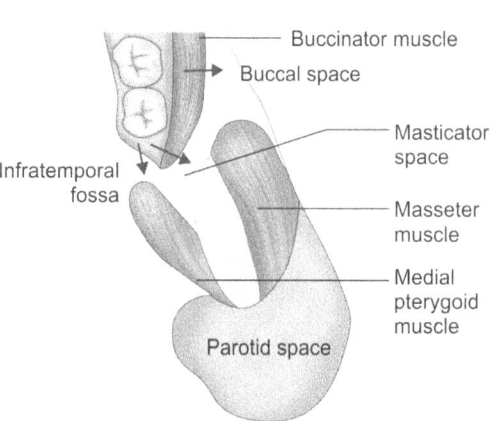

Fig. 5: Masticator space.

Lateral boundary: Mandible.

Superior boundary: Greater wing of sphenoid bone and squamous part of temporal bone.

Inferior boundary: Medial pterygoid muscle.

Anterior boundary: Posterolateral wall of maxilla.

Posterior boundary: Tympanic part of temporal bone.

Relations: Inferior orbital fissure, pterygomaxillary fissure.

Contents: Lower part of temporalis muscle, part of masseter, medial and lateral pterygoid muscles, internal maxillary artery, pterygoid venous plexus, branches of mandibular nerve, facial nerve, and otic ganglion.

Clinical relevance: ITF involvement can be either "high" or "low". Tumors involving the high ITF (involving lateral pterygoid and temporalis muscles) are considered unresectable because tumor can escape through the pterygomaxillary and inferior orbital fissures making the chances of complete (R0) resection remote **(Fig. 6)**.

Buccal Space

Medial boundary: Buccinator muscle.

Lateral boundary: Zygomaticus major muscle.

Contents: Mainly buccal fat pad which communicates posteriorly with the retroantral fat pad, Stensen's duct, minor or occasionally accessory salivary glands, facial and buccal arteries, facial vein, and branches of facial and mandibular nerves.

Clinical relevance: Tumor infiltration into the buccal space can potentially lead to spread to the ITF via the retroantral fat pad.

Surgical Principles Based on Anatomy

Resecting the Primary

Attention should be paid mainly to *the third dimension, i.e., deep resection margin*. This margin must contain at least one layer of

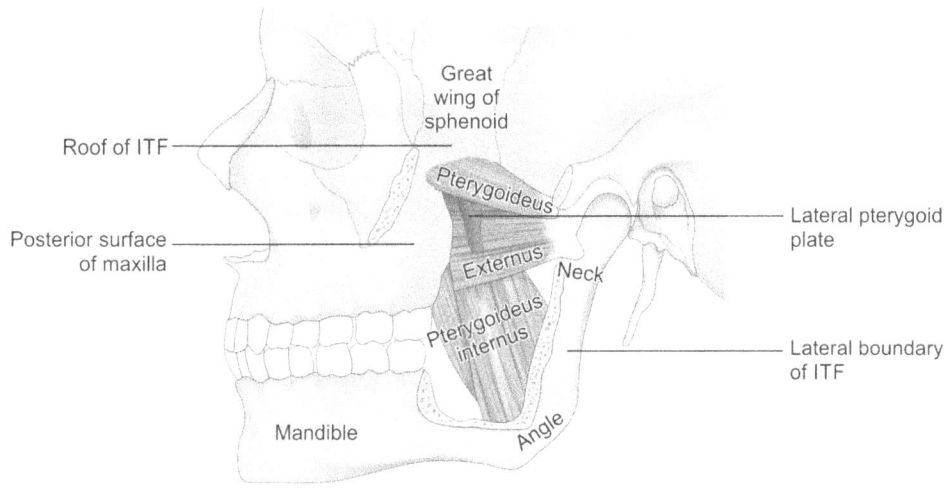

Fig. 6: Boundaries of infratemporal fossa (ITF).

normal tissue beyond the tumor. With this in mind, it should contain the buccinator muscle with superficial lesions and the buccal fat pad or the zygomaticus major muscle with deeper lesions. With lesions deeper than that, e.g., adhering to skin or causing *peau d'orange*, the overlying skin is excised to achieve an adequate margin. A vertical osteotomy is made about 2 cm anterior to the tumor with a powered saw, drill, or Gigli saw. This allows the surgeon to reflect the mandible laterally like opening a book and to expose the tumor.

If a bony reconstruction is to be done, then the mandible is preplated to ensure an accurate repair. If the RMT is not involved, then the posterior osteotomy is made 2 cm behind the posterior edge of the tumor. The coronoid process is exposed and released from its attachment to the temporalis muscle, remaining close to the bone to avoid injuring the vessels medial to the coronoid process.

Bite excision: This refers to excision of the superior and inferior alveoli with the intervening interalveolar tissue (like a bite). It is indicated for lesions involving the RMT extending to the superior alveolus. The specimen consists of the inferior as well as the superior alveoli in continuity with the overlying RMT mucosa and soft tissue formed by the pterygoid muscles.

Infratemporal fossa: If the lesion involves the medial pterygoid muscle, the pterygoid plate is included in the specimen to ensure adequate soft-tissue resection that includes the pterygoid muscles. "Bite excision" with resection of the entire medial pterygoid muscle is performed when the lower ITF is involved. If resection of the higher ITF is warranted, then "bite excision" encompassing the pterygoid plates is performed to include the entire medial and lateral pterygoid muscles. The temporalis muscle below the temporal fossa is resected in continuity with the coronoid up to the roof of the ITF.

Caution:
- Adequately expose all tumors margins before approaching the tumors.
- Mucosal, soft tissue and bone margins of >5 mm.
- Preserve function and avoid trismus with selection of appropriate reconstruction.
- Avoid obstruction of parotid duct; identify and stent it during major composite resections. May send cut end of duct for frozen section to check clearance.

Surgical approaches:
- Peroral
- Cheek flap
- Midline lip split
- Angle split

Management of Bone

Periosteum is a robust barrier to bone invasion. In alveolar lesions with intact dentition, the mandible is generally invaded via its occlusal surface. In the RMT or in edentulous mandibles, the occlusal surface corresponds to the junction of the attached and reflected mucosa (point of abutment). In irradiated mandibles and in large tumors, the mandible can be invaded at multiple points due to multiple breaks in the periosteum. With cancers of the FOM, mandible is infiltrated at the point of abutment. FOM cancer requires vertical or oblique marginal mandibulectomy to completely excise the lingual plate due to invasion occurring directly at the point of abutment.

Marginal Mandibulectomy

Marginal mandibulectomy is indicated when tumor abuts mandible without gross invasion, or when there is only superficial bony invasion. Three types of marginal mandibulectomy are described, i.e., *horizontal, vertical, and oblique.* As the lingual plate is weaker than the buccal plate, an isolated buccal plate excision may not withstand subsequent weight bearing and the bone may fracture. Hence, isolated buccal plate excision is risky in buccal mucosa lesions.

Right-angled cuts predispose to stress fractures and hence are avoided. Inferiorly a bony bridge of >1 cm in height should be retained to avoid a stress fracture. The bone is cut with sharp bone-cutting instruments, e.g., a powered saw. With marginal mandibulectomy for RMT cancer, the anterior aspect of the ascending ramus of the mandible is excised in continuity with the coronoid process, as releasing the attachment of the temporalis muscle avoids postoperative trismus.

Segmental/Hemimandibulectomy

This is indicated when there is gross bone erosion, either clinically or radiologically; for significant paramandibular disease; for postradiotherapy recurrence due to the multiple routes of tumor entry; or with a pipe stem mandible (inadequate bony remnant of <1 cm in height).

Tracheostomy

One should have a low threshold for tracheostomy. Midline alveolus lesions, postradiation (radical dose) oral cancers, bulky flaps, subtotal or total glossectomy are some of the indications of elective tracheostomy.

■ FLOOR OF MOUTH

The FOM is a horseshoe-shaped area that is confined peripherally by the inner aspect (lingual surface) of the mandible. It extends posteriorly to where the anterior tonsillar pillar meets the tonsillolingual sulcus, and merges medially with undersurface of the oral tongue. It has a covering of delicate oral mucosa through which the thin-walled sublingual/ranine veins are visible. The frenulum is a mucosal fold that extends along the midline between the openings of the submandibular ducts.

Anterior FOM: The mylohyoid muscle forms the diaphragm of the mouth and separates the FOM from the submental and submandibular triangles of the neck. The following structures are located between the mucosa and the mylohyoid muscle: paired geniohyoid muscles in the mid-line, submandibular ducts, oral component of submandibular salivary glands, genioglossus muscle and hypoglossal nerves. The paired sublingual salivary glands are located beneath the mucosa of the anterior FOM, anterior to the submandibular ducts, and above the mylohyoid and geniohyoid muscles. The glands drain via 8–20 excretory ducts of Rivinus into the submandibular duct and also directly into the mouth on an elevated crest of mucous membrane called the *plica fimbriata* and is located on either side of the frenulum of the tongue.

The submandibular duct is located immediately deep to the mucosa of the anterior and lateral FOM and opens into the oral cavity to either side of the frenulum. The lingual nerve provides sensation to the FOM. It crosses deep to the submandibular duct in the lateral FOM. In the anterior FOM, it is located posterior to the duct. Ranine veins are visible on the ventral surface of the tongue, and accompany the hypoglossal nerve.

Arterial supply to the tongue and FOM is derived from the lingual artery and its branches (ranine artery, dorsalis linguae, and sublingual arteries); and the mylohyoid and submental branches of the facial artery. The lingual artery arises from the external carotid artery between the superior thyroid and facial arteries. It courses obliquely forwards and medial to the greater cornu of the hyoid.

It then loops downward and anteriorly and crosses medial to XII nerve and the stylohyoid muscle. It then courses directly anteriorly below hyoglossus and finally ascends as the ranine artery (profunda linguae) submucosally on the undersurface of the tongue as far as its tip; it lies to either side of the genioglossus and is accompanied by the lingual nerve. Two or three small dorsales linguæ arteries arise beneath the hyoglossus and ascend to the posterior part of the dorsum of the tongue and supply the mucous membrane of the posterior FOM and oropharynx. The sublingual artery arises from the lingual artery at the anterior edge of the hyoglossus and runs forward between the genioglossus and mylohyoid and supplies the sublingual salivary gland and mucous membrane of the FOM and gingiva. The submental branch of the facial artery courses along the inferior, inner margin of the mandible. The mylohyoid artery and vein are encountered when the surgeon elevates the submandibular gland from the lateral surface of the mylohyoid (**Fig. 7**).

Surgical Principles based on Anatomy

- *Mandible in FOM lesion*: The mandible forms the peripheral border of the FOM and may be involved by FOM tumors or may have to be divided (mandibulotomy) or resected (alveolectomy/marginal mandibulectomy/segmental mandibulectomy/hemimandibulectomy). Important surgical features are the position of the mental foramina through which the mental nerves exit to innervate the lower lip, the mylohyoid line to which the mylohyoid muscle attaches, the height of the body of the mandible and the depth of the dental roots. The mental foramen and inferior alveolar nerve may be very close to the superior surface of a resorbed mandible such as is seen in older, edentulous patients. A marginal mandibulectomy may also not be possible in such a resorbed mandible due to the lack of residual bone.
- *Avoid postoperative orocervical fistulae*:
  - Maintain length and mobility of the tongue.

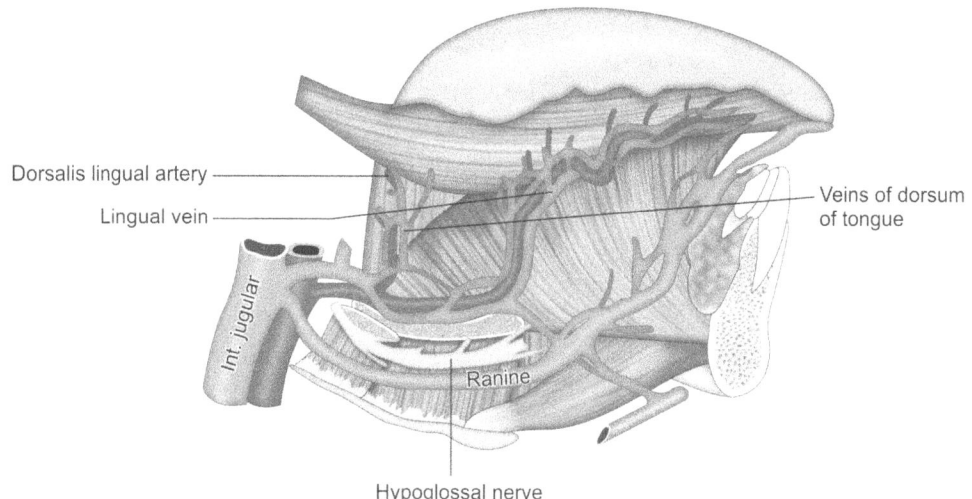

Fig. 7: Blood supply of tongue.

- Avoid pooling of secretions and food in the reconstructed FOM.
- Avoid obstruction of the submandibular ducts.
- Avoid injury to lingual and hypoglossal nerves.
- Maintain mandibular continuity and strength.
- Restore dentition.
- Tumors of the anterior FOM that approach the mid-line require bilateral END.
- Widening of the alveolar canal on mandibular orthopantomography (Panorex) may be seen. MRI can demonstrate peripheral nerve injury (PNI). Should there be evidence of PNI then the affected nerve should be dissected proximally until a clear tumor margin is obtained on frozen section. In the case of the inferior alveolar nerve, this would require a hemi- or segmental mandibulectomy that encompasses the entire inferior alveolar canal.
- Carious teeth seen on Panorex may be removed at the time of the surgery.
- A tumor of the FOM may invade the submandibular duct and cause a hard, fibrotic submandibular salivary gland that can be confused with a lymph-node metastasis.
- *Surgical access for FOM*: Transoral/midline lip-split/visor flap/pull-through.
- *Repair*: Following resection, the surgeon carefully assesses the defect to determine how best to restore form and function, i.e., mandibular integrity and contour, and oral competence, mastication, oral transport, swallowing, and speech.
  - Never suture the edge of the tongue to the gingiva; in such cases, always maintain tongue mobility with a flap.
  - Avoid tethering the tip of the tongue.
  - Some defects are best left open to heal by secondary intention to retain mobility.
  - Reduce the risk of orocervical fistula by approximating the mylohyoid to the digastric muscle in the neck, and ensuring that the suction drain is not placed in the upper neck.
  - No repair is required for small and/or superficial resections above the mylohyoid that do not communicate with the neck dissection, they may be left open to heal like a tonsillectomy wound.
- *Buccinator myomucosal flap*: This is an excellent flap for both anterior and lateral FOM defects as it has the same physical qualities as tissues of the FOM. The pedicle, however, crosses the mandible and is therefore best suited for edentulous patients, patients with missing teeth, or who have undergone marginal mandibulectomy.

ORAL TONGUE

The tongue is a mobile muscular structure for speech and swallowing. It is responsible in assisting mastication and turning over the food in the mouth propelling it onward. The mucous membrane covering the tongue varies in thickness and quality; this has relevance in terms of obtaining surgical margins and retaining tongue mobility. The undersurface of the tongue has a thin, smooth, and pliable mucous membrane. The mucous membrane covering the anterior two thirds of the dorsum is thin and quite smooth and adherent to the tongue muscle compared to the mucosa covering the base of tongue (BOT) behind foramen caecum and sulcus terminalis which is rough, thick, and fixed to the underlying muscles and contains a number of lymphoid follicles (lingual tonsil).

With BOT tumors, it is therefore difficult to determine the edge of a tumor making frozen section, especially useful to assess resection margins.

The tongue comprises eight muscles. Four extrinsic muscles: (1) genioglossus, (2) hyoglossus, (3) styloglossus, and (4) palatoglossus, control the position of the tongue and are attached to bone. Four intrinsic muscles modulate the shape of the tongue and are not attached to bone. Below the tongue are the geniohyoid and the mylohyoid muscles; the mylohyoid muscle serves as the diaphragm of the mouth and separates the tongue and FOM from the submental and submandibular triangle of the neck **(Fig. 8)**.

Vasculature: The tongue is a very vascular organ. The arterial supply is derived from the paired lingual arteries and its branches (ranine artery, dorsalis linguae, and sublingual arteries) and the mylohyoid and submental arteries. Additional blood supply to the tongue emanates from the tonsillar branch of the facial artery and the ascending pharyngeal artery.

Venous drainage is via lingual and ranine veins. The lingual veins originate on the dorsum, sides, and undersurface of the tongue and accompany the lingual artery and join the internal jugular vein. The ranine veins originate below the tip of the tongue and are visible on its ventral surface; they accompany the XII nerve as venae comitantes and either join the lingual vein or pass lateral to hyoglossus to join the common facial vein.

Innervation: Other than palatoglossus which is innervated by the X nerve, all intrinsic and extrinsic muscles are innervated by the XII nerve. The IX nerve provides somatic afferent and taste sensation to the posterior one third of the tongue. The lingual nerve provides general somatic sensation to the anterior two thirds of the mouth and FOM; taste is provided by the chorda tympani branch of the VII nerve via the lingual nerve. The lingual nerve crosses deep to the submandibular duct in the lateral FOM.

Surgical Principles Related to Anatomy

- Adequate resection margins (three-dimensional resection).
- Preserve at least one lingual artery to avoid infarction of tongue.
- Optimize cosmesis and function. Maintain length and mobility of tongue.
  - Avoid pooling of secretions and food.
  - Avoid obstruction of submandibular ducts.
  - Attempt to preserve lingual and XII nerves.
  - Maintain mandibular continuity and strength.
  - Maintain dental occlusion.
  - Restore dentition.
- Referred otalgia in oral malignancies via auriculotemporal nerve, branch of CN V3 **(Fig. 9)**.

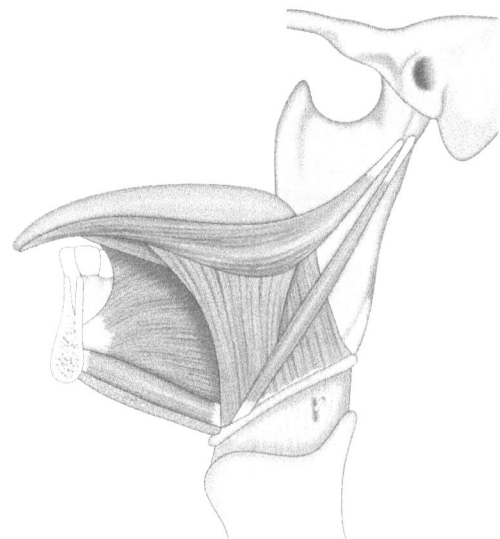

Fig. 8: Muscles of tongue.

Surgical Anatomy of Oral Cavity

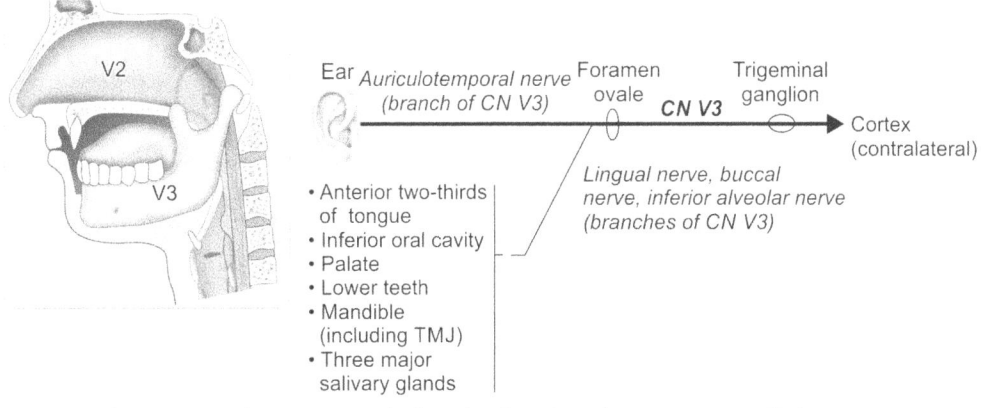

Fig. 9: Routes of transmission of referred otalgia. Cranial nerve V3—Mandibular nerve.
(TMJ: temporomandibular joint)
Source: Todd J Scarbough, MD.

KEY POINTS

- Reconstruction should suit resection and not the vice versa.
- Always aim at three-dimensional excision and obtain clear margins.
- Know the anatomy of oral cavity and neck well before surgery.
- Decisions are more important than incisions.

CHAPTER 2

Epidemiology and Etiology of Oral Cancer

Abhishek Singh, Mudit Agarwal

INTRODUCTION

Cancer of the oral cavity is today a major health problem all over the world due to its high morbidity and mortality. There are variations in the prevalence of this cancer in different parts of the world by as much as 20-fold among different countries, age groups, gender, races, and ethnicity. Globally, the incidence of oral cancer has been found to be higher in males than in females, and this risk increases with age. In 2013, oral cancer ranked 11th amongst all sites of cancer. The Indian subcontinent accounts for one-third of the entire oral cancer burden of the globe.

Squamous cell carcinoma is the most common histology to be diagnosed in oral and oropharynx accounting for 90% of oral and oropharyngeal malignancies.

INCIDENCE AND MORTALITY

The World Health Organization (WHO) in 2015 estimated cancer to be the first or second leading cause of death before the age of 70 years in 91 of 172 countries.

The mortality estimates in 2012 include an age-standardized rate (World) [ASR (W)] of 2.7 per 100,000 for oral and oropharyngeal cancers.

Indian statistics according to GLOBOCAN 2018 **(Fig. 1 and Table 1)**:
- Overall cancer statistics in India (GLOBOCAN 2018):
  - *Number of people estimated to be living with the disease*: Around 2.25 million
  - *New cancer patients registered each year*: Over 1,157,294
  - *Cancer-related deaths*: 784,821
  - Risk of developing cancer before the age of 75 years
    - *Male*: 9.81%
    - *Female*: 9.42%
  - *Cancer-related deaths in 2018*: 784,821
    - *Men*: 413,519
    - *Women*: 371,302
- Risk of dying from cancer before the age of 75 years is 7.34% in males and 6.28% in females.
- Over 200,000 cases of head and neck (H and N) cancers occur each year in India and nearly 80,000 oral cancers are diagnosed every year (2015).
- *India fact sheet*: GLOBOCAN 2018—huge increase in cancer of the lip and oral cavity—114.2% with 56,000 cases in 2012 to 119,992 in 2018.
- Population-based *5-year survival* for patients with oral cavity cancers—*approximately 50% in US, 45–49% in Europe, and approximately 30% in India*.
- 5-year survival rarely exceeds 40% for patients with regional disease and 15% for those with distant metastasis.

Although not listed among the top 10 cancers, some cancers are important within a particular regions or country.
- Cancers of the lip and oral cavity are common in Southern Asia (e.g., India and Sri Lanka) and in the Pacific Islands (Papua New Guinea, has the world's highest incidence rate in both sexes) **(Fig. 2)**.

Epidemiology and Etiology of Oral Cancer

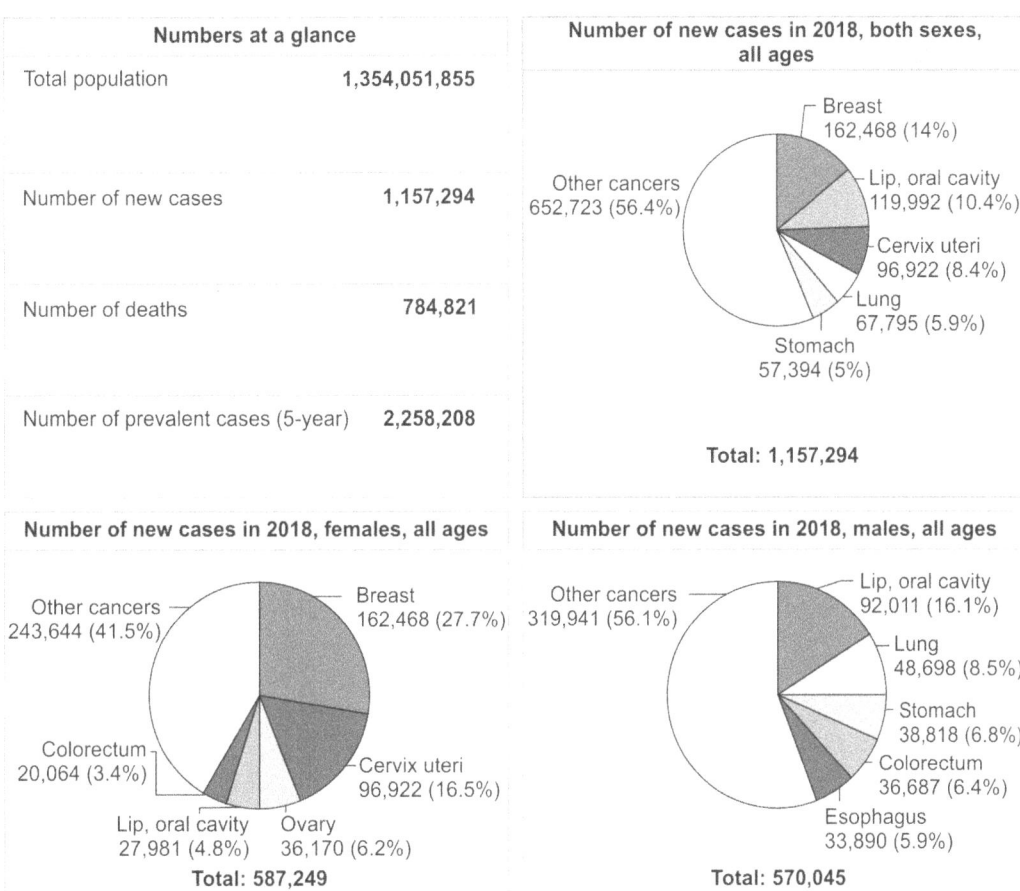

Fig. 1: GLOBOCAN 2018.

TABLE 1: GLOBOCAN 2018 data (India).

Summary statistic 2018			
	Males	Females	Both sexes
Population	701,546,980	652,504,878	1,354,051,855
Number of new cancer cases	570,045	587,249	1,157,294
Age-standardized incidence rate (world)	89.8	90.0	89.4
Risk of dying from cancer before the age of 75 years (%)	7.64	6.28	6.80
5-year prevalent cases	1,000,485	1,257,723	2,258,208
Top five most frequent cancers excluding nonmelanoma skin cancer (ranked by cases)	Lip, oral cavity	Breast	Breast
	Lung	Cervix uteri	Lip, oral cavity
	Stomach	Ovary	Cervix uteri
	Colorectum	Lip, oral cavity	Lung
	Esophagus	Colorectum	Stomach

Epidemiology and Etiology of Oral Cancer

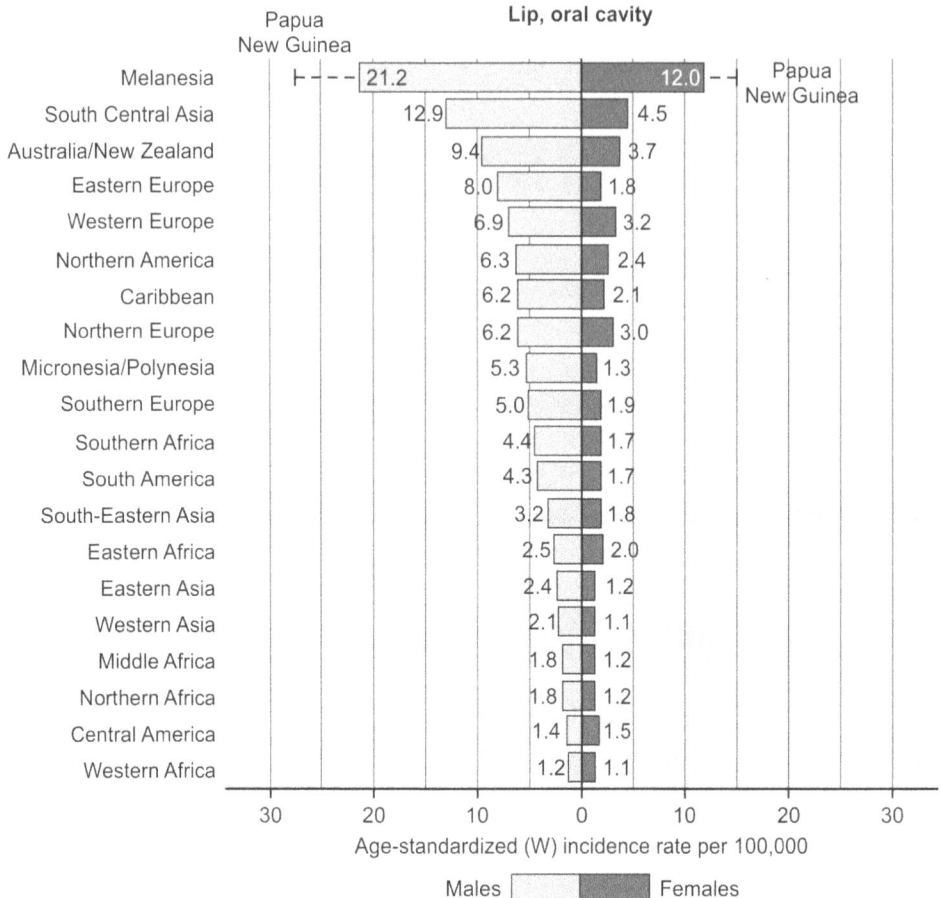

Fig. 2: Bar chart of region-specific incidence age-standardized rates by sex for cancers of lip and oral cavity in 2018.
Note: Rates are shown in descending order of the World (W) age-standardized rate among men, and the highest national rates among men and women are superimposed.
Source: GLOBOCAN 2018.

- It is also the most frequently encountered cause of cancer death among men in India and Sri Lanka.

The Global Initiative for Cancer Registry Development, an initiative of the major cancer organizations, is endeavoring to address inequities in the availability of robust data of incidence of cancer, by increasing its quality, comparability, and use. There are six International Agency for Research on Cancer (IARC) regional centers for cancer registration that have been established to include Africa, Asia, South and Central America, the Caribbean, and the Pacific Islands.

Nair et al., in his review of oral cancers from Regional Cancer Center, Trivandrum, noted that the prevalence of cancer of buccal mucosa was far more than that of tongue cancer (49.9% vs. 23.97%). Younger patients, without a history of smoking or chewing tobacco diagnosed with these cancers, had a worse outcome. Cancers of the gum and alveolar ridge on the contrary is uncommon before the age 50 and affect women more than men.

TABLE 2: Some established cancer registries in India.

Zones	Registries	ASR (male)	ASR (female)
North	Delhi	123.7	135.6
Central	Bhopal		
West	Ahmedabad	107.2	82.9
East	Kolkata	102.1	114.6
South West	Mumbai	116.3	122.4
	Poona	103.9	115.3
	Nagpur	118.4	118.8
South	Madras	108	118
	Trivandrum	87.8	81.1
	Bangalore	88.3	110.7
	Karunagappalli*	102.6	76
Rural	Barshi		

*HBCR: hospital-based cancer registry
(ASR: age-standardized rate)

However, according to a study by Shenoi et al. from Maharashtra, mandibular alveolar region was found to be the most common site. Unfortunately >80% of the patients had reported in an advanced stage (Stage III onward).

Age and Gender

Oral cancer is considered to be a cancer of the elderly. Most of the oral cancers occur between the age of 50 and 75 years. More recently, cancers are being reported in younger patients. A study in Asia found that about 17% of the younger patients are <40 years of age or in the early 40s. Overall, men are more commonly affected than women with a male-to-female (M/F) ratio ranging from 1.45 to 10.5 depending on the geographical region. Japan, for example, has the M/F ratio of oropharyngeal carcinoma as 1.45; similarly, the ratio is 1.5 in Pakistan; 1.9 in Iran; 2.2–2.4 in the United States and 10.5 in Taiwan. However, a reverse gender ratio was seen in Thailand and India (Bangalore) where M/F ratio is 1:1.56 and 1:2.0, respectively.

Site

It is a known fact the site of occurrence of a particular cancer is determined by the risk factors innate to that particular geographical region. The *tongue* is thus the most common site for oral cancer among Europeans, North Americans and Asians, constituting up to 40–50% of all the oral cancers.

The *buccal mucosa* is the next most common site of oral cancer, seen more in Asian population where areca nut/tobacco chewing is a common habit.

ETIOLOGY

Studies have reported strong association of oral cancer with the use of *tobacco (smoking or chewing)* or *alcohol intake*. According to studies, 57% of all men and 11% of women between the age of 15 and 49 years use some form of tobacco.

Use of smokeless tobacco (SLT) such as betel quid along with smoking is a common practice in many parts of India **(Table 3)**. Betel quid, is commonly known as *paan* which consists of leaf of piper betel vine wrapping pieces of areca nut, processed or unprocessed tobacco, aqueous calcium hydroxide (slaked lime). Other forms of tobacco used are, *gutka, zarda, kharra, mawa, and khaini* **(Table 4)**.

These are dry mixtures of lime, areca nut flakes, and powdered tobacco.

These days, sachets of premixed areca nut, lime, condiments with or without

TABLE 3: Classification of smokeless tobacco products by mode of use.

Oral			Nasal use (sniffing)
Sucking	**Chewing**	**Other oral use**	
Chimó	Betel quid	Creamy stuff	Dry snuff
Dry snuff	*Gutka*	*Gudhakhu*	Liquid snuff
Gutka	*Iqmik*	*Gul*	
Khaini	*Khaini*	*Mishri*	
Loose-leaf	*Khiwam*	Red tooth powder	
Maras	Loose-leaf	*Tuibur*	
Mishri	*Mawa*		
Moist snuff	Plug		
Naswar	Tobacco chewing		
Plug	Gum		
Shammah	Twist or roll		
Snus	*Zarda*		
Tobacco tablets			
Toombak			

TABLE 4: Some common forms of oral smokeless tobacco and their constituents.

Common/native name	Ingredients	Countries/populations
Toombak	Sodium carbonate and tobacco (*Toombak*-associated carcinogens have high prevalence of p53 protein aberration)	Sudan
Shammah	Tobacco, slaked lime, and ash	Saudi Arabia
Naswar	Tobacco, slaked lime, indigo, cardamom, oil, and menthol	Iran, Afghanistan, Pakistan, Central Asia
Nass	Tobacco, ash, cotton, and sesame oil	Iran, Afghanistan, Pakistan, Central Asia
Mawa	Areca nut, lime, and tobacco	India
Gudakhu	Tobacco and molasses	Central India
Zarda	Boiled tobacco	India and Arab countries
Paan/betel quid	Areca nut, betel leaf, slaked lime, spice, and catechu, with or without tobacco	Indian subcontinent, New Guinea, Southeast Asia, and South America
Mishri	Burned tobacco	India

powdered tobacco are available freely and are very popular among old and young alike. The *paan or gutka* is stored in the cheek and chewed or sucked for several minutes, or some users choosing to keep it overnight.

Addiction to tobacco typically starts early in life through company of family member or peers. Various researches carried out across the country indicate that at least a third of school children <15 years of age have used one or another of tobacco. However, with improved public health awareness, the use of tobacco is decreasing everywhere, including India. Recently, increased incidence of oral cancer, especially tongue cancer has been seen among young adults. In a study of 482 consecutive patients of H and N cancer at a tertiary care cancer center in India, 135 out of the 286 (47%) oral cavity cancer patients had no known habit of use of tobacco or alcohol.

Prevalence and pattern of SLT use:
- According to the population-based surveys, on an average currently nearly 25 crore Indians use SLT.
- Prevalence among men is higher, with more than one in every three using tobacco in some or the other form.
- A little over 14 crore men and almost 6 crore women use SLT in India.

More than one in every five urban Indians use tobacco products.

Smokeless tobacco is used commonly in Africa, North America, South-East Asia, Europe, and the Middle East in the following forms:

- Betel quid with tobacco, commonly known as *paan or pan* (**Fig. 3**). It consists of four main ingredients: (1) betel leaf (leaf of Piper betel vine), (2) areca nut (*Areca catechu*), (3) slaked lime, and (4) tobacco. Tobacco is the most important ingredient.
- *Gutka*: These are sun-dried, roasted, finely chopped tobacco, areca nut, slaked lime, and catechu mixed with some flavorings and sweeteners. It is kept in the mouth, sucked, and chewed.
- *Khaini*: This substance is made from sun-dried or fermented coarsely cut tobacco leaves. The tobacco used for this type is derived from *Nicotiana rustica* and/or *N. tabacum*. Areca nut are often added to khaini during use. It predominantly causes cancer of GBS (*gingivobuccal sulcus*) due to habit of pouching in the inferior GBS.
- *Zarda*: Tobacco, lime, spices and vegetable dyes. Tobacco leaves are broken up and boiled along with lime and spices until dry. This mixture is dried and later colored with vegetable dyes. Zarda is commonly chewed mixed with finely chopped areca nuts and spices. This is frequently used as an ingredient in the betel quid.

Tobacco products for smoking:
- *Cigarette*: This is a roll of tobacco wrapped in paper or any nontobacco material. It may be filter-tipped or untipped, about 8 mm in diameter and 70–120 mm in length.
- *Cigar*: Any roll of tobacco wrapped in leaf tobacco or in any other substance containing tobacco.

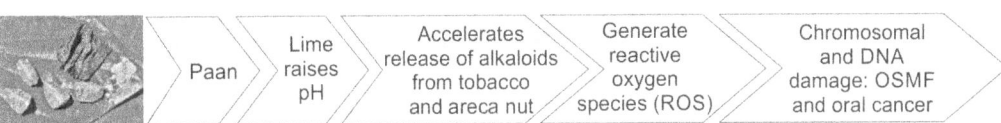

Fig. 3: Effects of *paan* consumption.
(OSMF: oral submucous fibrosis)

Types: Little cigars, small cigars ("cigarillos"), regular cigars, premium cigars. Some of the little cigars have filter tips and are shaped like cigarettes. Regular cigars are up to 17 mm in diameter and 110–150 mm in length.
- *Bidi*: Hand-rolled Indian cigarette. These are sun-dried temburni leaf rolled into a conical shape together with flaked tobacco and tied with a thread.
- *Chuttaa*: Hand-rolled cigarette used for reverse smoking. Used commonly by women in India (Rural and tribal—north coastal districts of Andhra Pradesh).

Advances in chemical analytical techniques have identified increasing number of carcinogens in tobacco smoke. The carcinogens identified include 10 species of polynuclear aromatic hydrocarbons (PAHs), six heterocyclic hydrocarbons, four volatile hydrocarbons, three nitrohydrocarbons, four aromatic amines, eight N-heterocyclic amines, 10 N-nitrosamines, two aldehydes, 10 miscellaneous organic compounds, nine inorganic compounds, and three phenolic compounds. Eleven compounds (2-naphthylamine, 4-aminobiphenyl, benzene, vinyl chloride, ethylene oxide, arsenic, beryllium, nickel compounds, chromium, cadmium and polonium-210) classified as IARC Group 1 human carcinogens have been in the smoke.

Since the last IARC Monograph on tobacco smoking (IARC, 1986a), the emphasis of research on carcinogens in tobacco and its smoke has primarily been on the following due to their established carcinogenic potency:
- Benzo[a]pyrene (a surrogate for all PAHs)
- Tobacco-specific N-nitrosamines (TSNA), especially N'-nitrosonornicotine (NNN) and 4-(N-nitrosomethylamino)-1-(3-pyridyl)-1-butanone (NNK).
- Aromatic amines, especially 4-aminobiphenyl (4-ABP)

Key Points
- *Heavy smokers of cigarettes*: 5–25-fold increase for developing oral cancer
- *>1 packet/day*: 13-fold increase for developing oral cancer
- Starting age below 18 years and duration over 35 years are high-risk factors.
- Tobacco contains over 50 known carcinogens.
- The risk of oral cancer is *reduced by 30%* in those who have discontinued its use for *1–9 years* and by *50%* in those who have stopped habit for *>9 years*.
- Pipe and cigar smokers have an increased *risk of oral cancer* compared to other head and neck subsites.
- Reverse smoking is commonly associated with cancer of the hard palate and palatine arch.
- Marijuana smoking is associated with release of carcinogenic agents such as polycyclic aromatic hydrocarbons, benzopyrene, phenols, phytosterols, acids and terpenes. A study from Memorial Sloan Kettering Cancer Center reported an overall risk of 2.6.

ALCOHOL (FIG. 4)

Alcohol has been implicated in the development of oral cancer. Alcoholic beverages have been reported to be carcinogenic to humans for cancers of the oral cavity, pharynx, larynx, esophagus, and liver but ethanol has not been found carcinogenic in animal studies.

Alcohol acts synergistically with tobacco to increase the risk of development of oral cancer.

A strong dose–response relationship has been observed in most studies. (Relative risks that range from 3.5 to 9.2)

Some substances that are thought to be carcinogenic to humans have also been seen in alcoholic beverages. A few of them are: N-nitroso compounds, mycotoxins, urethane, and inorganic arsenic.

The *major metabolite of alcohol is acetaldehyde*, which is transformed by the enzyme alcohol dehydrogenase (ADH). Acetaldehyde is then oxidized to acetate with

Epidemiology and Etiology of Oral Cancer

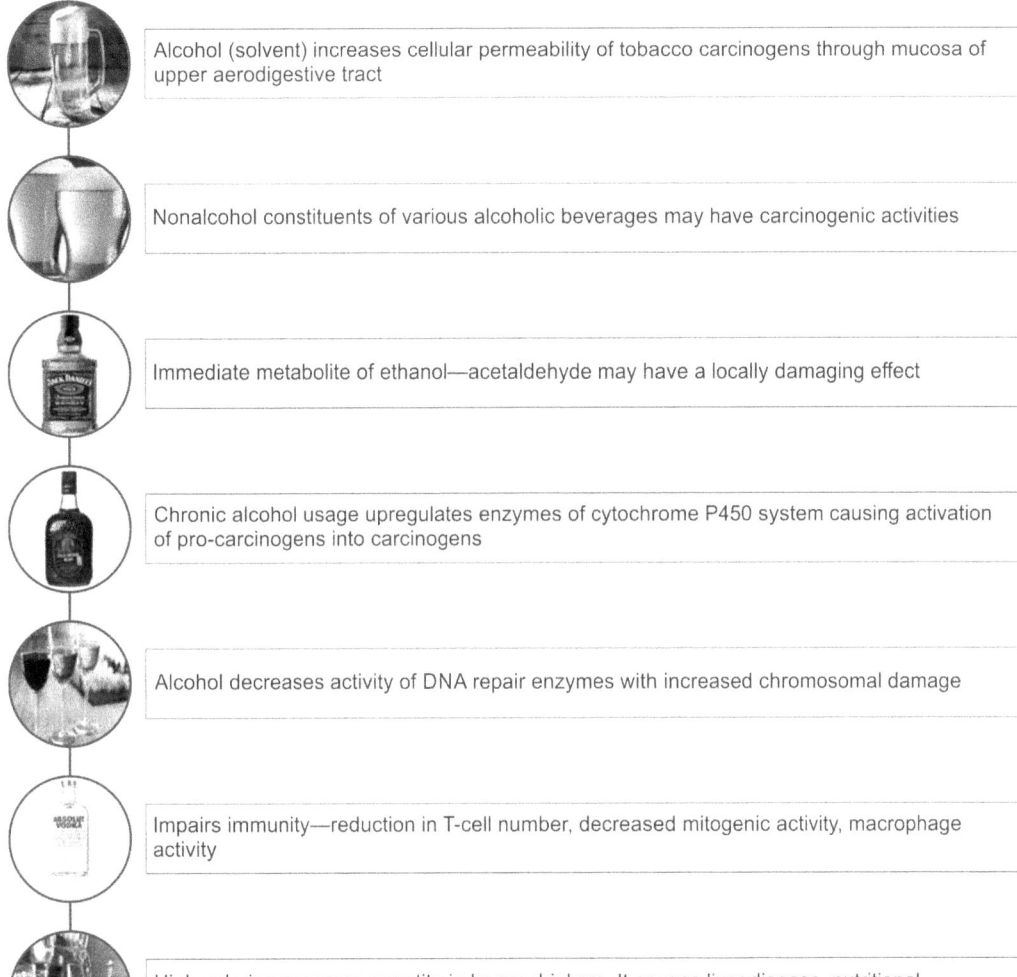

Fig. 4: Mechanism of action of alcohol.

the help of aldehyde dehydrogenase (ALDH). Toxic effects of acetaldehyde may be:
- Acetaldehyde causes damage to the DNA in cultured mammalian cells.
- It interferes with synthesis and repair of DNA.
- Acetaldehyde inhibits the enzyme 6-methyl guanine transferase which is needed for repairing damages caused by alkylating agents.
- Increased accumulation of acetaldehyde in the body whether due to increase in its production or decrease in its elimination, are deleterious.

HUMAN PAPILLOMAVIRUS

Human papillomavirus (HPV) infects the oral cavity of healthy individuals, and several HPV-related lesions have been described in literature.

Prevalence of HPV in oral and oropharyngeal squamous cell carcinoma (OSCC) has been reported to be 33.6% in Eastern India, 48% in South India, 15% in West India, 27.5% in Central India, and 28% in Northeast India.

DIET AND NUTRITION

Fruits and vegetables, particularly carrots, tomatoes, and green vegetables have been proved to reduce risks of oral and pharyngeal cancer. Other *food types that have a protective effect* are fish, cereals, legumes, protein, fat, fresh meat, chicken, liver, shrimp, lobster, vegetable oil, olive oil, bread, and fiber.

Many micronutrients and vitamins also decrease the risk of development of oral cancers. These are vitamins A (retinol), carotenoids (β-carotene), potassium; and selenium. β-carotene, retinol, retinoids, vitamin C (AA), and vitamin E (α-tocopherol), which are antioxidants that are useful in reducing free radical reactions which are responsible for DNA mutations, changes in enzymatic reactions, and lipid peroxidation of cellular membranes.

OCCUPATIONAL RISK

Exposure to excessive solar radiation/ultraviolet (UV) light are notorious in causing lip cancers. UV rays can also cause actinic cheilitis which may transform later to OSCC.

GENETIC FACTORS

Some individuals inherit inability to metabolize carcinogens or procarcinogens and/or an impaired ability to repair the DNA damage. Genetic polymorphisms in the genes coding for the enzymes (P450 enzymes and xenobiotics-metabolizing enzymes) that are causative for metabolism of the tobacco carcinogen are believed to play an important role in the genetic predisposition to tobacco-induced head and neck cancers.

DENTAL FACTORS

Chronic mechanical irritation of the mucosa of the oral cavity can arise due to following:
- Defective teeth (malpositioned with sharp or rough surfaces because of decay or fractures), (1.13 risk).
- Ill-fitting dentures (sharp or rough surfaces, lack of retention, stability, or overextended flanges) (Four-time risk)
- Parafunctional habits (e.g., oral mucosa biting or sucking, tongue interposition, or thrusting).

SEER 2016 ANALYSIS: LIFETIME RISK OF DEVELOPING CANCER

Based on 2014–2016 data, approximately 1.2% of men and women are likely to be diagnosed with cancers of oral cavity and pharynx at some point during their lifetime.

Survival (Fig. 5)

The outcome for cancers of the lip, appear to be best, with over 90% of patients surviving for 5 years. But in general, prognosis deteriorates with advanced stage of the disease. For cancers of oral cavity, women have been found to have higher survival rates than men. TNM stage at presentation significantly affects 5-year survival. For mobile tongue, 5-year survival for stage 1 disease is 80%, while, it drops to 15% for stage IV.

Recurrence is often an inevitable aspect of treatment outcome. It indicates poor prognosis. Recurrence may be local, regional, locoregional or distant metastasis. Recurrence rates vary between 25 and 40% after a follow-up period of 2–4 years.

Epidemiology and Etiology of Oral Cancer

Estimated new cases in 2019	53,000
% of all new cancer cases	3.0%
Estimated deaths in 2019	10,860
% of all cancer deaths	1.8%

Percent surviving 5 years
65.3%
2009–2015

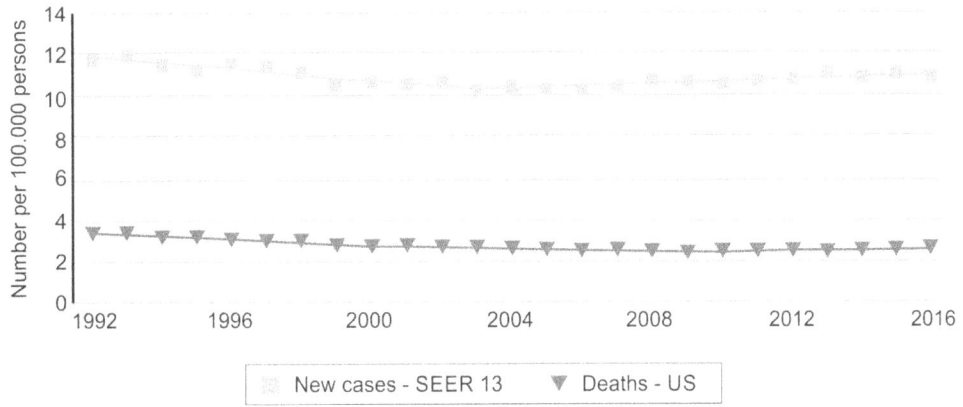

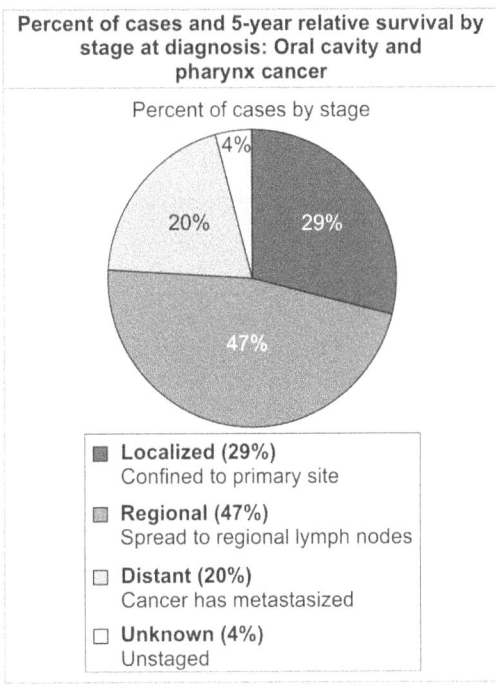

Fig. 5: Survival by stage.

Mortality

For most countries age-adjusted death rates from oral cancer have been estimated to be 3–4 per 100,000 men and 1.5–2.0 per 100,000 for women. Globally a low 5-year survival rate of 50% is seen among patients with oral cancer.

KEY POINTS

- Squamous cell carcinoma is the most common type of malignancy that is diagnosed in the oral and oropharyngeal regions.
- *India fact sheet*: GLOBOCAN 2018, cancer of the lip and oral cavity, huge increase of 114.2% with 56,000 cases in 2012 that increased to 119,992 in 2018.
- Population-based *5-year survival* for patients with the group of oral cavity cancers—*approximately 50% in US, ranges from 45 to 49% in Europe and approximately 30% in India.*
- *RCC, Trivandrum*: Highest prevalence of cancer of buccal mucosa (49.9%).
- Maharashtra has reported mandibular alveolus as the most common site of oral cancer.
- Estimates indicate 57% of all men and 11% of women between 15 and 49 years of age use some form of tobacco.
- 14 crore men and almost 6 crore women use SLT in India.
- *Heavy smokers of cigarettes*: 5–25-fold increase for developing oral cancer.
- *>1 packet/day*: 13-fold increase for developing oral cancer.
- *Other etiological factors*: Alcohol, genetic, diet and nutrition, occupation, and dental factors.

CHAPTER 3

Prevention and Chemoprevention

Kiran Joshi

INTRODUCTION

Very recently, enormous interest is being created in prevention of cancer and cardiovascular diseases using antioxidants. Epidemiological studies show that a diet rich in fruits and vegetables is associated with a diminished risk of cancer and cardiovascular disease. These studies suggest that antioxidants such as ascorbic acid (vitamin C), tocopherol (vitamin E), and β-carotene (provitamin A), selenium, and other bioactive micronutrients impart a protective effect against cancer.

PRIMARY CANCER PREVENTION

Prevention of cancer by avoiding known carcinogens is known as "Primary Prevention". It has been seen that after stopping smoking and use of alcohol, the risk of developing head and neck squamous cell carcinoma (HNSCC) reduces to a great extent. After avoiding smoking for 1–4 years, there has been a 30% reduction in risk for developing HNSCC compared to those who continue smoking. The risk reduces to that of never smokers for those who have quit smoking for >20 years.

SECONDARY CANCER PREVENTION

Secondary prevention of cancer involves detection of cancer early with the help of screening methods in a population at risk. Delays in diagnosing may give rise to decreased survival according to some studies. Hence, there is a need for increased awareness about early symptoms of potentially malignant diseases (PMDs) among public along with education of healthcare workers about these symptoms. This would enable early detection, increase in cure rates, and decrease treatment-related morbidity.

Cancers of the oral cavity are more likely to be detected early, during routine screening examination, or by self-examination. Regular dental examination by a dentist may be useful in detecting oral and oropharyngeal cancers and precancerous lesions early. Often, it is recommended that people have a scrutinizing look at their oral cavity in a mirror once every month. The American Cancer Society has also recommended that doctors must examine the oral cavity and throat, as part of a routine checkup. An exception may be the oropharyngeal cancers. These cancers are generally asymptomatic till late and hence may not be detected early like their counterpart. For adults who are asymptomatic but present with a large neck mass, must be approached with a high index of suspicion, especially when there is a history of use of tobacco and/or alcohol.

TERTIARY CANCER PREVENTION

Tertiary cancer prevention is the prevention and early detection of second primary tumors (SPTs) in patients already treated

for a malignancy. Regular follow-ups are strongly recommended by the National Comprehensive Cancer Network, for such patients after their curative treatment to detect:
- Recurrence
- A second primary cancer in the head and neck or lung
- Complications of treatment

CRITERIA FOR DIAGNOSIS OF MULTIPLE CANCERS

It was Warren and Gates who first introduced a set of criteria to diagnose multiple primary carcinomas. These were later modified by Hong et al., *for diagnosis of multiple cancers*, the criteria to be met are:
- The neoplasm must be distinct and anatomically separate. A tumor is known as multicentric when a dysplastic mucosa is present next to it.
- A potential second primary carcinoma which represents a metastasis or a local relapse to be excluded.
- It must have occurred 3 years after the first diagnosis or it should be separate from the first tumor by at least 2 cm from the normal epithelium.

FIELD CANCERIZATION

The concept of field cancerization was first introduced by Slaughter et al. in 1953. He suggested that multiple tumors could develop within an anatomically and histologically related site because of migration of a clonal lineage to an adjacent site or by separate clones in the area receiving critical genetic insults due to similar exposures.

CHEMOPREVENTION (FIG. 1)

The rationale behind the development of chemoprevention was the failure of conventional therapies such as surgery, radiation, and chemotherapy to prevent recurrence and the risk of second primary neoplasms in a number of patients. The interesting concept was first presented by Michel B Sporn. It refers to the prevention of reversal, suppression, or transformation of a premalignant form to an invasive lesion with the help of natural or synthetic chemicals. Chemoprevention for head and neck cancer denotes prevention of development of both synchronous and metachronous second primary tumor within the exposed epithelium of the upper aero digestive

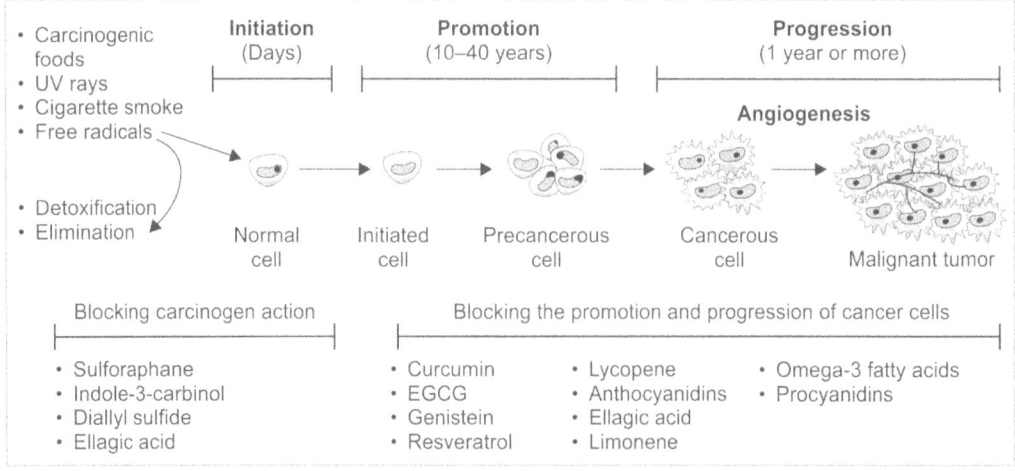

Fig. 1: Model of chemoprevention.
(EGCG: epigallocatechin gallate)

tract and lung. Different classes of natural products, targeted agents such as retinoid receptors ligands, selective cyclooxygenase inhibitors, p53-targeted agents, peroxisome activator receptor gamma (PPARγ) agonists, and epidermal growth factor receptor (EGFR) inhibitors, have been studied in great detail.

Retinoids (Fig. 2)

Retinoids are naturally occurring and synthetic vitamin A (retinol) metabolites and analogs that bind to retinoic acid receptors (RAR and RXR types) and promote cell differentiation and decrease cell proliferation and apoptosis. The loss of nuclear RARβ is an early event observed in premalignant dysplastic lesions. Targeting the retinoid signaling pathway therefore could act as a strategy for chemoprevention. Retinoids cause a characteristic, mucocutaneous toxicity syndrome with dryness, itching, peeling, alopecia, and photosensitivity which is dose related. These toxicity and the rapid reversal of their beneficial effects after stopping the retinoids have prevented them from being used as the standard of care.

Curcumin (Flowchart 1)

Curcumin (diferuloylmethane) is a polyphenol compound which plays anticancer roles due to its properties of inhibition of tumor initiation and tumor promotion. The pleiotropic activity of curcumin producing chemoprevention is through regulation of many intracellular signal transduction pathways at different levels such as transcriptions factors—nuclear factor (NF) transcription.

Lycopene (Flowchart 2)

Lycopene is an efficient biological antioxidizing agent with property of modifying intercellular exchange junctions, and thus preventing cancer.

Cyclooxygenase Inhibitors

Cyclooxygenase-2 (COX2) is commonly seen to be overexpressed in oral dysplasias and squamous cell carcinomas of the head and neck. Some preclinical research indicate that COX2 inhibitors could have some chemopreventive role. But due to the cardiovascular toxicities of these COX-2 inhibitors along with disappointing results, in chemoprevention studies of colonic polyps they are not being used for HNSCC prevention.

Green Tea

The polyphenol (-)-epigallocatevhin-3-gallate (EGCG), a known antioxidant, has been found in green tea extract. EGCG can modulate multiple signaling pathways including inhibition of receptor tyrosine kinases and their downstream pathways, inhibition of NF kappa-B, and activation of p53 pathway. They have used in several *cancer prevention* protocols in different preparations and along with other potentially active ingredients. Therefore, results from these studies have to be interpreted very cautiously.

p53-targeted Agents

p-53 mutations may be found in 47–62% of cancers of the head and neck region. Attempts have been made at restoring p53 function in premalignant lesions, or targeting the p53 mutant premalignant cells. ONYX-015 is an attenuated oncolytic adenovirus, which is supposed to be cytotoxic to cells with dysfunctional p53-dependant signaling pathways.

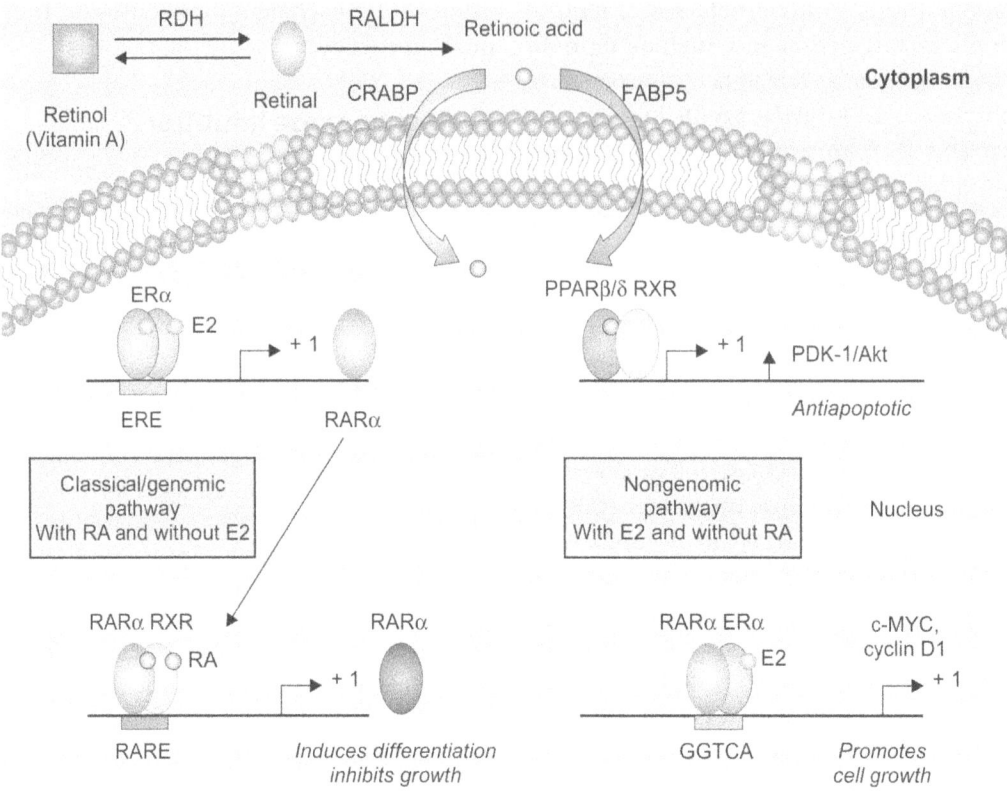

Fig. 2: Retinoid signaling pathways.
The retinoic acid receptors (RARs) and their action: Vitamin A (retinol) is metabolized through the oxidizing action of retinaldehyde (RDH) to retinal and by retinaldehyde dehydrogenase (RALDH) to retinoic acid (RA). RA has three different isomers: all-*trans*, 9-*cis*, and 13-*cis*RA. RA is transported to the nucleus by the protein cellular RA-binding protein (CRABP) and delivered to the RARα. RARα heterodimerizes with and binds to retinoic acid response elements (RARE) present most often in gene promoters. In the classical pathway of RA action, RA binds to dimers of RARα and RXRs (α, β, or γ) to induce expression of its downstream target genes, including *RAR*β. Upon activation, RARβ can regulate its own expression and that of its downstream genes, the function of which is mainly to inhibit cell growth. Alternatively, RA can be bound and transported to the nucleus by other factors such as FABP5. This delivers RA to other nonclassical receptors such as peroxisome activator receptor beta/gamma (PPARβ/δ) and estrogen receptor alpha (ERα) which activate nongenomic pathways such as phosphoinositide-dependent protein kinase 1 (PDK-1)/Akt or the ERα pathway. Contrary to the differentiation functions attributed to the classical pathway, the nongenomic pathways exert strong antiapoptotic and proliferative effects on cancer cells. It is believed that the classical and nongenomic pathways are controlled by the relative abundance of their own ligands. RA has a stronger affinity for RARs than for the other receptors, and the classical pathway plays a dominant role over the nongenomic pathways. Thus, if RA is present with other ligands such as estrogen, signaling through the classical pathway is preferred to result in cell differentiation and growth inhibition.

Thiazolidinediones

Thiazolidinediones, pioglitazone or troglitazone, have been studied in preclinical animal models. It was found that they decreased the tongue carcinoma multiplicity and incidence, respectively. They have

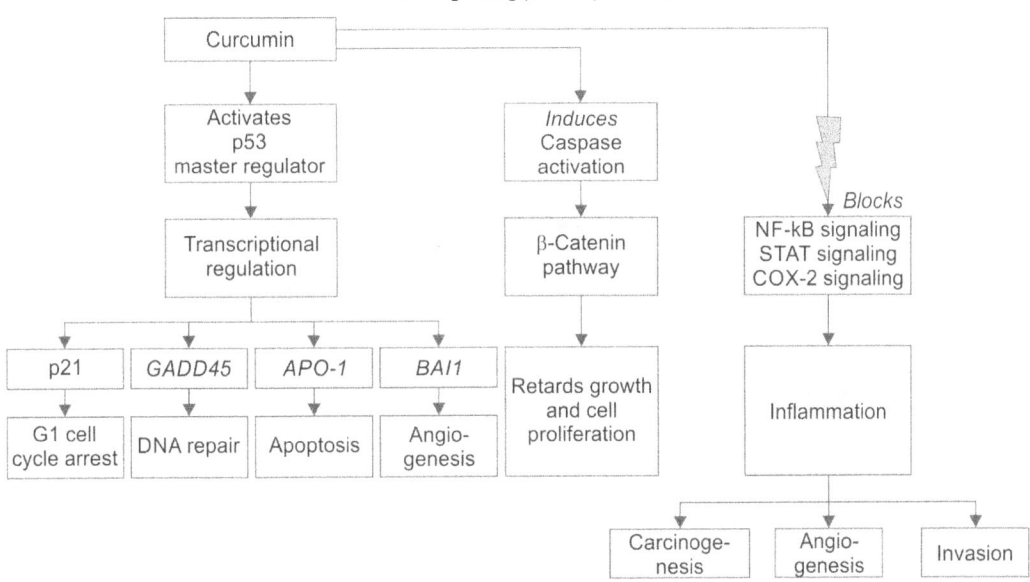

Flowchart 1: Signaling pathways—curcumin.

(APO-1: apolipoprotein 1; BAI1: brain-specific angiogenesis inhibitor 1; COX-2: cyclooxygenase-2; GADD45: growth arrest and DNA damage inducible; NF-κβ: nuclear factor kappa-light-chain-enhancer of activated B-cells; STAT: signal transducer and activator of transcription)

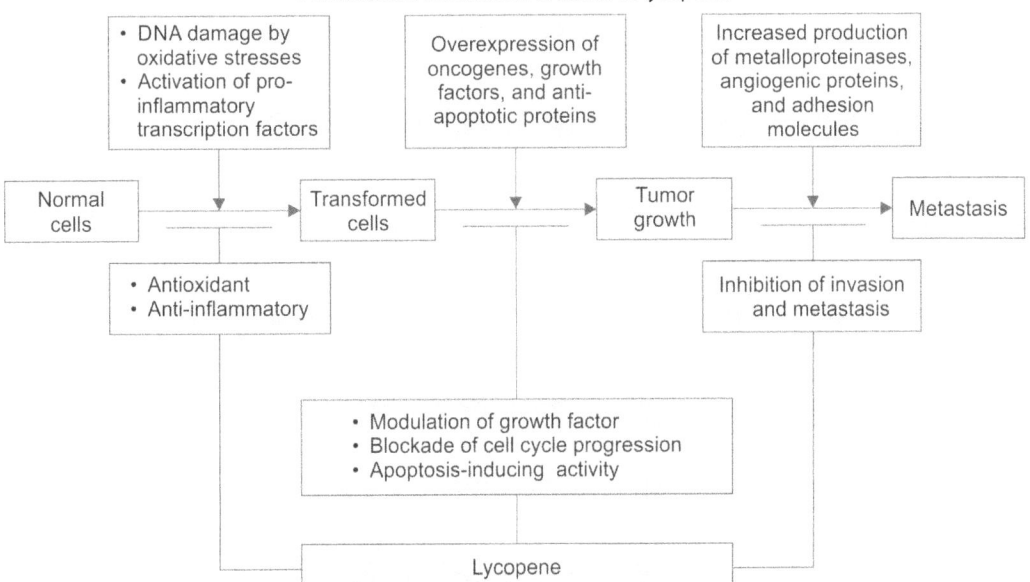

Flowchart 2: Mechanism of action of lycopene.

also shown a reduced incidence of lung and head and neck cancers in diabetic patients in retrospective epidemiologic studies in comparison to diabetic patients who have been treated with alternative oral hypoglycemic agents.

EGFR Inhibitors

Epidermal growth factor receptor is known to be overexpressed in malignant, premalignant, and also normal tissues of patients of *head and neck carcinomas*. Also, EGFR expression increases with increasing degree of dysplasia and is profoundly increased in >90% HNSCC. Erlotinib decreases the incidence of oral squamous cell carcinoma (OSCC) in a chemically-induced mouse model.

KEY POINTS

- There is a high incidence (15%) of second primaries in patients with oral cavity cancer.
- The main causative factors are tobacco and alcohol.
- There is synergistic interaction between tobacco and alcohol.
- There is a strong association with human papilloma virus, particularly in tonsil cancer.
- Leukoplakia, erythroplakia, and submucous fibrosis are important precancerous conditions.
- Genetic predisposition syndromes include Li–Fraumeni syndrome, Fanconi syndrome, Bloom syndrome and ataxia-telangiectasia.
- Oral cancer is largely a preventable public health problem.
- Chemoprevention refers to the use of natural or synthetic chemicals for the reversal suppression or prevention for conversion of a premalignant lesion to an invasive form.

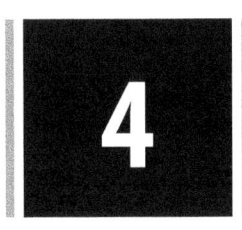

CHAPTER 4

Histopathology and Molecular Pathology of Squamous Cell Carcinoma of Oral Cavity

Sunil Pasricha, Meenakshi Kamboj

INTRODUCTION

Head and neck cancers are one of the most common cancers worldwide with significant health problems. More than 90% of these are squamous cell carcinomas (SCCs). Risk factors for oral squamous cell carcinomas (OSCCs) include smoking, tobacco chewing, and alcohol, with a strong synergistic effect. Human papilloma virus (HPV) infection is seen in only 3% of OSCCs, and sunlight exposure is a risk factor for lip cancers.

A list of epithelial tumors and premalignant lesions, as classified by the World Health Organization (WHO), is given in **Box 1**.

EPITHELIAL PRECURSOR LESIONS OF OSCC

Precursor lesions are mostly seen in the adult population and affect men more than women, with mean age for the first precursor lesion diagnosis reported from 48.0–56.5 years. The incidences vary worldwide with the magnitude and duration of carcinogen exposure. Risk factors for the precursor lesions are the same as those of invasive cancers.

Dysplasia is the premalignant lesion in mucosa showing altered architectural and cytological epithelium. It can be nonkeratinizing (classic) or keratinizing dysplasia.

Dysplasia is architecturally defined as irregular epithelial stratification with loss of polarity of basal cells, drop-shaped rete

Box 1: The WHO classification of epithelial tumors of the oral cavity and mobile tongue.

Oral potentially malignant disorders and oral epithelial dysplasia
- Oral potentially malignant disorders:
  – Erythroplakia
  – Erythroleukoplakia
  – Oral submucosal fibrosis
  – Dyskeratosis congenital
  – Chronic candidiasis
  – Lichen planus
  – Discoid lupus erythematosus
  – Actinic keratosis (lip only)
- Oral epithelial dysplasia
- Proliferative verrucous leukoplakia

Benign epithelial tumors
- Papillomas:
  – Squamous cell papilloma
  – Condyloma acuminatum
  – Verruca vulgaris
  – Multifocal epithelial hyperplasia

Malignant surface epithelial tumors
- Squamous cell carcinoma (SCC):
  – Subtypes of SCC:
    - Verrucous carcinoma
    - Basaloid SCC
    - Papillary SCC
    - Spindle cell carcinoma
    - Acantholytic SCC
    - Adenosquamous carcinoma
    - Carcinoma cuniculatum
- Lymphoepithelial carcinoma

ridges, premature keratinization in single cells (dyskeratosis), and keratin pearl within rete pegs (paradoxical maturation). Cytologic atypical features include abnormal variation in nuclear size (anisonucleosis), nuclear shape (nuclear pleomorphism), cell

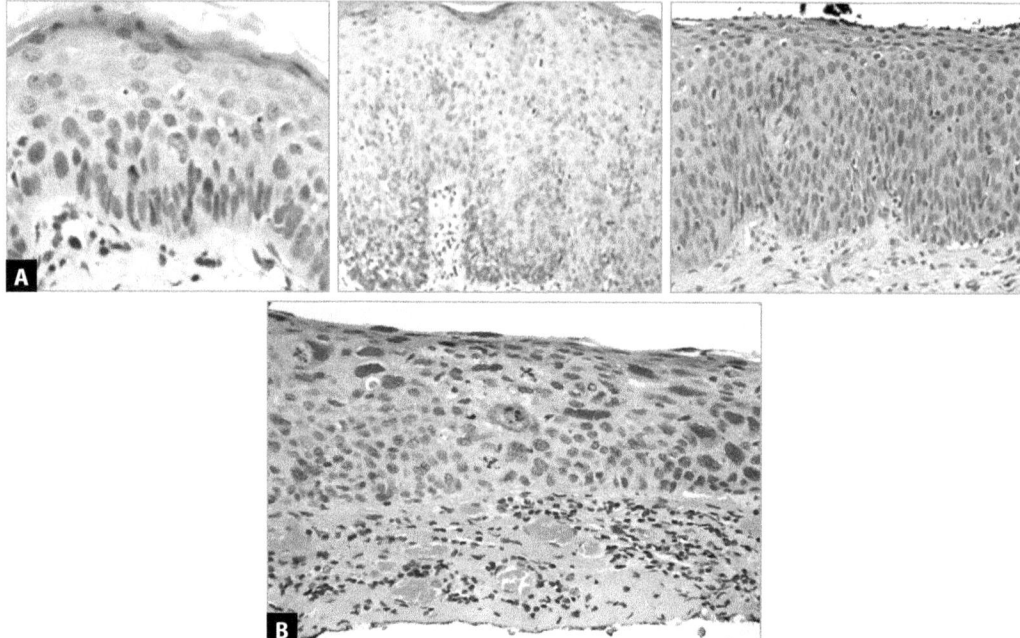

Figs. 1A and B: (A) Microphotograph showing mild, moderate, and severe squamous dysplasia; (B) Squamous carcinoma-in-situ; marked nuclear pleomorphism with atypical mitotic figures.

size (anisocytosis), and increased nuclear: Cytoplasmic ratio with nuclear enlargement, hyperchromasia, and prominent nucleoli. Atypical mitotic figures can be seen.

Dysplasia is graded as mild, moderate, and severe as per the WHO classification **(Fig. 1A)**. It can also be graded using binary system into low and high grade (includes moderate and severe) which is more relevant for decision-making in management.

Mild dysplasia shows these changes limited to the lower third of the epithelium while in *moderate dysplasia*, they extend into the middle third of the epithelium. *Severe dysplasia* shows greater than two-thirds of the epithelium showing architectural and cytologic atypia. Coexisting high degree of cytological atypia upgrades moderately dysplastic lesions to severe dysplasia.

Carcinoma-in-situ by definition show full-thickness architectural abnormalities accompanied by pronounced cytologic atypia, with frequent mitosis reaching superficial layer, including atypical mitosis. This lesion depicts malignant transformation without any invasion, and is synonymous with severe dysplasia **(Fig. 1B)**.

Risk of progression for mild, moderate, and severe dysplasia is estimated to be 6%, 18%, and 39%, respectively.

Leukoplakia is clinically a keratotic white plaque that cannot be scraped off, cannot be given another specific diagnostic name and has no known etiology, except tobacco use. A large number of these lesions are found in close proximity to mucosal carcinomas. It forms 85% of oral precancerous lesions and the most common chronic lesion of the oral mucosa. Histologically, it shows acanthosis and hyperkeratosis. Approximately 90% of these lesions are benign, with a low rate of dysplasia (8–9%) and transformation to invasive carcinoma (6.5–17.5%) over prolonged periods. Lesions of long duration have a greater risk of malignant transformation than those of short duration.

When clinically white leukoplakic lesions are interrupted by red lesions, they are called *erythroleukoplakia* or *speckled leukoplakia*. They carry an extremely high risk of malignant transformation.

Erythroplakia is a chronic red mucosal patch which, like leukoplakia, cannot be given another specific diagnostic name and cannot be attributed to traumatic, vascular, or inflammatory causes. They are frequently seen in association with early invasive oral carcinomas. Most cases of erythroplakia are diagnosed on the mucosa of the lateral and ventral tongue, floor of mouth and soft palate. Histologically, they typically present as carcinoma in situ, severe epithelial dysplasia, or superficially invasive carcinoma.

In general, leukoplakia has a lower risk of malignant transformation than speckled leukoplakia, which has an intermediate risk, and pure erythroplakia has the highest risk of invasive cancer development.

Proliferative verrucous leukoplakia is a multifocal and progressive premalignant lesion, involving gingiva, alveolar mucosa, and palate. In early stages, they show verrucous hyperorthokeratosis without any dysplasia and band-like submucosal chronic lymphoplasmacytic infiltrate, with later progression to dysplasia and invasive carcinomas in 70% of cases. They have better prognosis than the conventional cancers.

Oral lichen planus is a chronic mucocutaneous immune inflammatory condition, with controversial malignant transformation. Oral lichenoid lesions are considered as lesions at risk if associated with dysplasia.

SQUAMOUS CELL CARCINOMA

Squamous cell carcinoma is microscopically seen as keratinization with variable amount of "pearl" formation and presence of intercellular desmosomes. Invasive growth shows disruption of the basement membrane and extension of nests and islands of tumor cells into the underlying tissue, often accompanied by stromal reaction (desmoplasia).

Squamous cell carcinomas are graded as well, moderate, or poorly differentiated. As the tumor grade increases, it shows decrease in keratinization, increase in cellular and nuclear pleomorphism, hyperchromasia, and mitotic figures. However, the grading does not correlate well with prognosis.

Well-differentiated SCC show minimal atypia, pleomorphism, and mitosis, with presence of keratinization and pearl formation. *Poorly differentiated SCC* shows sheets of immature cells, numerous typical and atypical mitosis, with minimal keratinization (individual cell). *Moderately differentiated SCC* show intermediate features between both these, and lesser degree of keratinization than the well-differentiated SCC **(Fig. 2)**.

Conventional SCC is locally invasive, aggressive lesion, with early lymph node metastasis. The most significant prognostic factors of SCC are tumor size, nodal status

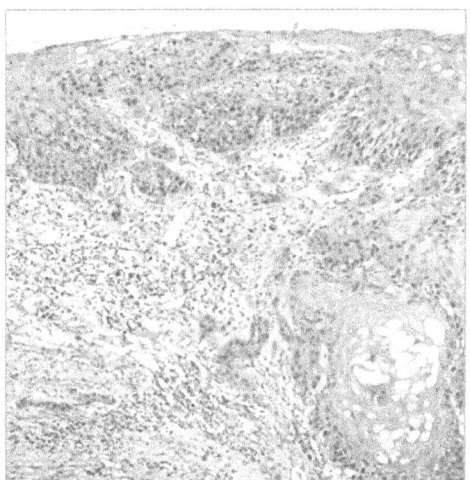

Fig. 2: Moderately differentiated squamous cell carcinoma.

and distant metastasis, which form part of the pathologic (p) TNM staging classification **(Box 2)**. Various other parameters, such as depth of invasion (DOI) and extranodal extension (ENE), are also part of the staging system.

Box 2: Pathological stage classification (pTNM).

Primary tumor (pT):
- *pTx*: Primary tumor cannot be assessed
- *pTis*: Carcinoma in situ
- *pT1*: Tumor ≤ 2 cm with depth of invasion (DOI) ≤ 5 mm
- *pT2*: Tumor ≤ 2 cm with DOI > 5 mm or tumor > 2 cm and ≤4 cm with DOI ≤ 10 mm
- *pT3*: Tumor > 2 cm and ≤4 cm with DOI > 10 mm
  or tumor > 4 cm with DOI ≤ 10 mm
- *pT4*: Moderately advanced or very advanced local disease
- *pT4a*: Moderately advanced local disease—Tumor > 4 cm with DOI > 10 mm or tumor invades adjacent structures only (e.g., through cortical bone of the mandible or maxilla or involves the maxillary sinus or skin of the face)
- *pT4b*: Very advanced local disease—Tumor invades masticator space, pterygoid plates, or skull base, and/or encases the internal carotid artery

Regional lymph nodes (pN):
- *pNx*: Regional lymph nodes cannot be assessed
- *pN0*: No regional lymph node metastasis
- *pN1*: Metastasis in a single ipsilateral lymph node, 3 cm or smaller in greatest dimension and extranodal extension (ENE)(−)
- *pN2*:
  - Metastasis in a single ipsilateral lymph node, 3 cm or smaller in greatest dimension and ENE(+)
  - *or* larger than 3 cm but not larger than 6 cm in greatest dimension and ENE(−)
  - *or* metastases in multiple ipsilateral lymph nodes, none larger than 6 cm in greatest dimension and ENE(−)
  - *or* in bilateral or contralateral lymph node(s), none larger than 6 cm in greatest dimension and ENE(−)
- *pN2a*:
  - Metastasis in single ipsilateral node 3 cm or smaller in greatest dimension and ENE(+)
  - *or* a single ipsilateral node larger than 3 cm but not larger than 6 cm in greatest dimension and ENE(−)
- *pN2b*: Metastases in multiple ipsilateral nodes, none larger than 6 cm in greatest dimension and ENE(−)
- *pN2c*: Metastases in bilateral or contralateral lymph node(s), none larger than 6 cm in greatest dimension and ENE(−)
- *pN3*:
  - Metastasis in a lymph node larger than 6 cm in greatest dimension and ENE(−)
  - *or* metastasis in a single ipsilateral node larger than 3 cm in greatest dimension and ENE(+)
  - *or* multiple ipsilateral, contralateral or bilateral nodes any with ENE(+)
  - *or* a single contralateral node of any size and ENE(+)
- *pN3a*: Metastasis in a lymph node >6 cm in greatest dimension and ENE(−)
- *pN3b*:
  - Metastasis in a single ipsilateral node >3 cm in greatest dimension and ENE(+)
  - *or* multiple ipsilateral, contralateral or bilateral nodes any with ENE(+)
  - *or* a single contralateral node of any size and ENE(+)

Note: Measurement of the metastatic focus in the lymph nodes is based on the largest metastatic deposit size, which may include matted or fused lymph nodes

Distant metastasis (pM) (confirmed pathologically):
- *pM1*: Distant metastasis

Source: Amin MB, Greene FL, Edge SB, Compton CC, Gershenwald JE, Robert KB, et al. The eighth edition AJCC Cancer Staging Manual: Continuing to build a bridge from a population-based to a more "personalized" approach to cancer staging. CA A Cancer J Clin. 2017;67(2):93-9.

Subtypes of SCC

- *Verrucous carcinoma (VC)* is a non-metastasizing, locally invasive, slow-growing variant of well-differentiated SCC, and 75% occur within the oral cavity. Clinically VC is a white, sharply circumscribed, broad-based, firm, and exophytic warty tumor. Microscopically they show thickened club-shaped papillae with pushing superficial invasion, marked keratinization of cells, lack cytologic atypia, and rarely show mitosis. They may show dense lymphoplasmacytic host response and foreign body reaction to abundant keratin. Differential diagnoses include exophytic SCC, papillary SCC, keratinizing squamous cell papilloma, and verruca vulgaris.

  Grading of VC is not required as biologically they are low-grade tumors, and have excellent prognosis, with 5-year survival of 85–95%. *Hybrid VC* is a controversial entity with features of VC showing foci of conventional SCC and potential to metastasize.

- *Basaloid SCC* is an aggressive, high-grade variant of SCC. They are uncommon within oral cavity, and are usually seen in the oropharynx, pyriform sinus, and supraglottic larynx. Grossly they show an ulcerated mass with submucosal induration. Microscopically they show basaloid cells with small hyperchromatic nuclei without nucleoli, and scant cytoplasm. These cells are in solid lobular pattern with peripheral palisading and comedonecrosis. Differential diagnoses include neuroendocrine carcinoma, poorly differentiated adenoid cystic carcinoma, and adenosquamous carcinoma.

  They have a poor prognosis, with regional lymph node metastasis seen in two-thirds and distant metastasis in 35–50% at the time of diagnosis. Grading is not required as biologically they are high-grade tumors.

- *Papillary SCC* often arises in gingiva within oral cavity. Grossly they are soft, friable, polypoid, papillary outgrowth, frequently arising from a thin stalk.

  Microscopically they can be keratinizing or nonkeratinizing with predominant papillary growth pattern and less depth of infiltration. Papillae with thin fibrovascular cores are covered by atypical cells or immature basaloid cells, with minimal keratosis, foci of necrosis and hemorrhage. Stromal invasion by single or multiple nests of tumor cells with dense lymphoplasmacytic infiltrate is seen at the interface. Differential diagnoses include squamous papilloma, VC and exophytic SCC. They have a better prognosis than conventional SCC, probably due to limited stromal invasion.

- *Acantholytic SCC* is an uncommon variant, with a false glandular appearance. It is seen over lip, and other sun exposed areas of head and neck. Microscopically it shows SCC with foci of acantholysis in tumor nests, creating pseudolumina. Differentials include adenosquamous carcinoma, adenoid cystic carcinoma, and mucoepidermoid carcinoma. Prognosis of this subtype is similar to conventional SCC.

- *Adenosquamous carcinoma* is a rare aggressive neoplasm characterized by both SCC and true adenocarcinoma. It is seen in larynx and oral cavity. Histopathology shows distinct SCC and adenocarcinoma components in close proximity. Squamous component can be either as in-situ or invasive SCC, and adenocarcinomatous component shows tubular structures with glands, mucin production, as well as signet ring cells.

On immunophenotyping, both components express high molecular weight keratin (HMWK), while carcinoembryonic antigen (CEA) and low molecular weight keratin (LMWK) (CK7+, CK8+/CK20−) are seen in glandular component. Differentials include mucoepidermoid carcinoma, acantholytic SCC, SCC invading or entrapping seromucinous glands. Prognostically they are worse than conventional SCC with 5-year survival rate of 15–25%.

- *Sarcomatoid carcinoma*, also known as spindle cell SCC is a biphasic tumor, more commonly seen in larynx (glottis). It is composed of variable proportion of SCC and malignant spindle cell component with a mesenchymal appearance, but of epithelial origin. It is seen in elderly males in 7th decade, and may develop after radiation exposure. Grossly they are usually polypoidal with ulcerated surface, and rarely ulceroinfiltrative.

On microscopy tumor bulk is formed by spindle cell component, and foci of heterologous differentiation may be seen. An identifiable squamous component as either in-situ or invasive SCC may be present. On immunohistochemistry (IHC), the spindle neoplastic cells can variably express both epithelial [cytokeratin (CK)] and mesenchymal markers (vimentin), and p40 positivity confirms squamous origin of tumor **(Figs. 3A and B)**. This tumor needs to be differentiated from fibrosarcoma and myoepithelial carcinoma.

Favorable prognostic factors for sarcomatoid carcinoma include polypoid growth and shallow depth of sarcomatous component with a 5-year survival of 65–95%.

MIMICKERS OF MALIGNANCY

Pseudoepitheliomatous hyperplasia is a reactive epithelial hyperplasia seen in response to a variety of persistent stimuli. Common causes include chronic ulcer, bacterial/fungal infection, degenerative changes, retained foreign material, trauma, and malignancy **(Fig. 4)**.

Necrotizing sialometaplasia is a benign, reactive inflammatory process most commonly involving salivary glands of the palate region, and mimics SCC both clinically as well as on histology. Etiology includes compromised vascular supply to salivary gland, leading to ischemic necrosis which can be iatrogenic, trauma related, or associated with neoplasm and radiotherapy.

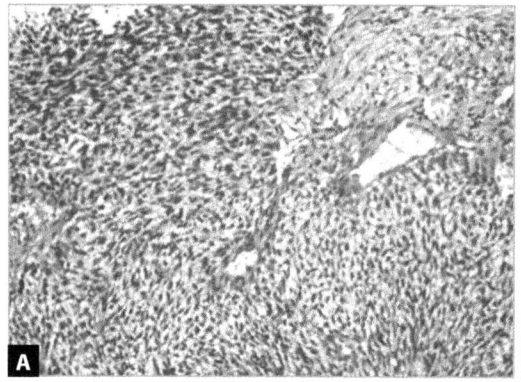 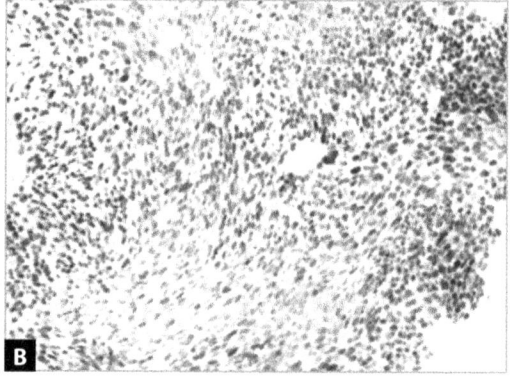

Figs. 3A and B: Sarcomatoid carcinoma showing sheets of neoplastic spindle cells. On immunohistochemistry (IHC), the tumor cells diffusely express p40.

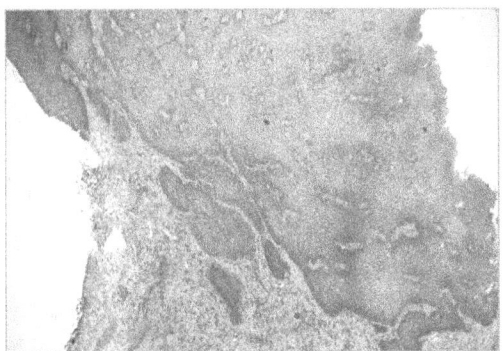

Fig. 4: Pseudoepitheliomatous hyperplasia.

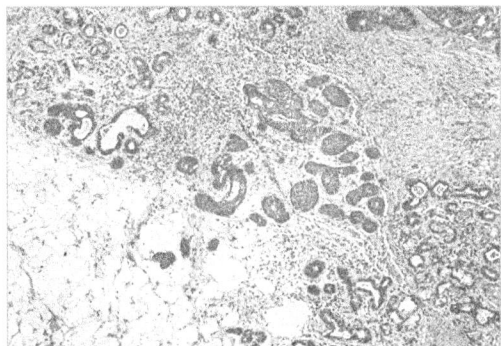

Fig. 5: Necrotizing sialometaplasia.

Lobular necrosis of the salivary gland with preservation of the lobular architecture and squamous metaplasia of residual acinar and ductal elements is seen. Squamous cells are usually bland with uniform nuclei and abundant eosinophilic cytoplasm; however, they can show atypia with mitosis. It commonly mimics SCC and mucoepidermoid carcinoma. Identification of lobular pattern of growth is the clue for diagnosing necrotizing sialometaplasia **(Fig. 5)**.

HISTOLOGICAL PROGNOSTIC FACTORS

- *Depth of invasion*: The DOI is an important predictor of regional nodal involvement and survival in OSCC, and thus dictates the staging in current guidelines. Evaluation of DOI during FS also helps decide subsequent neck dissection (neck nodes addressed if DOI ≥ 4 mm).
  Microscopically tumor thickness is measured from the mucosal surface of the tumor to the deepest point of tissue invasion, while DOI is measured from the basement membrane of adjacent normal epithelium to the deepest point of invasion **(Fig. 6)**.
- *Lymphovascular invasion*: LVI is defined as the presence of neoplastic cells within an endothelial cell lined channel. It occurs in 50% of head and neck SCC. It correlates

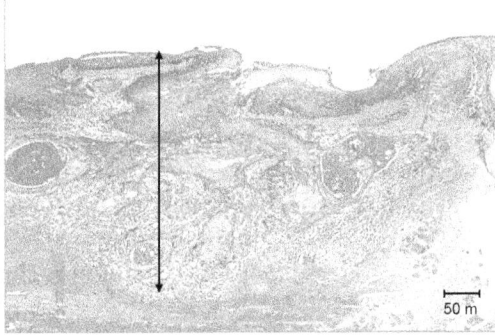

Fig. 6: Measurement of depth of invasion in a moderately differentiated squamous cell carcinoma (MDSCC).

with the presence of concomitant cervical nodal metastasis and show an increased risk of distant metastasis.

- *Perineural invasion (PNI, neurotropism)*, defined as wrapping of tumor around the nerves, is a poor prognostic factor, and is associated with metastasis to regional lymph nodes, irrespective of the size of nerve. PNI is also associated with decrease in disease-specific survival and overall survival. Some have shown increased association of PNI with distant metastasis. Extent of PNI, intratumoral or extratumoral, should also be documented. Extratumoral PNI is a parameter for worst pattern of invasion (WPOI) 5 **(Fig. 7)**.
- *Worst pattern of invasion* is a validated prognosticator for OSCC, divided into five patterns. WPOI alone is also predictive for locoregional recurrence. WPOI-1,

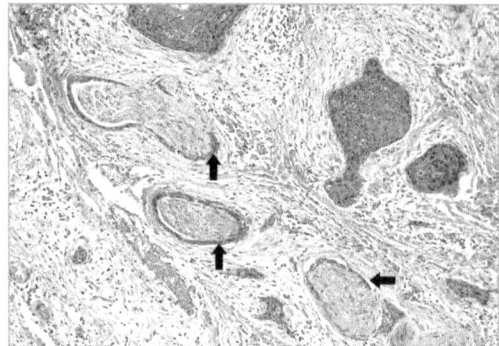

Fig. 7: Perineural invasion in a squamous cell carcinoma.

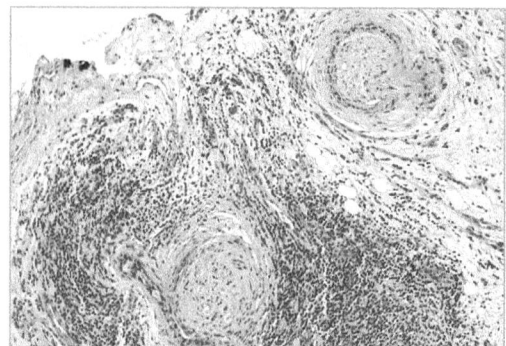

Fig. 8: Extratumoral perineural invasion (PNI) (top left) and worst pattern of invasion (WPOI).

2, and 3 form the "nonaggressive POI," defined as broad-pushing fronts, finger-like pushing fronts, or large (15 cells) separated islands, respectively. WPOI-4 tumors are defined as having small discontiguous tumor islands (<15 cells per island). WPOI-5 tumors are recognized by a dispersed, discontiguous growth pattern with satellite tumor ≥1 mm away, dispersed/extratumoral PNI or dispersed lymphovascular tumor emboli. With a WPOI-5, the probability of developing locoregional recurrence has been shown to be 42% **(Fig. 8)**.

- *Bone invasion*: Patients with OSCC and bone invasion have widely variable outcomes depending on the depth of bone invasion and tumor size. The current American Joint Committee on Cancer (AJCC) staging system classifies all tumors invading through cortical bone as T4. Only superficial erosion of bone/tooth socket by gingival primary is not sufficient to classify as T4. Only medullary bone invasion is considered as T4 lesion, which by definition is stage-IV disease. A significant association between bone involvement and risk of distant metastases with treatment failure exists.
- *Lymph node metastasis*: Measurement of size of largest contiguous metastatic tumor deposit in lymph node (not the size of lymph node itself) is a prognostic and staging parameter.
- *Extranodal extension*: Reporting of lymph node metastasis should include presence or absence of ENE, which is now part of staging. It consists of extension of metastatic nodal tumor through the lymph node capsule into the surrounding connective tissue, with or without associated stromal reaction. Documentation of distance of extension from capsule has also been suggested, ENE (>2 mm) and ENE (≤2 mm).
- *Lymphocytic host response (LHR)* at the advancing tumor with formation of dense lymphoid nodule is also one of the prognostic parameters under consideration; however, no demonstrable association with tumor grade or prognosis is yet elucidated.
- *Status of surgical margins in resection specimen*: Evaluation of margin clearance should be calculated from both gross and microscopic distance from the tumor (mucosal and soft tissue). Sections from margins can be taken as radial (perpendicular to the mucosa) or shaved (tangential).

Radial margins give precise microscopic distance between tumor and margin.

They are preferred for evaluation of deep resection soft-tissue margin, and grossly close mucosal margins (≤1 cm). However, it allows a limited evaluation of area/length of margin. *Shaved margins* allow evaluation of larger area/length of margin; however, precise microscopic distance from tumor cannot be estimated. They are preferred for grossly good clearance between tumor and the mucosal margins (>1 cm).

Positive margins are defined as "microscopic cut-through the tumor/lesion" showing invasive tumor or moderate/severe dysplasia or carcinoma-in-situ at the margin. Mild dysplasia at margins has low risk for progression, and is considered negative. The definition of a *"close margin"* is not standardized. Commonly used cutoff points are 5 mm or less for OSCC, and are associated with considerable risk of local recurrence.

Resection specimen margins (RSM) are obtained from the main resection specimen by the pathologist, while the *tumor bed margins (TBM)* are taken separately as additional or revised margins by the surgeons. TBM have a less reliable prognostic value than the RSM due to their uncertain origin and lack of precise orientation with respect to the main specimen. The interpretation and orientation of TBM requires close coordination between the surgeon and pathologist in order to give a final margin. Positive RSM is as an adverse independent prognostic factor for recurrence, irrespective of subsequent negative TBM (additional margin).

MOLECULAR PATHOGENESIS OF OSCC

Oral squamous cell carcinoma is a complex disease, usually characterized by accumulation of genetic and epigenetic alterations. In spite of advances in medical oncology care and operative skills, mortality of head and neck SCC (HNSCC) has not significantly improved in the last few decades. Therefore, investigation of the molecular biology of OSCC and elucidating the various underpinnings can strongly enhance the development of modern chemotherapy agents, which in turn will improve and prolong the lifespan of OSCC patients.

There are several critical steps during OSCC development, such as progressive allelic loss of 9p, 3p, 17p, 11q, 3q, 14q, 6p, 8p, 4q, accommodated by mutation and inactivation of *CDKN2A*, multiple mutations of *TP53*, mutations in and amplification of *CDH1* and inactivation of *PTEN*. Until recently, *TP53* was the only known recurrent mutation, with frequencies ranging from 60 to 80%. Recently revealed *NOTCH1* mutation by whole-exome sequencing, seen in up to 15% of patients, has opened new avenues of investigation.

Later data demonstrated additional mutation events in *PIK3CA/PIC3R1*, *RB1*, and *EGFR*.

HPV-negative tumors feature novel coamplifications of 11q13 (*CCND1*, *FADD*, and *CTTN*) and 11q22 (*BIRC2*, *YAP1*) which also harbor genes implicated in cell death/ nuclear factor kappa B (NF-κB) and Hippo pathways. HPV-negative tumors also feature novel focal deletions in the *nuclear SET domain protein 1 (NSD1)* gene and tumor suppressor genes (e.g., *FAT1*, *NOTCH1*, *SMAD4*, and *CDKN2A*).

Recently identified tumor suppressor *FAT1*, which is the third most frequently inactivated gene, like *NOTCH1*, is a large transmembrane protein involved in cell–cell signaling. *FAT1* has been shown to control migration and invasion in OSCC, and recent work has linked FAT1 to Wnt signaling. Recurrent focal amplifications in receptor tyrosine kinases [e.g., epidermal growth factor receptor (EGFR), *ERBB2*, and fibroblast growth factor receptor 1 (FGFR1)] also predominate in HPV-negative tumors.

The Cancer Genome Atlas Network has recently profiled 279 HNSCCs to provide a comprehensive landscape of somatic genomic alterations. Unsupervised clustering analysis of copy number alterations (CNAs) identified a mutually exclusive subset of predominantly oral cavity tumors with reduced CNAs, a pattern recently described in cancer as "M" class (tumors driven by mutation rather than CNA). This subset in particular harbored a novel three-gene pattern of activating mutations in *HRAS*, frequently with inactivating *CASP8* mutations, and wild type TP53 which portends a favorable clinical outcome in tumors with few CNAs. Frequent mutation of *CASP8* defines a new molecular subtype of OSCC with few copy number changes.

FIELD CANCERIZATION: A GENETICALLY ALTERED FIELD

The phenomenon of field cancerization has often been brought up to explain the occurrence of second primary tumor (SPTs) and local recurrences despite resection of tumor with adequate margins. Molecular analysis in terms of loss of heterozygosity (LOH), microsatellite alterations, chromosomal instability, and mutations in the *TP53* gene have been performed on tumor-adjacent "normal tissue" and surgical margins to assess the presence of a field lesion. Genetically altered cells could be found in the histologically normal surrounding area and margins of a specimen, which may lead to recurrences or SPTs.

Distinct Molecular Alterations considering Age and Sites within Oral Cavity

Few studies comparing young and old patients with tongue SCC using high-fidelity DNA histograms revealed that tumors from young patients were more likely to be aneuploid and tetraploid. Also, other parameters related to DNA content abnormalities and genomic instability [DNA index (DI), the percentage of cells with DNA exceeding 5N (5N-EC), and heterogeneity index (HI)] were consistently higher in young patients. Young patients with SCC represent a distinct clinical entity. The high incidence of DNA ploidy abnormalities suggest that they may have increased genomic instability.

The India Project Team of the International Cancer Genome Consortium evaluated mutational landscape of gingivobuccal (GB) SCC which revealed new recurrently mutated genes and molecular subgroups. GB OSCC, an anatomical and clinical subtype of HNSCC, is prevalent in regions where tobacco chewing is common. Exome sequencing and recurrence testing reveals that some significantly and frequently altered genes are specific to GB OSCC (*USP9X, MLL4, ARID2, UNC13C,* and *TRPM3*), while some others are shared with HNSCC (e.g., *TP53, FAT1, CASP8, HRAS,* and *NOTCH1*). It was found that a high proportion of C > G transversions exist among tobacco users with high numbers of mutations. Many pathways that are enriched for genomic alterations are specific to GB OSCC. These findings open new avenues for biological characterization and exploration of therapies.

Therapeutic Implications

Although genomic alterations are dominated by loss of tumor suppressor genes, 80% of patients harbor at least one genomic alteration in a targetable gene, suggesting that novel approaches to treatment may be possible for this debilitating disease. Discovery of the overexpressed EGFR due to EGFR high polysomy and gene amplification in HNSCC led to the development and application of EGFR-specific cetuximab-based immunotherapy for HNSCC treatment.

Aberrations of PI3K pathway have important clinical implications in the treatment of OSCC. PI3K plays a key role in the progression of OSCC and they frequently constitute "gain of function" mutations which trigger oncogenesis. PI3K mutations can also lead to emergence of drug resistance after treatment with EGFR inhibitors. Genomic alterations affecting PI3K are common in OSCC and serve as an attractive target for the treatment of HNSCC. Early clinical trials evaluating PI3K inhibitors have shown disappointing results, but further evaluation with more potent agents and careful patient selection may show a hope of some promising results and which might lead to development of effective PI3K inhibitors in HNSCC.

KEY POINTS

- *Squamous cell carcinoma variants*:
  - Conventional SCC
  - Papillary SCC
  - Verrucous carcinoma
  - Spindle cell squamous carcinoma
  - Basaloid SCC
  - Adenoid SCC
  - Adenosquamous carcinoma
  - Others
- *Risk factors for OSCC*:
  - Smoking, tobacco chewing, and alcohol (with a strong synergistic effect).
  - HPV infection is seen in only 3% of OSCC.
  - Sunlight exposure is a risk factor for lip cancers.
- *Necrotizing sialometaplasia* and *pseudoepitheliomatous* hyperplasia mimic SCC.
- Field cancerization explains the occurrence of SPTs and local recurrences.
- p53 mutations are associated clinically with resistance to radiotherapy and chemotherapy.
- Overexpression of EGFR has also been shown to correlate with radioresistance.

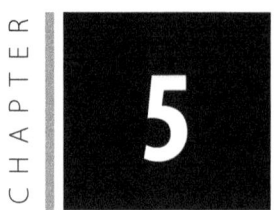

Evaluation and Staging of Oral Cancer

Vikas Arora

EVALUATION OF AN ORAL CANCER PATIENT

All patients should be examined and evaluated by a head and neck surgeon or oncologist and discussed in multidisciplinary team before starting treatment in the following sequence.

History

The clinician should take:
- Complete history related to the current disease
- Detailed history of risk behaviors such as use of tobacco and alcohol
- Past history of radiotherapy, especially to the head and neck
- Review the social, familial, and medical history
- Familial history of head and neck cancer
- Personal history of cancer

Clinical Examination

Local Examination
- Inspect facies, mention grade of trismus if any, submucous fibrosis (SMF), orodental condition, and hygiene.
- Inspect and measure the size of the lesion in all the dimensions.
- Palpate the depth of the lesion (bimanual palpation of the floor of mouth and tongue).
- Define and describe the exact location and local extensions.
- Simultaneously look for synchronous primary tumor. Indirect laryngoscopy (IDL) to be done.
- Clinical staging and documentation of the subsite(s) involved.
- Assess for performance status and nutritional status.

Neck Examination
- Palpate the right and left side of the neck to clinically assess for any lymph nodes present.
- Do clinical staging as per TNM classification system.

Dental Examination
- It should be routinely done, especially if radiation is a part of the treatment plan.
- Dental opinion regarding need for replacements of prosthesis to help restore cosmesis, comfort, and function once the treatment is over.

Endoscopic Examination
- This can be done when the entire lesion cannot be assessed during the clinical oral examination in the OPD due to gagging reflex or physical limitation because of severe trismus.
- The patient is then examined in the operating room with examination under anesthesia (EUA) and direct laryngoscopy.
  - For mapping of disease
  - For procuring biopsy if needed
  - For assessment of resectability

ANKYLOGLOSSIA

Etymologically, "ankyloglossia" originates from the Greek words "agkilos" (curved) and "glossa" (tongue). In the history of medical literature, the term ankyloglossia had probably been used for the first time in the 1960s, when Wallace defined tongue tie as "a condition in which the tip of the tongue cannot be protruded beyond the lower incisor teeth because of a short frenulum linguae, often containing scar tissue." The term free-tongue is defined as the length of tongue from the insertion of the lingual frenum into the base of the tongue to the tip of the tongue. Clinically acceptable, normal range of free tongue is >16 mm.

The ankyloglossia can be classified into four classes based on Kotlow's assessment as given in **Table 1**.

A normal range of motion of the tongue is described as:

- The tip of the tongue should be able to protrude outside the mouth without clefting.
- The tip of the tongue should be able to sweep the upper and lower lips easily without straining. When the tongue is retruded, it should not blanch the tissues lingual to the anterior teeth.
- The lingual frenum should not create a diastema between the mandibular central incisors.

- Common cause of ankyloglossia is tongue tie; however, in carcinoma of tongue ankyloglossia is a sign of:
  - Extrinsic muscles of tongue involvement
  - Floor of mouth muscles involvement
  - Neurovascular bundle involvement
  - Base of tongue involvement

The 7th edition of tumor staging by the American Joint Committee on Cancer (AJCC) has defined stage T4a for those tongue carcinomas with extrinsic muscle involvement. The extrinsic muscles of the tongue are likely to be involved early even in superficial tumors because they are not deep and even superficial thin tumors may involve these muscles according to many studies. However, AJCC, 8th edition, has included DOI and hence excluded extrinsic muscle invasion (EMI) as a criterion for the T4 category.

CONFIRMATION OF DIAGNOSIS

- *Biopsy*: A lesion within and around the oral cavity, which does not respond to the conventional treatment, should be considered suspicious until histologically proved otherwise. A duration of 2–3 weeks may be allowed as an appropriate period to evaluate the response to the treatment before attempting a definitive

TABLE 1: Kotlow's classification.

Type	Movement of the tongue
Clinically acceptable, normal range of free tongue movement	>16 mm
Class I: Mild ankyloglossia	12–16 mm
Class II: Moderate ankyloglossia	8–11 mm
Class III: Severe ankyloglossia	3–7 mm
Class IV: Complete ankyloglossia	<3 mm

tissue diagnosis. The types of biopsies for diagnosing oral cancers are:
- *Incisional/punch biopsy*: A tiny piece of tissue is punched out from the abnormal-looking area including normal area. This is a simple in office procedure but may sometimes require general anesthesia if the lesion is located in an inaccessible area.
- *Exfoliative cytology*: The suspicious-looking area is gently scraped and sample of cells collected on a glass slide. It is then stained and visualized under a microscope that if any abnormal looking cells would call for a deeper biopsy.

  One should always review the adequacy of biopsied material; it should be a representative sample.
- *Fine-needle aspiration cytology (FNAC)*: It is a simple procedure, done by trained personal, indicated where patient presents with palpable lesion in neck of high suspicion.
- *Slide review*: If biopsy has been done elsewhere.

RADIOLOGIC ASSESSMENT FOR STAGING

Imaging has an important role for assessing the primary tumor, the regional lymph nodes, and also to rule out any distant metastasis. This helps in establishing the clinical stage of the cancer. The type of imaging needed depends on the site of the tumor, its stage, and or institutional preference.
- *Panoramic radiograph/tomogram*:
  - *Orthopantomogram (OPG)*: To assess the status of the dentition and mandible.
  - *X-ray mandible*: Determination of cortical erosion.
  - *Chest X-ray*: An initial assessment of a patient in preparation for surgery or chemotherapy.
- *Cross-sectional imaging*: For staging
  - To assess the primary site, location, its deeper extension, and perineural spread
  - To assess status of regional lymph nodes
  - Decision regarding management strategy
  - To assess resectability and operability
  - To evaluate for residual/recurrent disease.

  The most common imaging modalities used are magnetic resonance imaging (MRI) or contrast-enhanced computed tomography (CECT) of the neck and oral cavity. While subtle cortical erosions of the bones are detected with CT, the extent of marrow involvement is perhaps better assessed with the help of MRI.

  In advanced and recurrent cancers, positron emission tomography (PET)-CT has become the imaging of choice due to its higher rate of detection of distant metastasis when compared with other imaging modalities.
- *Ultrasound (US) neck* for N0 neck in selected cases to determine node characteristics.

ASSESSMENT FOR RESECTABILITY

Involvement of the following sites by the tumors harbingers poor outcome. T4b tumors are unresectable due to technical inability to obtain clear margins. Involvement of these sites although is not an absolute contraindication to surgery in selected cases where total resection is possible.

- Involvement of the pterygoid muscles, especially when associated with severe trismus or involvement of the pterygopalatine fossa causing cranial neuropathy.
- Direct extension to the superior nasopharynx or deep extension into the Eustachian tube and lateral pharyngeal walls.
- Invasion or encasement of the common carotid or the internal carotid artery (>270°).
- Gross extension of the tumor to the skull base causing erosion of the pterygoid plates or sphenoid bone, widening of foramen ovale.
- Direct extension of disease to involve the skin.
- Direct extension to mediastinal structures, prevertebral fascia, or cervical vertebrae.
- Presence of subdermal metastasis (satellite nodules).

How does imaging resolve resectability issues?

Perineural spread: Tumors that involve one third of the circumference of a nerve in close proximity, and or the presence of tumor cells within any of the three layers of the nerve sheath.

Trigeminal nerve is known to be most vulnerable of all for perineural invasion (PNI) because it supplies the skin over the major sites of the head and neck. Tumor cells travel to the skull base through foramen rotundum, foramen ovale, superior and inferior orbital fissures.

Intracranial extension is also seen along the jugular foramen and the hypoglossal canal. Spread to cavernous sinus, infiltration of the cranial nerve, and the skull base are associated with poor outcome and make the tumor unresectable.

Tumors in the cephalic region which are >2 cm, have a greater likelihood for PNI due to its rich cutaneous innervation. These tumors initially invade the peripheral cutaneous nerves and then metastasize along the larger nerves.

Perineural invasion is divided as "incidental PNI" and "clinical PNI":

- PNI which have no preoperative symptoms is called as "incidental" or microscopic (mPNI). The diagnosis of such PNI is made on biopsy.
- *Clinical PNI (cPNI)*: Patients develop symptoms such as paresthesia, hypoesthesia, pain in the distribution of a trigeminal nerve branch or facial weakness.

Contrast-enhanced MRI is the modality of choice for detection of such lesions.

Orbital Invasion

Locally advanced malignant lesions of oral cavity, especially hard palate, upper alveolus, and upper gingivobuccal sulcus invade skull base and may reach the orbit through the orbital fissures and orbital apex. Findings on imaging with CT or MRI are equivocal to identify the invasion of periorbita. Surgical extent may include orbital exenteration with sacrifice of orbital nerve.

Cavernous Sinus Invasion

Clinical findings consisting of neurological disturbances related to cranial nerves III to VI, especially diplopia due to involvement of abducens nerve (CN VI), together with radiological findings of MRI, suggest invasion of cavernous sinus. MRI depicts well about loss of contrast enhancement of cavernous sinus and lateral bulge of cavernous sinus also indicates unresectable disease. In most cases, treatment is palliative with radiotherapy and/or chemotherapy as prognosis is poor.

TREATMENT PLAN (FLOWCHART 1)

- All cases should be discussed in multi-specialty clinic (MSC), especially those in which organ preservation is a possibility.
- Hemogram, biochemical profile, viral markers, and cardiopulmonary assessment should be done as appropriate. Carotid Doppler in elderly, frailty index, and morbidity status should be assessed.
- Prospective surveillance plan should be made that includes adequate dental, nutritional, health behavior evaluation and intervention (tobacco, alcohol, and other addictions).
- Review of slides or radiological images, already procured by the patient, should be done whenever available.
- Patients undergoing surgery should be evaluated beforehand for the type of procedure and reconstructive plan. Patients should be counseled for same.
- Evaluate for potential surgical options, look for resectability (especially borderline resectable lesions), and review those patients who were previously unresectable.
- Patients may be appropriately referred to *palliative care team, rehabilitation team,* or other caregivers.

TUMOR-NODE METASTASIS STAGING OF ORAL CANCER

The staging process of a cancer is dynamic and modifiable with clinical and pathologic information gathered during the workup and treatment process. The following prefixes are commonly used in cancer staging:

- "r" for recurrent tumor and "R" for residual disease.
- "y" after radiation therapy and/or chemotherapy have been rendered.
- Of note, "r" and "y" prefixes are placed before "c" and "p" prefixes.

However, when a diagnosis of invasive squamous cell carcinoma (SCC) has been made, T1, T2, and T3 describe the greatest surface dimension primary lesion. In the 7th edition of the AJCC staging system, T1 was denoted for a lesion less than or equal to 2 cm, T2 for a lesion that was greater than 2 and less than or equal to 4 cm, and T3 for a lesion greater than 4 cm.

The 8th edition of the AJCC staging system has included depth of invasion (DOI) too

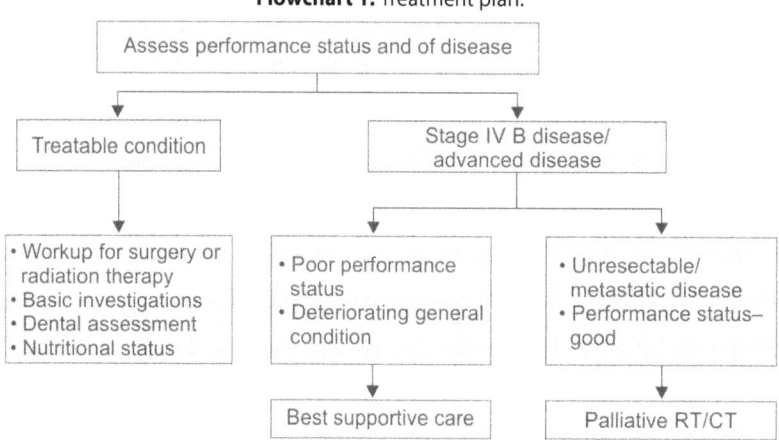

Flowchart 1: Treatment plan.

(CT: chemotherapy; RT: radiotherapy)

in its classification **(Table 2)**. In pathology, DOI is defined as a measurement from the basement membrane relative to an area of intact squamous mucosa, which is denoted as the horizon. The distance from the horizon to the area of greatest invasion denotes DOI (Depth of Invasion). DOI is not the same as tumor thickness.

The thickness of the tumor has not been incorporated into the TNM staging system for oral cavity SCC. The rationale for including DOI for oral cavity SCC was based on strong evidence of DOI predicting the risk for metastasis to the cervical lymph nodes, as also the prognosis, especially in early stage oral SCC.

The T4 stage is now divided into T4a, which is moderately advanced local disease and T4b, which is very advanced local disease, and predicts the local invasiveness of the primary tumor.

The T4a and T4b categories do not consider the surface dimensions of the lesion or the DOI.

T4 is divided into two subgroups:
1. *T4a*: When the tumor grows into surrounding structures and the oral cancer is considered as moderately advanced local disease. The cells may invade structures according to the location and type of oral cancer.
   - For oral cavity cancers, the tumor may invade into bones of the jaw or face, deep muscle of the tongue, skin of the face, or maxillary sinus.
   - For lip cancers, the tumor may grow into nearby bone, the inferior alveolar nerve, the floor of the mouth, or the skin over the chin or nose.

According to the previous staging, invasion of the extrinsic muscles of the tongue would upstage the tumor to T4a.

TABLE 2: TNM staging classification (8th edition).

Tumor category for non-human papilloma virus-associated (p16 negative) oral squamous cell carcinoma, 8th edition cancer staging manual

T category	Tumor size	Additional criteria
TX	Not applicable	Primary tumor cannot be assessed
Tis	Not applicable	Carcinoma in situ
T1	≤2 cm, ≤5 mm DOI	Not additional criteria
T2	≤2 cm, DOI ≥5 mm, and ≤10 mm or tumor >2 cm but ≤4 cm and DOI ≤10 mm	No additional criteria
T3	≥4 cm or any tumor ≥10 mm DOI	No additional criteria
T4	Not applicable	Moderate-to-advanced local disease
T4a	Not applicable	Oral cavity, lip, chin, or nose tumor invading cortical bone or involving inferior alveolar nerve, floor of the mouth, facial skin, bones of mandible, or maxilla affecting basal bone
T4b	Not applicable	Advanced local disease in which tumor invades masticator space, pterygoid plates, or skull base, and may or may not encase internal carotid artery

(DOI: depth of invasion)

But the 8th edition of the staging manual does not consider invasion of any of the extrinsic muscles of the tongue in the staging process.
2. *T4b*: The tumor has grown through the surrounding structures into deeper tissues. At this stage, the cancer is considered locally very advanced.

The tumor may grow into nearby bones of the pterygoid plates and of the skull base. The tumor may also encroach upon the internal carotid artery. For lip and oral cavity cancers, the tumor may invade into the masticator space.

Malignant tumors of the minor salivary glands are staged based on their anatomic site of origin. The tumors of the major (submandibular, sublingual, and parotid) salivary glands follow the same TNM staging.

Mucosal melanoma has a distinct T criteria:
- Tx similar to SCC denoted a situation in which the primary tumor cannot be assessed.
- T1 and T2 categories do not exist for mucosal melanoma.
- T3 refers to a mucosal melanoma that is limited to the mucosa.
- T4a refers to a lesion that invades the deep tissues (overlying skin, muscles, bone, and cartilage).
- T4b refers to a lesion that invades the masticator space, prevertebral space, mediastinal structures, carotid artery, brain, dura, skull base, and lower cranial nerves (CNs), such as glossopharyngeal nerve (CN IX), vagus nerve (CN X), spinal accessory nerve (CN XI), and the hypoglossal nerve (CN XII).

Surgical Margins

Definition of a positive margin is invasive carcinoma or carcinoma in situ/high-grade dysplasia present at the margins (microscopic cut through of tumor). Reporting of surgical margins should also include information regarding the distance of invasive carcinoma, carcinoma in situ, or high-grade dysplasia (moderate-to-severe) from the surgical margin.

Regional Lymph Node Classification

The neck nodes are grouped as levels I to VII. They serve as the first sites of metastasis of oral SCC and of all minor salivary gland cancers (excluding adenoid cystic carcinoma). Any metastasis found in the neck nodes is considered to be the most important prognostic factor for all *head* and *neck* SCC.

Salient features:
- Metastatic spread of oral cancer usually occurs in an orderly pattern, beginning with the uppermost lymph node groups and spreading down the cervical chain. The jugulodigastric nodes are most likely to develop early metastasis.
- Carcinomas involving the lower lip and floor of the mouth tend to spread to the submental nodes.
- Lymph node metastasis has been found in 40% of cases of oral cavity SCC.
- About 15–34% of these cases will have occult cervical nodal metastasis.

Occult nodal metastasis are deposits of tumor which are not detectable with standard clinical or radiographic methods based on the criterion of metastatic lymphadenopathy; however, cancer cells are identified on histologic analysis of lymph nodes.

Extranodal Extension

Extranodal extension (ENE) is defined as tumor cells invading beyond the lymph node capsule into the perinodal tissues **(Table 3)**.

Pathological regional lymph nodes (pN):
- *NX*: Regional lymph nodes cannot be assessed.
- *N0*: No regional lymph node metastasis.

TABLE 3: Nodal status in TNM staging.

Node category	Node criteria
NX	Regional lymph nodes cannot be assessed
N0	No regional lymphadenopathy
N1	Metastases in a single ipsilateral lymph node ≤3 cm and ENE negative (–ve)
N2	• Ipsilateral node ≤3 cm, ENE positive (+ve) • 3–6 cm with ENE(–ve) • Multiple ipsilateral metastatic lymph nodes none >6 cm and ENE(–ve) • Metastatic bilateral or contralateral node ≤6 cm, ENE(–ve)
N2a	• Ipsilateral single metastatic node ≤3 cm, ENE(+ve) • Ipsilateral single metastatic node ≥3 cm but ≤6 cm, ENE(–ve)
N2b	Metastatic multiple ipsilateral nodes ≤6 cm, ENE(–ve)
N2c	Metastatic bilateral or contralateral lymph node ≤6 cm, ENE(–ve)
N3	Metastatic lymph nodes ≥6 cm, ENE(–ve); metastatic single ipsilateral lymph node ≥3 cm, ENE(+ve); metastatic multiple ipsilateral, contralateral or bilateral lymph nodes, ENE(+ve)
N3a	Metastatic lymph node ≥6 cm, ENE(–ve)
N3b	Metastatic single lymph node ≥3 cm, ENE(+ve) or metastatic multiple ipsilateral, bi- or contralateral lymph nodes, ENE(+ve)

(ENE: extranodal extension)

- *N1*: Metastasis in a single ipsilateral lymph node, ≤3 cm in greatest dimension and ENE(-ve)
- *N2*: Metastasis in a single ipsilateral lymph node, ≤3 cm in greatest dimension and ENE(+ve) or >3 cm but ≤6 cm in greatest dimension and ENE(-ve); or metastases in multiple ipsilateral lymph nodes, none >6 cm in greatest dimension and ENE(-ve); or in bilateral or contralateral lymph nodes(s), none >6 cm in greatest dimension and ENE(-ve)
- *N2a*: Metastasis in either:
  - Single ipsilateral lymph node, i.e., ≤3 cm and ENE(+ve) or
  - Single ipsilateral lymph node, i.e., >3 cm but ≤6 cm in greatest dimension and ENE(-ve)
- *N2b*: Metastasis in multiple ipsilateral lymph nodes, none >6 cm in greatest dimension and ENE(-ve)
- *N2c*: Metastasis in bilateral or contralateral lymph node(s), none >6 cm in greatest dimension and ENE(-ve)
- *N3*: Metastasis in a lymph node >6 cm in greatest dimension and ENE(-ve); or in a single ipsilateral node >3 cm in greatest dimension and ENE(+ve); or multiple ipsilateral, contralateral or bilateral nodes, any with ENE(+ve); or a single contralateral node of any size and ENE(+ve)
- *N3a*: Metastasis in a lymph node that is >6 cm in greatest dimension and ENE(-ve)
- *N3b*: Metastasis in either:
  - Single ipsilateral lymph node, >3 cm and ENE(+ve)
  - Multiple ipsilateral, contralateral or bilateral lymph nodes, any with ENE(+ve), or
  - Single contralateral lymph node of any size and ENE(+ve).

Salient features:

- Designation of "U" or "L" may be used for any N category to indicate metastasis above the lower border of the cricoid (U) or below the lower border of the cricoid (L).

- As per the AJCC, 8th edition, for pN, a selective neck dissection ordinarily includes 10+ lymph nodes and a comprehensive neck dissection (radical or modified radical neck dissection) ordinarily includes 15+ lymph nodes.
- Negative pathologic examination of a smaller number of nodes still mandates a pN0 designation.
- Midline nodes are considered ipsilateral nodes.

Distant Metastasis Classification

Distant metastasis is associated with high mortality and low chances of survival. The incidence of distant metastasis for oral cavity SCC has been reported to occur in 10–18% of patients at time of initial diagnosis in various studies.

Advanced T and N classifications predict the presence of any distant metastasis. Distant metastatic disease is commonly detected by whole-Body PET-CT or CT neck, US abdomen, and chest radiograph and sometimes indicated by blood tests such as liver function test. The designation "Mx" is used until the completion of the entire metastatic workup investigations have been performed. Mx denotes unknown metastatic status. M0 is used for absence of distant metastasis and M1 for presence of any distant metastasis.

Distant Metastasis (M)

- *M0*: No distant metastasis
- *M1*: Distant metastasis
- Metastasis found on imaging is considered cM1.
- Biopsy-proven metastasis is considered pM1.

TABLE 4: Changes in TNM classification of 7th and 8th editions.

Change	7th edition (2010)	8th edition (2017)
T-stage	T0: No primary T1: Size ≤ 2 cm T2: Size 2–4 cm T3: Size > 4 cm T4: • T4a: Moderately advanced (extrinsic tongue muscle involvement constituted T4a) • T4b: Very advanced	• T0 deleted • T1: Size ≤ 2 cm and DOI ≤ 5 mm • T2: Size ≤ 2 cm and DOI 5–10 mm or size 2–4 cm and DOI ≤10 mm • T3: Size > 4 cm or >10 mm DOI • T4a extrinsic tongue muscle infiltration now deleted
N-stage	N0: No LN involved N1: Single ipsilateral LN ≤ 3 cm in size N2: • N2a: Single ipsilateral LN, 3–6 cm in size • N2b: Multiple ipsilateral LNs, all <8 cm in size • N2c: Any bilateral or contralateral LNs, all <8 cm in size N3: Any LN > 6 cm in size	*Clinical N-stage*: • N1–N2 is same as previous and ENE(–ve) • N3 now with subcategories: – N3a is previous N3 (size: 6 cm) and ENE(–ve) – N3b is any ENE(+ve), either clinical or radiographic *Pathological N-stage*: Microscopically evident ENE(+ve) LNs results in upstaging
Stage grouping	Clinical or pathological TNM used for same grouping system	Same as previous

(DOI: depth of invasion; ENE: extranodal extension; LN: lymph node)

TABLE 5: Staging of oral squamous cell carcinoma.

Stage 0	Tis	N0	M0
Stage I	T1	N0	M0
Stage II	T2	N0	M0
Stage III	T3	N0	M0
	T1, T2, T3	N1	M0
Stage IV A	T4a	N0, N1	M0
	T1, T2, T3, T4a	N2	M0
Stage IV B	Any T	N3	M0
	T4b	Any N	M0
Stage IV C	Any T	Any N	M1

KEY POINTS

- Complete history and detailed locoregional examination should be a routine in oral cavity cancer patients and look for any skip lesions and synchronous primary.
- MRI is a better chosen modality for oral soft-tissue lesions, especially tongue malignancies. Bone involvement is best commented by CT scan.
- The 8th edition of the AJCC staging system incorporates DOI as a third dimension of the primary tumor and ENE is now part of the TNM classification.
- In 8th edition of the AJCC staging system, T0 has also been removed, and also the invasion of any of the extrinsic muscles of the tongue is not considered in the staging.
- The clinical suspicion of N3b mandates the oncologist to order whole body PET CT to rule out distant metastasis and is also considered to be poor prognostic feature.
- All cases should be discussed in MSC.
- The staging provides important information about the extent of cancer in the body and anticipated response to treatment.

CHAPTER 6

Imaging in Carcinoma of Oral Cavity

Vivek Mahawar

INTRODUCTION

Oral cavity is a challenging area for radiological analysis due to its complex anatomy. Osseous, glandular, and soft-tissue structures are in close proximity in oral cavity. Imaging has direct impact on patient management as it provides information about resectability, extent of resection, and reconstruction in surgical planning.

Oral cavity cancer is different from oropharynx cancer because:
- Squamous epithelium within oral cavity originates from ectoderm and is usually well differentiated.
- Squamous epithelium within oropharynx originates from endoderm and is usually poorly differentiated.

Imaging plays a crucial role in oral cavity squamous cell carcinoma (SCC) as it:
- Provides information regarding resectability of disease
- Provides accurate information regarding extent and spread of disease, and thus helps to decide appropriate management strategy
- Provides information regarding prognosis
- Differentiates between post-treatment changes and tumor recurrence in follow-up

ANATOMY

Oral cavity is divided into two parts (**Fig. 1**):
1. *Central part (oral cavity proper):* It consists of oral tongue, hard palate (forms roof), upper and lower alveolus, and lingual surface of gingival mucosa (forms lateral wall), mylohyoid (forms floor), circumvallate papillae, tonsillar pillars and soft palate (forms posterior wall). Circumvallate papilla serves as a demarcation between oral tongue and base tongue (**Fig. 2**).

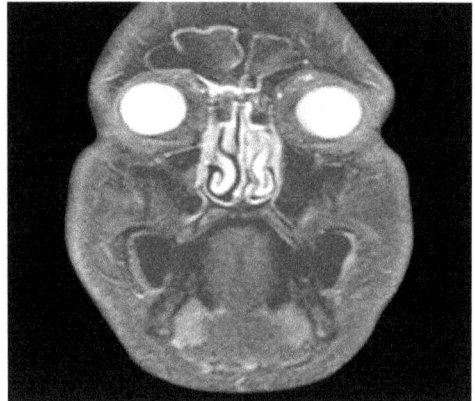

Fig. 1: Oral cavity proper.

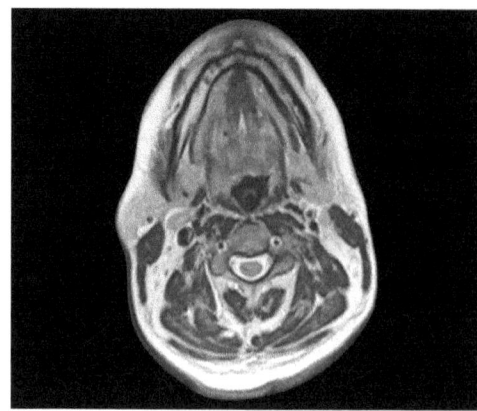

Fig. 2: Demarcation between oral tongue and base tongue (BT).

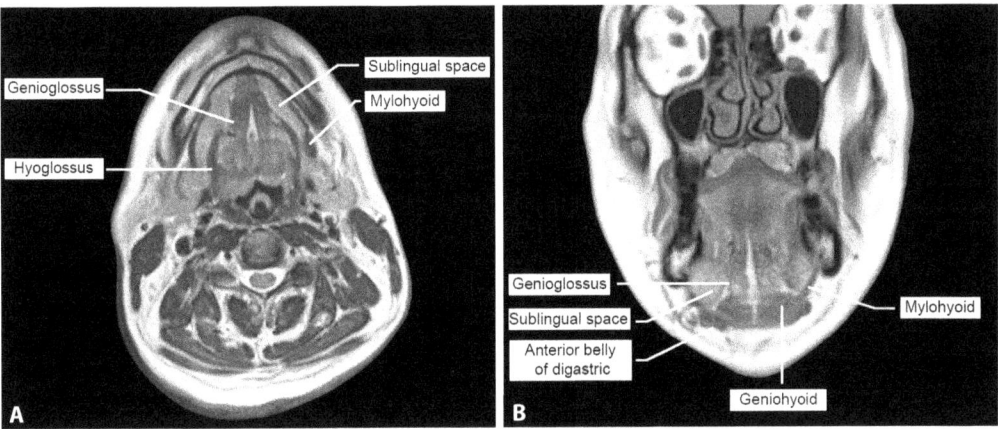

Figs. 3A and B: Floor of mouth (FOM).

The oral tongue consists of the intrinsic and the extrinsic muscles. The sling-like mylohyoid along with the paired geniohyoid on its upper surface and the anterior belly of digastric on its lower surface form the radiological floor of mouth (FOM) **(Figs. 3A and B)**. The genioglossus, hyoglossus, mylohyoid, and anterior belly of digastric are well seen on T2-weighted (T2W) magnetic resonance imaging (MRI) sequences. The sublingual space is a fat-filled space between the genioglossus located medially and mylohyoid situated inferiorly and laterally. The lingual artery is seen as a flow void at MRI or enhancing structure at computed tomography (CT) within this space, but the lingual and hypoglossal nerves (lateral to the artery) may not be visualized on imaging.

2. *Lateral part (vestibule)*: It consists of buccal mucosa laterally, upper and lower gingivobuccal sulcus (superiorly and inferiorly) and buccal surface of gingival mucosa (medially), lips (anteriorly), and retromolar trigone (RMT) (posteriorly).

Salient features of staging of oral cancer: The 8th edition of the American Joint Committee on Cancer (AJCC) staging of oral SCC, published in 2017 and revised in 2018, are provided in the **Box 1**.

Routes of Spread of Oral Cavity SCC

- Direct extension in mucosal/submucosal surface, muscle and bone.
- Via lymphatic drainage pathway.
- By extension along neurovascular bundle.

Direct Extension

Superficial mucosal ulcer or induration may not be evident on imaging. However, imaging is needed to detect submucosal spread, direct invasion of adjacent structure, and overall extent of tumor.

Direct extension of oral cavity SCC to adjacent bone is seen as: (1) Subtle cortical erosion (best seen on CT scan); (2) periosteal reaction; and (3) abnormal marrow attenuation/signal intensity (better seen on MRI).

The osseous involvement requires varying degrees of mandibulectomy or maxillectomy. Imaging should ideally record the presence or absence of cortical, marrow, and inferior alveolar canal invasion; the depth and length of erosion; the height of the intact mandible at the site of erosion and/or the height of

Imaging in Carcinoma of Oral Cavity

Box 1: Staging of oral squamous cell carcinoma (SCC).

Primary tumor (T):
- *TX*: Primary tumor cannot be assessed.
- *Tis*: Carcinoma in situ
- *T1*: Tumor ≤ 2 cm in greatest dimension with depth of invasion (DOI) ≤ 5 mm
- *T2*: Tumor ≤ 2 cm with DOI >5 mm, or tumor > 2 cm and ≤ 4 cm with DOI ≤ 10 mm
- *T3*: Tumor > 2 cm and ≤ 4 cm with DOI > 10 mm, or tumor > 4 cm with DOI ≤ 10 mm
- *T4*: Moderately or very advanced
- *T4a*: Moderately advanced local disease: Tumor > 4 cm with DOI > 10 mm, or tumor invades adjacent structures (e.g., through cortical bone of mandible or maxilla, into the maxillary sinus, into the skin of face)*
- *T4b*: Very advanced local disease: Tumor invades masticator space, pterygoid plates, or skull base, and/or tumor encases the internal carotid artery. T4b disease is further subdivided into—supranotch and infranotch diseases. Mandibular notch between coronoid and condyloid process of mandible used as a line of demarcation for supranotch and infranotch disease.
  - *T4b infranotch disease* has more favorable prognosis with local control of 74%.
  - *T4b supranotch disease* has less favorable prognosis with local control of 42.9% (**Figs. 4A and B**).

*Superficial erosion alone of bone/tooth socket by gingival primary is not sufficient to classify as T4.

Note: T4a and T4b diseases are now referred to as moderately advanced and very advanced cancer in place of resectable and unresectable cancer, as many of the patients with masticator and lower pterygoid plate involvement (T4b disease) are considered resectable now.

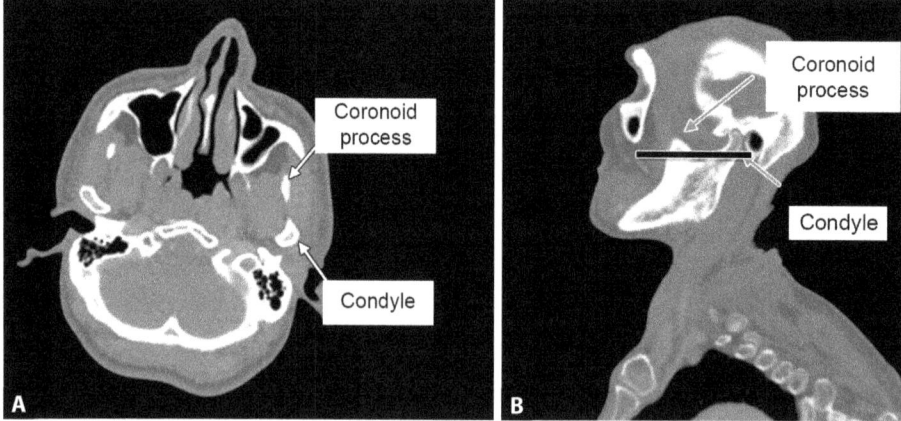

Figs. 4A and B: Axial computed tomography scans: (A) At the level of the mandibular notch; (B) Bone window shows *black line* demarcating supra- and infranotch levels.

the mandible free from paramandibular soft tissue. The latter information is obtained by measuring the height from the inferior border of the mandible to the inferior limit of the paramandibular soft-tissue component.

Although the positive predictive value of CT for mandibular invasion is considered satisfactory, the sensitivity is still considered inadequate by some who advocate intraoperative periosteal stripping when CT is negative. On the other hand, MRI has high negative predictive value but less specificity. Major reasons for inadequate sensitivity or specificity of imaging methods are failure to visualize the alveolar crest of the mandible and coexistent odontogenic infections, respectively.

- If lesion abuts mandible but is freely mobile—wide local excision of lesion with resection of periosteum is sufficient.
- If a lesion is fixed or adherent with minimal of subtle cortical involvement—marginal mandibulectomy is performed. After marginal mandibulectomy, vertical length of remaining mandible should be at least 1 cm for strength, otherwise it is predisposed bony fracture.
- In presence of gross cortical invasion, involvement of mental foramina or inferior alveolar nerve, extensive paramandibular soft tissue spread, edentulous mandible (mandible without teeth) and previously irradiated mandible, segmental mandibulectomy is performed **(Figs. 5A to D)**.

Lymphatic Dissemination

Nodal involvement is the single most important prognostic indicator **(Table 1)**.

In RMT and floor of mouth SCC: 50% with nodal disease, oral tongue: 40%, hard palate: 10–25%, and lips: 10% patients present with

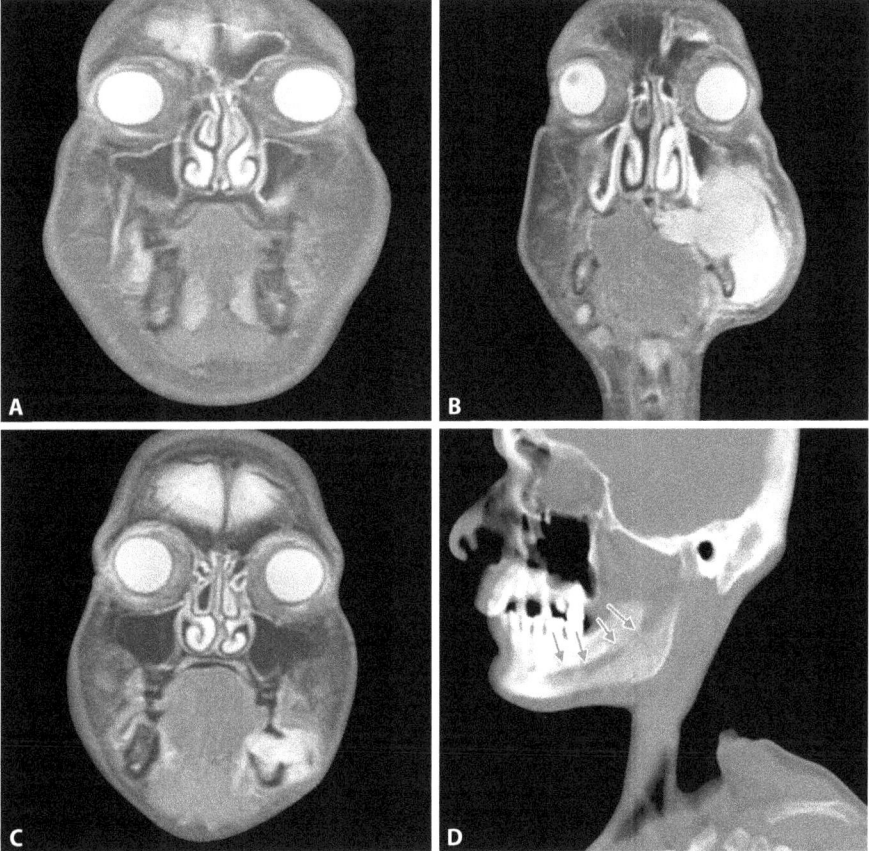

Figs. 5A to D: (A) Lower GB sulcus involved—needs only marginal mandibulectomy; (B) Gross paramandibular extension—needs segmental mandibulectomy; (C) Involvement of bony mandible—needs segmental mandibulectomy; (D) Perineural extension along inferior alveolar nerve—needs segmental mandibulectomy.

TABLE 1: Imaging features of pathological lymph nodes.

- *Nodal size (considered suspicious)*   Short axis
  - Jugulodigastric node   11 mm
  - Other nodes   >10 mm
  - Retropharyngeal node   >8 mm **(Figs. 6A and B)**
- *Morphological features*: Suspicion is increased if node is
  - Round in shape
  - Necrotic

Note: Cystic (fluid density/intensity) node can be seen with HPV-positive SCC and should not be confused with brachial cleft cyst.

- *Extracapsular spread*: Best seen on T2-weighted (T2W) fat-suppressed and contrast-T1-weighted (T1W) images as high signal intensity/edema in tissue surrounding node, poorly defined nodal border, irregular rim-like enhancement of node and large nodal size.
  Reporting of extracapsular extension of nodal disease is important because it is associated with 3.5-fold increase in the local recurrence rate **(Fig. 7)**.
- *Neurovascular/perineural spread*: Leads to inadequate locoregional control by allowing tumor extension beyond the expected treatment margin. On CT imaging, perineural spread is seen as foraminal enlargement and replacement of normal fat density within the neural foramen. MR is imaging of choice to look for perineural spread and shows diffuse enhancement and thickening along involved nerve.

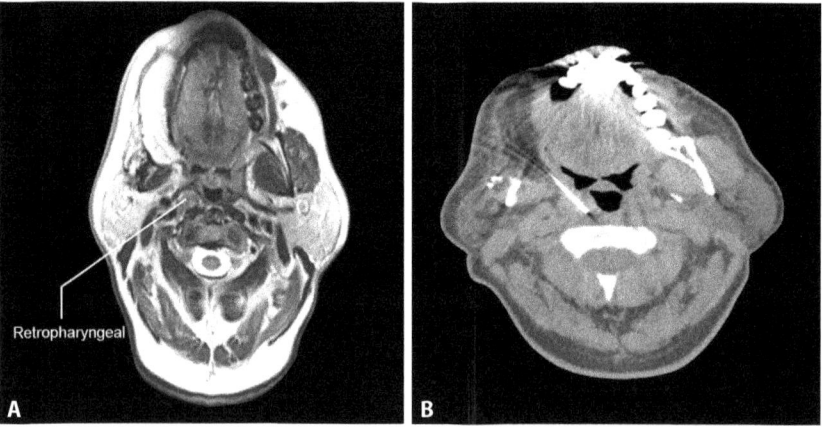

Figs. 6A and B: (A) Retropharyngeal (RP) node; (B) CT-guided fine-needle aspiration cytology (FNAC) from RP node.

nodal disease; however, in lip SCC either side of neck lymph node may be involved due to bilateral lymphatic drainage of lip.

Lateral Part of Oral Cavity (Vestibule)

It consists of buccal mucosa, upper and lower gingivobuccal (GB) sulcus, buccal surface of gingival mucosa, lips, and RMT.

Due to habit of tobacco chewing lower GB complex SCC is prevalent in Indian subcontinent and also known as Indian oral cancer. Special sequence, puffed cheek sequence (puffing the cheek outward) is taken for assessment of vestibule. Reporting should include extent of primary lesion, lymph node, and osseous involvement. Most commonly levels I and II lymph nodes are involved.

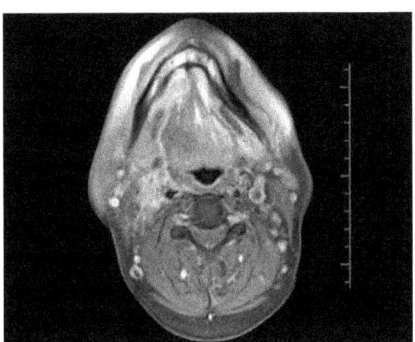

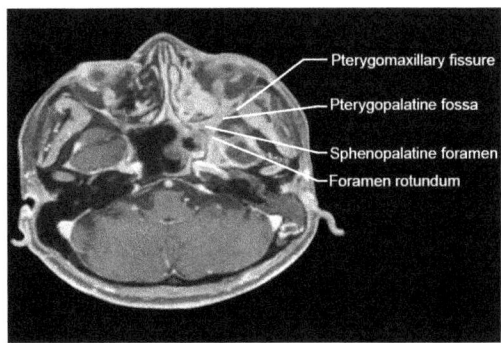

Fig. 7: T1 postcontrast MRI axial section reveals an enhancing right upper deep cervical (UDC) node with irregular margins and extranodal extension (ENE).

Fig. 8: Axial contrast MRI shows disease in the pterygopalatine fossa.

Mandibular involvement in lip and buccal mucosa SCC may lead to perineural invasion along inferior alveolar nerve and should be seen carefully. SCC of buccal mucosa that involves high infratemporal fossa (ITF) may have perineural extension along foramen ovale or pterygopalatine fossa **(Fig. 8)** at base of pterygoid plate.

Retromolar Trigone

Retromolar trigone is a triangular shaped mucosal fold extending behind the mandibular last molar, cranially along the ascending ramus up to the maxillary last molar.

RMT needs special mention, because it provides numerous route of spread **(Fig. 9)**.

Central Part (Oral Cavity Proper)

It consists of oral tongue, FOM, and hard palate.

Oral Tongue

Oral tongue SCC most commonly arises from lateral border and few arise from ventral surface. Contrast-enhanced magnetic resonance is imaging of choice in tongue SCC. The following points must be covered in tongue SCC reporting:
- *Depth of invasion*: Depth of invasion decides type of treatment **(Fig. 10)**.

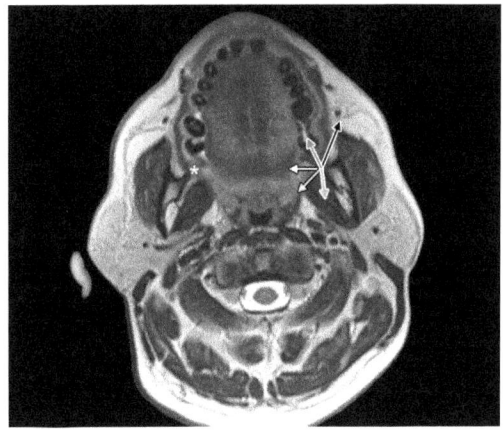

Fig. 9: Possible pathways of spread of retromolar trigone (RMT) cancers in axial T2W MRI, buccal mucosa maxillary, and mandibular alveolus, base tongue/floor of mouth (FOM), tonsil, masticator space, and through pterygomandibular raphe (*) superiorly to pterygopalatine fossa.

- Lesion crossing/not crossing midline
- FOM and neurovascular involvement
- Tip/base of tongue involvement
- Lymph node involvement
- Bone involvement

Intrinsic muscles of tongue: Superior longitudinal, inferior longitudinal, transverse and vertical muscles **(Figs. 11A and B)**.

Extrinsic muscles of tongue: Genioglossus, hyoglossus, styloglossus, and palatoglossus muscles.

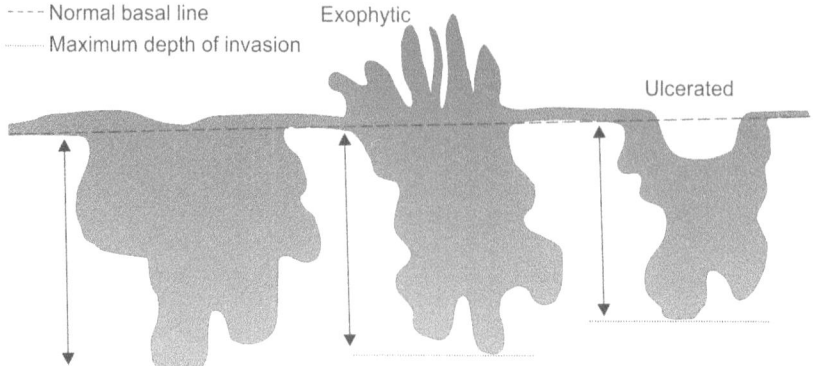

Fig. 10: Different types of squamous cell carcinoma (SCC).

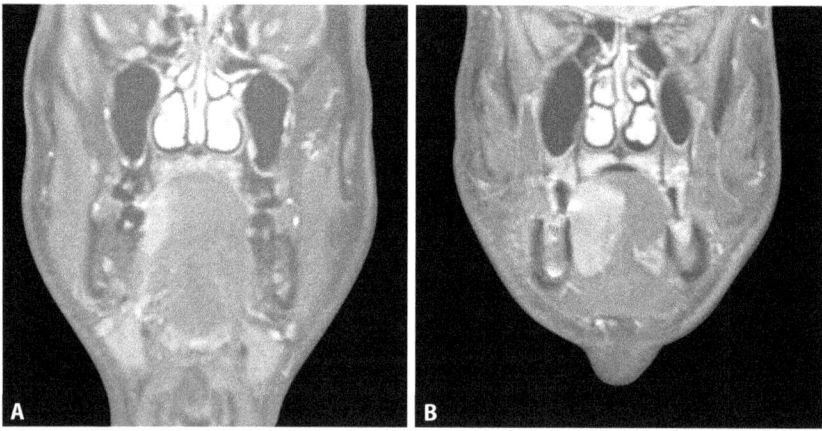

Figs. 11A and B: (A) Coronal subsequent coronal short tau inversion recovery (STIR) image shows right lateral oral tongue lesion; (B) Coronal STIR image shows right oral tongue lesion reaching midline with right floor of mouth (FOM) involvement.

Due to relative difference in size and bulk of tongue in different patients, tongue volumetry with ratio of total tumor volume and total tongue volume could be more helpful.

Floor of Mouth

It is formed by mylohyoid muscle (seen as U-shaped sling on coronal images from mylohyoid ridge of one side of mandible to other side), geniohyoid, anterior belly of digastric muscle, sublingual space that contains sublingual gland, Wharton's (submandibular duct) and lingual neurovascular bundle through which perineural extension may occur.

Hard Palate

It is better visualized on coronal and sagittal images.

Primary SCC of hard palate is rare and usually involved by extension of upper GB sulcus/upper gingival lesion. Perineural spread from hard palate tends to occur along the greater and lesser palatine nerves, which may further extend upward to pterygopalatine fossa **(Fig. 12)**.

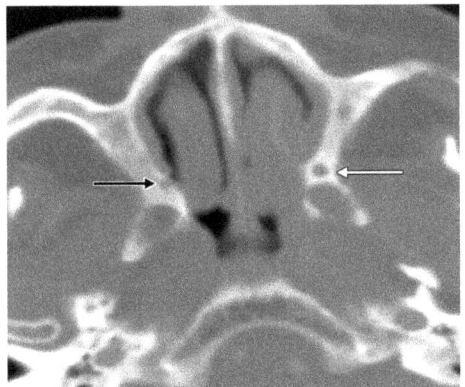

Fig. 12: Axial CT image demonstrates asymmetric enlargement of the left greater palatine foramen (white arrow) in comparison with the right (black arrow) suggestive of tumor extension along the greater palatine nerve.

POST-TREATMENT IMAGING IN ORAL CAVITY SCC

Post-treatment imaging in oral cavity cancer is complicated and difficult to understand because of postsurgical changes superimposed with postradiation changes. Visualization or palpation of tumor recurrence deep to the flap reconstructions is often not possible on clinical examination. MR is imaging of choice for evaluation of post-treatment follow-up in oral SCC.

Post-treatment imaging findings can be divided into following four groups:
1. Altered anatomy secondary to flap reconstruction
2. Tumor recurrence
3. Postsurgical complications, e.g., serous retention, infection, hematoma, abscess, fistula formation
4. Postradiation changes, e.g., edema, inflammation, fibrosis, scarring, osteoradionecrosis

In oral cavity cancer usually wide local excision of tumor is performed, followed by flap reconstruction. Sharp boundary between flap and adjacent normal structure helps to differentiate it from tumor recurrence.

KEY POINTS

- On CT scan, tumor recurrence has attenuation similar to muscle; hence, any lesion that has lower attenuation than that of muscle is unlikely to be malignant.
- On MRI, tumor recurrence seen as an infiltrative mass with intermediate signal on T1WI, intermediate-to-high signal on T2WI and reveals restricted diffusion with low apparent diffusion coefficient (ADC) values and nodular enhancement on contrast administration.
- Good quality T2WI is most useful in differentiating tumor signal from postsurgery/postradiotherapy changes with diffusion-weighted imaging (DWI) with ADC map and contrast-enhanced MRI further aids in diagnosis.
- Lymph node recurrence/metastases in postoperative neck is detected by their expansive nature, higher and nodular enhancement, and restricted diffusion with low ADC value.
- Perineural tumor spread is unique form of tumor recurrence and best seen on MRI.
- Comprehension of the patterns of disease spread at each subsite in oral cavity, with the impact on treatment and prognosis requires a deeper interpretation of the role of imaging.
- Imaging information helps in accurate staging, assessing resectability, and planning appropriate treatment.
- Mandibular erosion, posterior soft-tissue extent, and perineural spread influence treatment and prognosis in gingival, buccal, and RMT cancers.
- Multidetector computed tomography (MDCT) with multiplanar reformations provide the highest specificity for bone erosion.
- Contrast-enhanced MRI is the modality of choice for tongue, FOM, hard palate lesion, and skull base due to its superior soft-tissue resolution and for detection of perineural spread.
- For nodal staging (N staging), all imaging methods are equivalent.
- Positron emission tomography (PET)/integrated PET/CT has a role in pretreatment assessment of advanced oral cavity SCC for depicting distant metastases and for mapping nodal extent in the clinically positive neck.
- Diffusion-weighted MRI, dynamic contrast-enhanced MRI, and CT perfusion have a role in baseline pretreatment studies, post-treatment follow-up and for response assessment to chemoradiation in advanced oral cavity SCC and recurrent disease.

Principles of Oral Cancer Treatment

Vishal Yadav

INTRODUCTION

Head and neck cancers are a complex group of cancer sites characterized by varying histopathology, each with its own distinct natural history and clinical behavior.

All patients with suspected carcinoma of the oral cavity should be evaluated by an oncologist specialized in head and neck. The following should be recorded:
- *History*:
  - Information related to the disease
  - Detailed information of his habits, addictions, and occupation
  - Medical and family history, including any prior malignancy
  - Comorbidities if any
- *Clinical examination*:
  - Assessment of performance and nutrition status
  - *Histological diagnosis*: Fine-needle aspiration cytology (FNAC)/biopsy/review of any slides
  - Appropriate imaging for the extent of disease and assessment for resectability
  - Clinical staging and documentation of the subsite(s) involved
- *Investigations*:
  - Chest X-ray
  - Computed tomography (CT) scan/magnetic resonance imaging (MRI) for extent of disease (appropriate sequences, with and without contrast)
  - Examination under anesthesia/endoscopy for accurate disease mapping
  - Ultrasonography (USG) for select cases of N0 neck
  - Positron emission tomography (PET)–contrast-enhanced CT (CECT) in advanced cancers to rule out distant metastasis

All treatment decisions should be taken in a multidisciplinary joint clinic with the aim of maximizing survival and preservation of form and function **(Flowchart 1)**.

GENERAL GUIDELINES FOR SELECTING A TREATMENT MODALITY

- *Stage I/II*: Single modality [surgery or radiotherapy (RT)]
- *Stage III and IV*: Combined or multimodality
  - Surgery + RT ± chemotherapy
  - Chemotherapy + RT

Selection of a particular treatment modality depends on the subsite of cancer:
- When different treatment options are available, the one that gives maximum chance of cure is selected.
- When different treatment modalities have similar results, the one that gives better quality of life (QOL), with organ function preservation, is selected.

Principles of Oral Cancer Treatment

Flowchart 1: Decision-making in management of oral cancer.

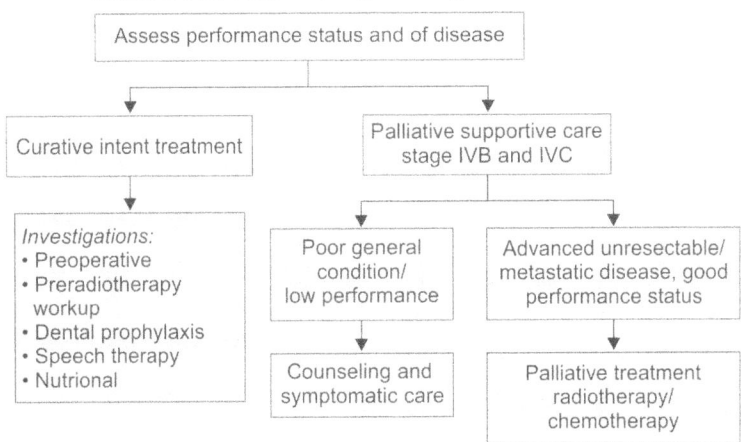

As a single modality, surgery is preferred over RT in:
- Sites where surgery is not cosmetically and functionally morbid
- *Lesions that involve or lie close to bone*: In order to prevent radionecrosis of the bone
- Young patients as there could be a possibility of a subsequent second primary
- Presence of submucous fibrosis (SMF)

As a single modality, RT is preferred over surgery where:
- Severe impairment of function/cosmesis expected with surgery, e.g., cancers of the vocal cord, selected base tongue.
- Surgery is technically difficult with high morbidity and poor outcome expected, e.g., carcinoma of the nasopharynx.
- Patient refuses to undergo surgery.
- Risk of surgery is high.

For patients planned for surgery:
- A tumor-free resection margin and appropriate reconstruction for restoration of form and function should be aimed and planned in detail.
- The plan should not be changed later, based on response to any planned prior chemotherapy.
- Plan may be modified for wider resection, when there is progression of the disease during waiting.

Assessment of Resectability

Involvement of the following structures by tumor is generally considered as unresectable:
- Erosion of pterygoid plates, sphenoid bone, widening of foramen ovale.
- Extension to superior nasopharynx or deep extension into Eustachian tube or lateral nasopharyngeal wall.
- Encasement of internal carotid artery, defined radiologically as tumor surrounding the carotids > 270°.
- Involvement of prevertebral fascia or cervical vertebrae.
- Dermal nodules may appear resectable but are poor surgical candidates.

Principles of Resection

- Complete resection of the primary tumor whenever possible

- Dissection of the neck if there is involvement of primary to the neck.
- Third dimension or the base must be considered before excision.
- *Adequate margin*: 1.5–2 cm; *Clear margin*: > 0.5 cm; *Close margin*: < 0.5 cm
- Confirmation of the margins by frozen section may be done when facility is available.
- Addressing the neck for tumors of these sites is a function of the site, extent of disease, and histology.
- When the chances of bilateral/contralateral metastases are high, e.g., in tumors that cross the midline/midline tumors, contralateral neck should also be addressed.

OPTIONS FOR RECONSTRUCTION

- *Mucosal defects*:
  - In a small defect, primary closure or local flap or soft-tissue coverage (SSG) or leave area raw according to the site involved.
  - In a large defect, try to replace the tissue loss with similar type of tissue.
- *Soft-tissue loss*: [Pedicled flaps, e.g., pectoralis major myocutaneous (PMMC)] or free tissue transfer
  - Skeletal defects +/− soft-tissue and skin loss:
    - *Anterior or midline*:
      - Free fibula/deep circumflex iliac artery (+/− Skin paddle)
      - Regional osteomyocutaneous flaps
      - Metallic plate
    - *Posterior segment*:
      - PMMC
      - Free fibula
  - *Skin defects can be covered with*:
    - Local flaps/forehead flap
    - Deltopectoral flap/PMMC
    - Free flap

INDICATIONS OF POST-OPERATIVE RADIOTHERAPY

- *Primary*:
  - Large primary – T3/T4
  - Deep infiltrative type of tumor
  - High grade of the tumor
  - Lymphovascular invasion and perineural invasion
- *Lymph nodes*:
  - Bulky nodal disease N2/N3
  - Extranodal extension
  - Multiple level of involvement
  - Multiple lymph nodes
- *Chemoradiotherapy*:
  - Positive or close margin after curative resection
  - Nodes with perinodal extension
  - Unresectable disease

RADICAL RADIOTHERAPY

- *T1-4 N0-2*:
  - *Concomitant chemoradiation*: 66–70 Gy/33–35#/6–7 weeks + concomitant cisplatin, 30 mg/m^2 for 6–7 weeks or 3-weekly cisplatin, 100 mg/m^2 × 3 cycles
    or
  - *External RT*: 66–70 Gy/33–35 fractions/6–7 weeks (reducing fields).

Doses and volumes of radiation in adjuvant setting:

- *Primary and involved nodal disease*: 56–60 Gys/28–30 fractions/6 weeks, with reducing fields

- *Site of residual disease, positive margins*: 4–10 Gys Boost
- *Uninvolved nodal areas*: 45–50 Gys

Dose of chemotherapy in the adjuvant setting in combination with RT: 30 mg/m² weekly with hydration and antiemetic prophylaxis.

Specific to the subsites, there is a need for pretreatment assessment of eye and auditory functions, nutritional assessment, dental prophylaxis, speech and swallowing assessment.

REHABILITATION

- Quitting tobacco/alcohol
- Good oral hygiene
- Physiotherapy of the shoulders in all cases of neck dissections
- Bite guide prosthesis after mandibulectomy
- Jaw stretching physiotherapy to prevent postoperative trismus
- Swallowing and speech therapy
- Ophthalmologic and auditory rehabilitation

FOLLOW-UP

- Every 2–3 months during the first 2 years
- 6-monthly for the next 3 years
- Annually after 3 years
- On every follow-up thorough clinical examination of the head and neck, for locoregional relapse, second primary tumor and late toxicities of the treatment. Investigation indicated only when symptoms and positive clinical findings are present.
- Serum T3, T4, and TSH annually for all patients receiving RT
- Imaging advised at follow-up if necessary
- Participation for suitable patients in clinical trials is encouraged.

IMAGING IN ORAL CANCERS

Imaging has an important role in:
- Delineating the deeper extent of disease.
- Guides the clinicians in deciding appropriate management strategy, assessing resectability, and estimating precise extent of resection.
- Image guidance can be used for targeting difficult/multiple negative biopsies and to plan radiation therapy (image-guided RT dose-painting).
- Imaging findings also help prognosticate disease.
- Evaluation for residual/recurrent disease.

Imaging provides information that helps in planning the therapy:
- To differentiate benign from malignant tumors
- To detect the location and surrounding extension of the lesion
- To evaluate perineural spread
- To assess for resectability, invasion of orbit, cavernous sinus or vascular structures, or of meningeal or brain parenchymal.

Which imaging modality to be used?
- *General principle*:
  - MRI is the modality of choice for tumors of the peripheral nervous system (PNS), nasopharynx, base skull, salivary gland, and parapharyngeal space.
  - Bone detail is a major strength and make CT scanning a complimentary imaging modality for temporal bone and paranasal malignancies.
  - In certain instances, multimodality approaches are complementary to each other.
  - Ultrasound is used for:
    - Evaluating salivary glands
    - Lymphadenopathy in the neck
    - Image-guided FNAC

- PET-CECT is valuable:
    - For evaluation in the staging workup in advanced cancers
    - Planning RT portals (especially reradiation)
    - Evaluation of malignant cervical adenopathy from an unknown primary
    - Post-therapy setting for response assessment and differentiating treatment changes versus residual disease
- Chest imaging is advocated for metastatic workup of the patient and at least chest radiograph must be performed as a part of staging workup of patients. However, there is more and more evidence supporting chest CT is far superior for staging workup, especially in patients that have a high risk of pulmonary metastasis at presentation, e.g., heavy smokers, advanced cancers.

Resectability Issues and Imaging

- *Perineural spread*: Perineural spread usually has a bad prognosis since it is associated with infiltration of the cavernous sinus, cranial nerves, skull base invasion. Perineural spread is found commonly along the cranial nerves V, III, IV, and VI through foramen rotundum, foramen ovale, and superior and inferior orbital fissures. It is also seen along the cranial nerves IX, X, XI, and XII with extension to the intracranial compartments along the jugular foramen and the hypoglossal canal.
- *Orbital invasion*: Lesions of the sinuses may infiltrate the orbit wall easily, through the lamina papyracea, which is the weakest wall of the orbit. Lesions of the central skull base invade the orbit through the orbital fissures or the orbital apex. Invasion is indicated by loss of fat and abnormal enhancement within these neural foramina. These can be better appreciated on an MRI. Strong fibrous periorbita attached along the orbital medial wall at its superior and inferior aspect may limit the spread of the tumor. Tumors which invade the periorbita and extend into the orbital apex merit orbital exenteration with consequent sacrifice of the optic nerve. Both CT and MRI are equivocal for detecting invasion of periorbita. Tumors spreading to the orbital apex may enter into the middle cranial fossa through the superior orbital fissure.
- *Cavernous sinus invasion*: Complete resection of a lesion is contraindicated with invasion of the cavernous sinus. Signs of cavernous sinus invasion on imaging are compression, or encasement, or stenosis, or irregularity of the cavernous carotid artery. Other signs may be loss of contrast enhancement of the cavernous sinus, best seen on a dynamic coronal MRI, and bulging of the lateral sinus wall, which under normal conditions, is concave.
- *Dural invasion*: When there are nodular or linear dural enhancement, thicker than 5 mm they indicate dural invasion. Any such enhancement <5 mm may be seen in reactionary fibrovascular changes and does not indicate dural invasion.
- *Cervical nodes*: CT and MRI are the usual imaging modalities for the assessment of metastatic nodes. There are defined by specific size criteria and presence of necrosis. PET-CT is superior for nodes that is less than 1 cm. But both false-negative and false-positive results are also commonly seen. US-guided FNAC

seems to have the highest accuracy in diagnosing metastatic nodes and, hence, may be used in institutes where expertise is available. Diffusion-weighted (DW) MRI and dynamic contrast-enhanced MRI also have an emerging role.
- *Post-treatment issues*: MRI and PET-CT have a very important role for differentiating between posttreatment changes and recurrent or residual disease after completion of treatment. PET-CT is useful for patients on long-term surveillance. DW MRI also has a promising role.

RECURRENT/METASTATIC ORAL CANCER

Factors affecting the prognosis are:
- *Patient-related factors*:
  - Performance score and presence or absence of comorbidities
  - QOL and functional outcomes
  - Treatment expenses
- *Disease-related factors*:
  - Stage and extent of disease
  - Site of recurrence
  - Disease-free interval (DFI) (Patients with disease recurrence within 1 year of initial treatment have significantly worse survival than patients who recur later).
- *Treatment-related factors*: History of previous treatment

SALVAGE SURGERY

Surgical salvage offers good survival rates in selected recurrent/metastatic cancers of head and neck, depending on the respectability of the volume and location of recurrent disease. Salvage surgery may also provides good long-term survival. 5-year overall survival rates after surgical salvage generally range between 11 and 39%.

Salvage Surgery in Curative Setting

- Isolated recurrence in the neck when the primary has already been treated but neck not addressed or has been treated with single modality.
- Recurrence in the neck following definite treatment with chemoradiation or radiation in undissected neck.
- Locoregional recurrence after single modality treatment for early-stage disease with surgery or radiation.
- When surgery does not cause functionally morbidity.

Salvage Surgery with Palliative Intent

The aim is to relieve symptoms such as airway obstruction, oral bleed or difficult feeding, tracheostomy/gastrostomy.

RERADIATION

Reirradiation may be considered for patients who are not suitable for salvage surgery, but who have locally recurrent disease after previous definitive treatment. Reradiation can be offered in both curative and palliative intent to patients with recurrent/metastatic cancers.

Reradiation with curative intent:
- Preferred for cancers which have not been radiated earlier.
- When surgery is extensive and associated with functional morbidity and more worse QOL.
- When surgery is not technically possible.

Re-radiation with palliative intent:
- Where surgery is not an option.
- When RT with radical doses is not possible due to short *disease-free interval*, or poor general condition of the patient and

extensive late sequelae following previous radiation.
- For palliation of symptoms such as fungating, bleeding, and pain.

SYSTEMIC CHEMOTHERAPY

In recurrent or metastatic patients, the role of systemic chemotherapy is palliative with a median survival of 6-8 months. Systemic chemotherapy may be planned as combination chemotherapy or single-agent chemotherapy. The general condition of the patient and his performance status play an important role in deciding the optimum management.

Factors determining systemic chemotherapy:
- Performance status [Eastern Cooperative Oncology Group (ECOG)] and comorbidities
- Disease extent and stage
- History of any prior chemotherapy

Chemotherapy can be administered as single-agent or as a combination chemotherapy.
- *Combination chemotherapy*: Cisplatin remains the cornerstone of treatment in recurrent and metastatic squamous cell carcinomas of the head and neck (SCCHN). Platinum-based combination chemotherapy produced higher response rates than those of single-agent therapy. Addition of cetuximab to combination has improved overall survival in this group of patients.
- *Single-agent chemotherapy*: A large number of conventional single agents have been investigated in the past in patients with recurrent/metastatic SCCHN. The most active and most extensively used agents are methotrexate, cisplatin and 5-fluorouracil (5-FU). Weekly methotrexate may be considered as the accepted treatment.

IMMUNOTHERAPY/TARGETED THERAPY

- *Immunotherapy with PD-L1 checkpoint inhibitors (e.g., pembrolizumab, nivolumab)*: First-line treatment for recurrent and metastatic tumors.
- Molecularly targeted agents [e.g., epidermal growth factor receptor (EGFR) inhibitors e.g., Cetuximab].

Metronomic therapy consisting of oral methotrexate, celecoxib, and erlotinib may give symptomatic relief. It may be continued till disease progression.

BEST SUPPORTIVE CARE

Patients with severe comorbidities or poor performance status may be best treated with supportive care at home.

METASTATIC DISEASE

Oligometastasis

Role of surgery:
- *Metastatectomy*: Not indicated in patients with short DFI, extensive nodal burden, and when the previous surgery was not curative.

Role of RT:
- *Bony metastasis*: Pain, compression, and fracture
- Brain metastasis
- *Pulmonary metastasis*: Bleeding, chest pain, etc.

KEY POINTS

- Treatment decisions for all patients should be made in a multidisciplinary joint clinic with the goal for maximizing survival and preservation of form and function.
- *Stage I/II disease*: Single modality (surgery or RT)
- *Stage III and IV disease*: Combined modality
  - Surgery + RT ± chemotherapy
  - Chemotherapy + RT
- Surgery is preferred over RT as a single modality in sites where surgery is not cosmetically and functionally morbid, lesions involving or close to bone (to prevent radionecrosis), in young patients due to possibility of a subsequent second primary and in presence of SMF.
- MRI is the modality of choice for tumors of the PNS, nasopharynx, base skull, salivary gland, and parapharyngeal space.
- Systemic chemotherapy is essentially palliative with a median survival of 6–8 months in recurrent/metastatic settings.

CHAPTER 8

Management of Oral Premalignant Lesions

Vishal Yadav

"The best prevention is early detection."

INTRODUCTION

Sir James Paget first described malignant transformation of an oral lesion into tongue carcinoma in the year 1870. Squamous cell carcinoma (SCC) is the most common cancer of the oral cavity. Normal tissues progress to dysplasia or carcinoma due to multiple genetic mutations. Overexpression of some markers such as ALDH1 and CD133 also increases the risk for progression of oral leukoplakia (OL) to invasive SCC. There are other predictive markers such as chromosomal allelic imbalances, loss of heterozygosity in chromosome 3p, 9p, 17p, polysomy, mutations in EGFR, p53, cyclin D and specific DNA methylation sites, which suggest the presence of a shared pathway of conversion of normal mucosa to premalignant lesions and invasive carcinoma.

TERMINOLOGY AND DEFINITIONS

The World Health Organization (WHO) proposed in 1978 that potentially malignant disorders should be classified into two broad groups, as lesions and conditions with the following definitions **(Table 1)**:
1. A precancerous lesion is "a morphologically altered tissue in which oral cancer is more likely to occur than its apparently normal counterpart."

TABLE 1: Precancerous lesions and conditions.

Precancerous lesions	Precancerous conditions
Leukoplakia	Oral submucous fibrosis
Erythroplakia	Lichen planus
Proliferative verrucous leukoplakia	Discoid lupus erythematous
Palatal lesions of reverse smoker	Epidermolysis bullosa

2. A precancerous condition is "a generalized state associated with significantly increased risk of cancer."

DIAGNOSIS (TABLE 2)

Leukoplakia, erythroplakia, and erythroleukoplakia are those lesions that can be appreciated on clinical examination and need further diagnostic steps to confirm dysplasia or invasive carcinoma. Biopsy is the gold standard procedure to diagnose such lesions. Incisional biopsies may underdiagnose underlying invasive carcinoma because of missing the biopsy site, inadequate depth of the biopsy taken or poor handling, and poor preparation of the specimen. Excisional biopsy of the suspected area should be obtained whenever feasible.

Recently some noninvasive procedures such as narrow band imaging and chemiluminescence have been used effectively in identifying markers that may predict

TABLE 2: Diagnostic methods.	
Noninvasive	*Invasive*
Supravital staining	Incisional/wedge biopsy
Chemiluminescent light	
Tissue autofluorescence	
Oral cytology/brush	
Positive predictive value of brush biopsy: 58% *Sensitivity of Brush:* 43%	

Box 1: Types of leukoplakia.

- *Based on clinical types*:
  - *Homogeneous*: Smooth, furrowed, ulcerative
  - *Nonhomogeneous*: Speckled, nodular
- *Based on etiology*:
  - Tobacco associated
  - Idiopathic
- *Based on extent*:
  - Localized
  - Diffuse
- *Based on histology*:
  - Dysplastic
  - Nondysplastic

dysplastic or invasive changes. Staining with toluidine blue helps in selection of the site for biopsy. These dyes have shown to reduce the chances of benign tissue biopsies and can identify lesions that are at higher risk for malignant transformation. Hence, staining with toluidine blue could prove to be helpful in diagnosis of premalignant lesions of the oral cavity.

ORAL LEUKOPLAKIA

Oral leukoplakia is a clinical diagnosis, referring to any white patch on the oral mucosa that cannot be scraped out, and not attributable to any other disease. The words "leuko" mean white and "plakia" mean patch. It may be thin or thick, well-defined, slightly elevated or wrinkled appearance (homogeneous) or speckled or nodular appearance (nonhomogeneous) **(Box 1)**.

The global prevalence of OL is estimated as 0.5–3.4%, with a transformation rate to malignancy, of approximately 1%. Range of variations have been found in the reported rate of malignant transformation (0.13–17.5%). The rate is seen to be higher in:
- Nonhomogeneous OL
- Lesions that demonstrate moderate-to-severe dysplasia
- Lesions on the tongue or FOM
- Lesions > 200 mm^2
- Age > 60 years
- Nonsmokers

Dysplasia is known to be the strongest indicator of malignant transformation with rates between 15 and 30% over a long duration of follow-up. The rate may also depend on the degree of dysplasia. Those lesions that have high grade of dysplasia may be 4.5-times more predisposed to malignant transformation as compared with mildly dysplastic lesions. It needs to be emphasized that oral epithelial dysplasia is a histological diagnosis and has no particular clinical appearance.

Based on the clinical appearance, Sharp described three stages/phases of leukoplakia:
- *Phase I*: A white, slightly translucent non-palpable lesion
- *Phase II*: An opaque white, slightly elevated plaque with irregular outline. The lesion may be localized or diffuse and may have a granular texture.
- *Phase III*: Thickened white lesions that show fissuring, induration, and ulcer formation.

Management

A detailed history and thorough clinical examination are mandatory to rule out any other causes such as trauma, smoking, and smokeless tobacco. If a causative factor is identified, then lifestyle modifications should be encouraged. 4–6 weeks' observation period is given to determine any spontaneous regression of the lesion.

TABLE 3: Surgical and nonsurgical interventions.

Surgical therapies	Nonsurgical therapies
Wide local excision	Vitamin A and C
Laser ablation	Beta-carotene
Electrocauterization	Lycopene
Cryosurgery	Bleomycin
	Photodynamic therapy

If the lesion does not subside, a biopsy needs to be obtained to confirm the presence or absence of dysplasia. In cases of multifocal leukoplakia, a series of "mapping" biopsies should be carried out to examine the entire site. There are numerous classification systems developed to characterize the premalignant mucosal lesions of the head and neck. The classification recommended by the WHO is most commonly used. When the biopsy reveals dysplasia, further management is determined by patient characteristics, size and location of the lesion and institutional factors. The treatment options include surgical and nonsurgical interventions, which are given in **Table 3**.

Surgical Therapies

Wide local excision of the lesion with a cuff of normal tissue is the standard treatment if the lesion is small, for both the primary and also for recurrent lesions. There is no consensus about the optimal surgical margin, but is generally accepted as a few millimeters.

Laser ablation is done for wider lesions when the large resection could compromise his functions. Morbidity for lase ablation is minimum.

After treatment with laser surgery, approximately 20% recur and a have malignant transformation rate of 10.4%. Moreover, patients undergoing CO_2 laser excision experience lesser pain and swelling, as compared with cold knife excision.

Nonsurgical Therapies

- *Vitamin C* (L-ascorbic acid) is a water-soluble vitamin that is needed for formation of collagen and mediates redox reactions with its antioxidant properties. It has been shown that smokers may have lower levels of L-ascorbic acid. Currently, there is no evidence, to demonstrate the efficacy of vitamin C as monotherapy.
- *Vitamin A*: This constitutes a family of fat-soluble vitamins such as retinol, carotenoids, and beta-carotene (pro-vitamin A). The antioxidant properties of Iso-tretinoin (13-cis-retinoic acid) have been used for treating of OL. This alone has shown to give a complete response in 52–71% of the patients, though after discontinuing the treatment, most of the lesions would recur. Side effects such as headaches and bodyaches are commonly seen with therapeutic doses of vitamin A. Long-term treatment with vitamin A is expensive.
- *Beta-carotene* is a hydrophobic precursor of vitamin A found in many colored (orange, yellow) fruits and vegetables. The protective effect of beta-carotene is due to its antioxidant properties. Studies have revealed a complete response rate of 4–33%, recurrence rate of 54%, and risk of malignant transformation of 5%.
- *Lycopene* is another carotenoid that is found in tomatoes. This too have shown efficacy in treating OL.
- *Bleomycin* is a chemotherapeutic agent. It acts by inducing breaks in the DNA strands. Topical use of 1% bleomycin has been studied in the treatment of OL in dimethyl sulfoxide (DMSO). About 75% of the patients showed complete resolution of dysplasia and 94% achieved a partial or complete clinical response in a small study. Malignant transformation was seen in two patients (11%).

- *Photodynamic therapy* is a nonsurgical unique method that utilizes a nonthermal photochemical reaction. It needs oxygen, a visible light and a photosensitizing drug. Illumination of the lesion by the light source of appropriate wavelength activates the photosensitizing drug. Thus, it causes destruction of cells by non-free radical oxidative procedure. The tissue later heals by regeneration with minimal scarring and morbidity. The most commonly utilized photosensitizing drug is 5-aminolevulinic acid (5-ALA). With topical application of 5-ALA, the lesions get exposed to a light-emitting diode or the pulse-dye laser. Multiple treatments are generally needed to achieve a complete response. Currently, there are only some small case studies suggesting its safety and efficacy.

Key Points—Leukoplakia
- Low rate of malignant transformation
- *Treatment modalities are based on*:
  - Lesion factors (size, location, homogeneous vs. nonhomogeneous)
  - Patient factors (smoker, drinker, comorbid status)
  - Clinical factors (availability of different treatment options)
- Nonhomogeneous lesions (high-risk lesions) require aggressive treatment.
- Large or multifocal lesions may require several biopsies to provide a histologic map of the area.
- Leukoplakia is often a life-long disease process that will require careful follow-up.

ERYTHROPLAKIA

Erythroplakia is a bright red velvety plaque in the oral mucosa. It cannot be characterized clinically as any other recognizable lesion. Erythroplakia when seen close to the leukoplakias are termed as "erythroleukoplakia." Erythroplakia is less common than leukoplakia but has more chances to contain SCC in situ and invasive carcinoma. A majority of leukoplakic lesions show hyperkeratosis or epithelial hyperplasia instead of dysplasia or carcinoma in situ with erythroplakia. Majority of the prevalence studies have been conducted in Southeast Asia with prevalence ranging from 0.02 to 0.83%.

Erythroplakic lesions are rarely found to be multicentric. They present with well-defined margins without any diffuse involvement of large surface areas. They may appear throughout the oral cavity but are generally seen on the palate, buccal mucosa, and the FOM. Use of alcohol and tobacco are known predisposing factors. Chewing tobacco and betel quid (with or without tobacco) contributes more significantly than smoking and alcohol consumption.

Erythroplakia carries the highest risk for malignant transformation in comparison to other premalignant lesions such as leukoplakia, lichen planus (LP), and oral submucous fibrosis (OSMF). Because of the potential risk of carcinoma being present in erythroplakia as well the significant risk for malignant transformation, the recent recommendation for treatment is wide local excision. The risk of transformation is 95% at 20 years.

Areas of erythroplakia are generally small (<1.5 cm) with clear margins and are good for surgical excision.

Key Points—Erythroplakia
- Less common
- Highest risk for malignant transformation
- *Treatment of choice*: Surgical excision, especially for small-sized lesion
- *Other treatment option*: Photodynamic therapy (5-ALA)

ORAL SUBMUCOUS FIBROSIS

Oral submucous fibrosis is a chronic condition which is characterized by alterations in the fibroelastic qualities of the submucosal soft tissues. It is most commonly seen in the oral cavity. Pathogenesis of the disease has not been well understood. It is generally believed to be a disease of metabolism of collagen. Sensitivity to spicy foods and a burning discomfort are generally early symptoms. They may also present with painful mouth ulcerations or vesicles on the palate. In more advanced disease, atrophy of the oral mucosa, xerostomia, and severe submucosal fibrosis are also noted. The most common sites of involvement are the buccal mucosa. Clinical examination shows dense fibrotic bands which are painful to touch. Fibrosis may lead to severe trismus, which limits examination of the mucosal surfaces.

There is evidence that OSMF is caused by areca nut. Areca nut, with or without tobacco, is customarily chewed in parts of Southeast Asia. Betel quid and Gutkha are products that contain areca nut. Gutkha is a powder that is packaged in small sachets and contains higher quantities of areca nut.

Oral submucous fibrosis undergoes malignant transformation at a rate of 7–30%. One long-term follow-up study showed malignant transformation rate of 0.5% per annum. Both tobacco and areca nut are known carcinogens and are synergistic in the pathogenesis of OSMF.

Management of OSMF includes reducing symptoms, disease progression, and close surveillance for malignant transformation:

- Stopping chewing areca nut is not likely to reverse the fibrosis, but it reduces the burning pain.
- Steroids with or without enzymes such as hyaluronidase may be injected into scar bands. It helps improvement in pain, but has little effect on fibrosis and trismus.
- Antioxidants may be given to combat the reactive oxygen produced by areca nut.
- The administration of vitamins A, B complex, and E with other micronutrients such as iron, calcium, copper, zinc, and magnesium has shown improvement in symptoms.
- Lycopenes
- Peripheral vasodilators such as pentoxifylline, interferon-gamma (IFN-γ), aloe vera, and turmeric.
- Surgery and physical therapy may help release fibrotic bands and stretch the tissues to prevent scar recurrence.
- Different types of flaps have been designed to cover the surgical defect created by scar release. Some of these are split-thickness skin grafts, pedicled flaps (temporoparietal fascia, temporalis muscle, nasolabial), intraoral flaps (buccal fat pad, palatal island), and vascularized free-tissue transfer (radial forearm and anterolateral thigh flaps). Surgical intervention may improve trismus and provide symptomatic relief
- The goal of surgical intervention is relief of symptoms. It does not reduce risk of malignant transformation.

Key Points in Care of OSMF
- Discontinuation of the use of areca nut
- Symptomatic management, antioxidants, and surgery
- Close oncologic surveillance. Surgery gives symptomatic relief and does not reduce risk of malignant transformation.

LICHEN PLANUS

Lichen planus is an inflammatory condition of the skin and the oral mucosa affecting 1–2% of the global population. There is a proved association between hepatitis C and lichen planus but yet, the exact cause of LP is unknown.

Pathophysiological studies suggest that it is a T-cell-mediated autoimmune disorder.

However, the inciting antigen and triggering factors are unclear. Oral lichen planus (OLP) presents as a symmetric lesion on the buccal mucosa. Other sites of OLP are the tongue and the gingiva. There are six subtypes of OLP that may present individually or in combination.

Subtypes of OLP

Subtypes of OLP include:
- Papular
- Reticular (most common)
- *Erosive*: Malignant transformation—high
- Plaque like
- Bullous and atrophic
- *Atrophic*: Malignant transformation—high

The reticular subtype is most common and usually presents as symmetric, fine white, or gray, raised lesions on the buccal mucosa referred to as *Wickham striae*. The other subtypes of OLP need histopathologic confirmation to make a diagnosis.

There is no known cure for LP and aim of treatment consists of symptom management and surveillance for transformation to carcinoma. Majority of the patients of LP will be symptomatic at some point during the course of their disease with waxing and waning symptoms.
- Topical applications of *steroids and tacrolimus* are useful to relieve symptoms.
- *Steroids* are superior to agents such as cyclosporine for relief of symptoms. Systemic use of steroids may be required when there is no improvement.
- Treatments should be aimed at eradication of OLP that has associated dysplasia. This includes *surgical excision, laser evaporation, photodynamic therapy,* and topical or systemic retinoids. Isotretinoin therapy has been seen to reduce dysplasia on biopsy when used over several months in incremental doses.
- Lycopene and curcumin extracts in high doses
- *Photodynamic therapy* and *cryotherapy* provide similar outcome with regards to recurrence (27 vs. 24%) and clinical response (73 vs. 89%). The most important aspects of management are regular follow-up and patient education. SCC can arise at mucosal sites away from the site of OLP and hence, thorough clinical examination of the entire oral cavity is essential.

Key Points—Lichen Planus
- Inflammatory disease of the skin and oral mucosa
- *Pathophysiology*: T-cell-mediated autoimmune disorder
- Most commonly presents symmetrically on the buccal mucosa
- Reticular subtype is the most common; erosive and atrophic subtypes carry the highest risk of transformation.
- Rate of malignant transformation is 0–5.3%.
- Goals of treatment are symptom management and surveillance for evolution to carcinoma.

PROLIFERATIVE VERRUCOUS LEUKOPLAKIA

Verrucous leukoplakia is a nonhomogeneous leukoplakia that may not be differentiated from verrucous carcinoma. Proliferative verrucous leukoplakia (PVL) is a type of verrucous leukoplakia. This premalignant lesion commonly has a multifocal presentation and has a high risk for malignant transformation as compared with a typical leukoplakic lesion. It is prevalent among elderly women and is not known to be associated with tobacco exposure.

The etiology of PVL remains unknown. A relationship has been found with the Epstein-Barr virus and human papillomavirus. Many of these lesions are likely to develop into verrucous carcinoma or conventional SCC over years. The carcinomas may develop both within or adjacent to a site of PVL. About 40–75% of these patients will develop cancer. The most common sites of involvement are the alveolar ridge, tongue, and buccal mucosa.

- *Treatment*: Aggressive surgical resection for severely dysplastic or malignant lesions.
- Nondysplastic lesions can be managed with CO_2 laser ablation and photodynamic therapy.
- A field cancerization phenomenon has been proposed for PVL because of its tendency to recur in a multifocal distribution. Antiviral medications and retinoids are recommended to prevent recurrence, though results have not been encouraging.

Key Points—PVL
- Multifocal presentation and carries a high risk for malignant transformation.
- More prevalent among elderly women and is not associated with tobacco exposure.
- Association with the Epstein–Barr virus and human papillomavirus has been suggested.
- About 40–75% of patients with PVL will go on to develop cancer.
- *Treatment options*: Surgical resection, CO_2 laser ablation, and photodynamic therapy.

KEY POINTS

- Premalignant lesions of the oral mucosa include leukoplakia, erythroplakia, and premalignant conditions include LP and OSMF and their variants.
- Lesions often arise in the setting of shared risk factors and genetic alterations.
- Detection of visibly abnormal mucosal lesions should prompt surgical biopsies based on characteristics of lesion and patient risk factors.
- Continued surveillance of affected mucosa aids in early identification and management of lesions suspected to undergo malignant transformation.
- Dysplastic lesions should undergo excision with negative margins.
- Lesion ablation with laser, cryotherapy, electrocautery, or photodynamic therapy may be considered when a broad resection incurs unacceptable morbidity.
- Antioxidants, vitamin preparations, and antimetabolites may offer promise in refractory cases of leukoplakia, although there are limitations to data in support of their use.
- Erythroplakia is much less common than leukoplakia but carries a higher risk of malignant transformation.
- Surgical biopsies and excision remain the mainstay of erythroplakia management.
- Symptom improvement with topical steroids can be attained in OLP and OSMF.
- Surgical release of scar and adjunctive reconstructive strategies result in improved oral aperture in OSMF, allowing better patient satisfaction and clinical surveillance.
- Diagnosis of LP (particularly the erosive and atrophic subtypes) confers an increased risk of malignant transformation in affected and adjacent mucosa.
- PVL imparts a high risk for development of invasive carcinoma in affected and surrounding normal mucosa.

CHAPTER 9

Trismus in Head and Neck Cancers

Ghanashyam Mandal

INTRODUCTION

The word trismus originates from the Greek word *"trismos,"* which means grating, grinding, or squeaking. Historically, "trismos" was referred when a patient was unable to open the mouth like in tetanus. Presently, it is used to indicate severely restricted opening of the mouth due to any etiology.

Trismus occurs due to the persistent contraction of one or more muscles of mastication. It may be result of local inflammatory processes or involvement by malignant tumors into these muscles. It generally affects patients after intraoral surgical procedures, or after a stroke, and those who are undergoing radiation therapy for head and neck malignancies.

PREVALENCE

- Depending on the site and extension of the tumor, the reported prevalence of trismus in head and neck cancer ranges between 0 and 100%.
- 10–40% of those with head and neck cancer receiving radiation would develop trismus.
- Patients with carcinoma of tonsils are most prone to develop trismus.

TRISMUS AND ITS RELATION WITH RADIATION THERAPY

- A significant correlation has been found between the absorbed dose of radiation to the mastication structures and opening of the mouth. The prevalence of trismus increases with increasing doses of radiotherapy (RT); doses > 60 Gy are more likely to develop trismus. Trismus worsens as the dose of radiation to medial pterygoid muscles increases.
- The chances of trismus are found to increase 24% for every 10 Gy of additional radiation delivered to the medial pterygoid muscles.
- The incidence of trismus is associated with the radiation dose received by both pterygoid and masseter muscles.
- Previously irradiated patients being treated for a recurrence appear to be at higher risk of trismus than those who are receiving for the first time. This therefore suggests that there is cumulative effect of RT on tissues inside irradiated volume.
- About 1 year after RT, the deterioration of trismus gradually slows down.

Trismus as a Sign of Recurrence

- Recent-onset painful trismus after completion of treatment → suspect recurrence
- If mouth opening decreases in spite of exercises, especially when associated with pain and halitosis, then a recurrence should be suspected.

TRISMUS AND ITS RELATION WITH ALCOHOL

- Regular alcohol users have a smaller chance of developing trismus or of presenting with trismus before treatment.
- Alcohol acts as a muscle relaxant and counteracts the laying down of collagen.

INTRA-ARTICULAR VERSUS EXTRA-ARTICULAR CAUSES OF TRISMUS

- Intra-articular causes of trismus are associated with restricted horizontal movement of the mandible (toward the contralateral/unaffected side).
- Extra-articular causes are generally not associated with restricted horizontal movement of the mandible. Most cases of oncology-related trismus are extra-articular in nature.

PROBLEMS WITH TRISMUS

- Difficulty with oral intake
- *Compromise speech*: With limited jaw movement, it is painful to form proper words and sentences often leading to slurring and discomfort.
- Compromise oral hygiene and thus result in dental infections.
- Compromise tumor surveillance.
- *Compromise ability to safely secure an airway*: Difficult intubation, sometimes tracheostomy may be needed.
- Increase the risk of aspiration
- Limit proper postoperative maintenance of obturator
- Lack of intimacy, lack of self-esteem, depression and altered body image with nearly 60% of patients feeling discounted or stigmatized because of their cancer-related appearance.
- The normal act of swallowing requires to manipulate the food into a cohesive bolus initially. When the tongue cannot move normally, there may be postswallow excess residue. Such conditions with compromised mastication, poor bolus organization, and excess residue may to lead to aspiration of food. Restricted opening of the mouth can therefore has major consequences for proper food intake and communication. In advanced cases, patients are unable to take food of normal consistency and depend on mashed, liquidized food, or even on enteral tube feeding.

PATHOPHYSIOLOGY

- The muscles that close the mouth—the masseter, temporalis, and medial pterygoid muscles—exert a force which is 10 times stronger than exerted by the muscles that are responsible for opening the mouth—the lateral pterygoid, digastric and suprahyoid muscles.
- Most of these muscles are supplied by the mandibular division of the fifth cranial nerve.
- The muscle groups that control movements of the jaw act antagonistically. This is because of the neurogenic stimulation of one group results in reflex neural inhibition of the other.
- The causative insult may be unilateral, just as in a unilateral tumor but the reflex activated is bilateral resulting in restricted mouth opening.

TRISMUS MEASUREMENT AND CLASSIFICATION

How to Measure Mouth Opening?

- Ruler
- Sliding calipers with 1-mm gradations.
    - The instruments used should be made of materials which are easy to clean and sterilize.

- "Eyeballing" mouth opening
- Assessment with the number of fingers inserted between the teeth or alveolar ridges
  - Last two methods have less precision and hence less reliability.

Where to Measure Mouth Opening?

Maximal interincisal distance (MID) is measured.
- This is the distance between the incisal edges of the maxillary and mandibular incisors.
- In edentulous patients, the distance between the maxillary and mandibular alveolar ridges is measured.
- The measurement (MID) must be done twice with calipers, and the greatest value is recorded.

When to Measure Trismus?

- Prior to surgery
- After surgery
- Prior to RT
- After RT
- On every follow-up

What are the Grades of Trismus?

	Grade	Mouth opening (mm)
Normal	Normal	>35
I	Mild	35–26
II	Moderate	25–16
III	Severe	15–0

What is SOMA Classification of Trismus?

- The Radiation Therapy Oncology Group (RTOG) and the European Organization for Research and Treatment of Cancer have jointly developed "late effects in normal tissue" morbidity scales, and the National Cancer Institute consensus conferences introduced the *subjective, objective, management, analysis (SOMA) classification* for late cancer therapy toxicities. Trismus is included in these radiation-induced sequelae.
- The SOMA classification evaluates the radiation toxicities in grades:

Grade	Mouth opening (mm)
1	20–30
2	10–20
3	5–10

Recently, a mouth opening of ≤35 mm has been proposed as a cutoff point for defining trismus on the basis of sensitivity/specificity analyses of two external criteria:
1. Patients experience of limitation in mouth opening
2. Impairment of mandibular function assessed by means of the Mandibular Function Impairment Questionnaire (MFIQ).
- The MFIQ assesses perceived hindrance during 11 mandibular functions (i.e., speaking, taking a large bite, chewing hard food, chewing soft food, work and/or daily activities, drinking, laughing, chewing resistant food, yawning, and kissing) and perceived difficulty in eating food with different consistencies (i.e., a hard cookie, meat, a raw carrot, French bread, peanuts/almonds and an apple).

TREATMENT OF TRISMUS

- Conservative (with either medical or physical therapy)
- Surgical

Conservative Medical Treatment

- *Pentoxifylline*: Generally ineffective
- *Hyperbaric oxygen*: Generally ineffective
- Injection of *botulinum* toxin into the muscles of mastication is effective as an

analgesic, and also has potential benefit in the management of some selected cases of the radiation fibrosis syndrome.
- Microcurrent electrotherapy has limited effect in mouth opening.
- Physiotherapy

Conservative Physical Therapy

- Exercise therapy is the mainstay of the treatment of trismus although its effectiveness is limited.
- Exercising must be started as soon as possible after surgery and should begin during RT.
- Exercising should be performed as frequently as possible.
- It must include both vertical and horizontal ranges of motion.

Mechanical Methods

Mechanical methods of physical therapy may use any of the following:
- Tongue depressors
- Finger stretching
- Spring appliances
- Acrylic cones/wedges
- Clothes pegs
- Dynamic bite openers

Goal Setting

Goal setting for the patient (i.e., the number of tongue blades or the size of the plug):
- Generally begun with simple exercises that are acceptable by the patient.
- During the exercise period, serial measurement of mouth opening is important for evaluating the degree of improvement in trismus.
- Encourage adherence to the exercise
- The goal set is to strive for a mouth opening of >35 mm. Once this is achieved, then the frequency may be decreased.

Exercises for Trismus

The simplest form of exercise for trismus is called as *"active jaw movement exercises"* and involves the following:
- Opening and closing of the mouth repeatedly.
- Opening the mouth slightly, and then slowly moving the lower jaw to the left and then to the right.
- Stretching the chin downward and forward and then back to the original position just like a moving ball.
- Puffed cheek, as if blowing balloon

Passive Jaw Movement Exercises

Separating the maxillary and mandibular jaws manually by patient's own hands wrapped with gauze.

Rationale: Motion exercises and resistance exercises may strengthen the muscles, improve the blood circulation, and increase mobility and improve flexibility and elasticity of the temporomandibular joint (TMJ).

Jaw opening devices (**Figs. 1A to C**):
- Stacked wooden tongue depressors
- Corkscrew devices
- The TheraBite Jaw Motion Rehabilitation System:
  - This is a jaw mobilization device which is patient controlled and uses anatomically correct, repetitive passive movements and stretching to help restore jaw opening.
  - The improvement in jaw movements occurs due to a combination of stretching of connective tissues, mobilization of joints, and strengthening of the muscles across their entire range of motions.
  - After TheraBite exercises, mouth opening increases approximately 5.4 mm, provided the time from

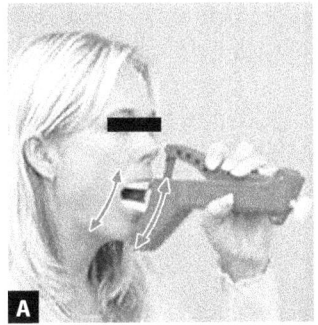 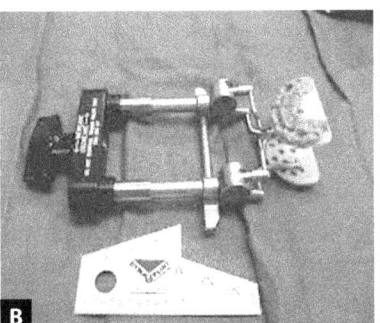 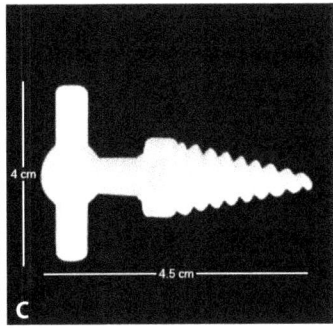

Figs. 1A to C: Jaw opening devices: (A) TheraBite; (B) Dynasplint Trismus System; (C) Corkscrew device.

oncological treatment is soon enough.
- *TheraBite protocol*: Follow the 5-5-30 protocol which is:
    - Five sessions per day
    - Five openings/closing per session
    - 30 seconds stretch for each opening
- The Dynasplint Trismus System (DTS)
- This system works on the principle of a low-torque, prolonged duration stretch.
- Forced mouth opening under general anesthesia (GA) can improve trismus but the effect is likely to be short lived. This may be complicated by fractures of the alveolus and injury of adjacent soft tissue.

Surgical Treatment

Surgical treatment may be considered for patients with good prognosis and when conservative treatment fails.
- *Coronoidectomy*: Coronoidectomy is beneficial in some selected patients. It is an invasive procedure with considerable surgical risks, especially in previously irradiated patients. Hence it should be used with caution. It is often recommended that a coronoidectomy is performed during tumor resection to prevent the development of trismus, especially when a curative surgery is performed, and when the tumor is close to the coronoid process.
- Dental extractions may be done in severe trismus to provide passage of food/spoon into mouth and maintain oral hygiene plus proper inspection of oral cavity.

PREVENTION OF TRISMUS

- Once radiation-induced trismus has set in, treatments may not be effective. Therefore, the prevention of trismus, rather than its treatment, should be the goal.
- Minimizing the dose of radiation to the TMJ and the muscles of mastication is the best way to prevent radiation-induced trismus. During the era of conventional RT which was delivered with parallel opposed or wedge fields, this was difficult to achieve. Intensity-modulated radiation therapy (IMRT) has been greatly beneficial in reducing the dose without compromising on therapeutic dose.
- Patients with tumour close to TMJ and masticatory muscles are at risk of trismus. It is important to identify these patients and inform them about the risk of developing trismus, the consequences of trismus, and the importance of ongoing exercising.
- Prevention exercises involve massaging masseter muscles from the outside two to three times a day for 30 seconds.

- Exercises in movement of your jaw, including moving mouth up and down and side-to-side to help stretch the jaw muscles avoiding restricted mouth movement.
- Passive stretching exercise, which involves stretching your mouth with your forefinger and thumb, can help.
- Maintaining good posture is another key in prevention of trismus. Simple exercises can help with posture such as neck stretches in the forward, backward, left, and right positions, holding stretches for 30 seconds and performing them twice a day.
- Maintain proper oral hygiene.

KEY POINTS

- Trismus can result from local invasion into critical structures of mastication including the masseter and pterygoid muscles, their neural innervations, and the TMJ.
- When a patient presents with trismus after tumor treatment, it is important to determine whether the trismus is the result of the treatment, or is the first sign of a recurrence.
- Higher the RT dose delivered to the relevant structures, the greater is the severity of trismus.
- Devices such as the TheraBite may show efficacy in achieving improved jaw opening.
- Forced mouth opening under GA can improve trismus but the effect is often short-lived.
- Coronoidectomy may be effective if conservative measurements fail.
- Botulinum toxin injection into the muscles of mastication is effective as an analgesic modality in particular.
- As treatment of trismus is difficult, prevention is important. Therefore, reduction in the RT dose delivered to structures involved in mastication using IMRT reduces the incidence and severity of radiation-induced trismus after RT.
- Exercising therapy should be performed as often as possible and should particularly involve vertical and horizontal range of motion exercises.

Jaw Tumors

Vishal Yadav

ODONTOGENIC TUMORS

These are rare tumors that may have originated from the tooth-forming elements of the jaws.
- Most of these tumors are benign or aggressive locally, with only few malignant variants reported.
- There are several tumors which only appear to arise in the jaws and though they do not contain odontogenic tissue, they are considered odontogenic because of the site of origin.
- Some lesions of the jaws have giant cells, and their differentiation may present a problem. The diagnosis of such jaw lesions that contain giant cells depends on a combination of its histological examination, clinical history, and ancillary laboratory tests (**Table 1**). Treatment must be customized to the biological behavior of the lesion.

BENIGN EPITHELIAL ODONTOGENIC TUMORS

Ameloblastoma

It is a benign tumor arising exclusively in the jaws.
- It has a typical histological appearance. They are columnar, basally staining cells arranged in a palisading pattern along the basement membrane.
- The tumor derives its name from the cells closely resembling ameloblasts and are believed to be the cells of origin.
- These cells are epithelial in origin and may express amelogenin, which is a precursor of enamel.
- Ameloblastomas are divided into three types:
  1. Solid ameloblastomas
  2. Cystic ameloblastomas
  3. Peripheral ameloblastomas

Solid Ameloblastomas

These tumors have various histological patterns such as follicular, plexiform, and granular cell variants. They are believed to be of histological interest only and the treatment or prognosis is unaffected.
- They are benign tumors but locally aggressive and can sometimes metastasize.
- They generally occur in the mandible, especially around the angle of the mandible.
- They are most commonly found in the third to fifth decades of life.
- The male-to-female ratio is approximately equal.
- Imaging of these lesions is initially done with plain radiography such as Panorex radiographs. Computed tomography (CT) scans are advised, when there is any suspicion of lingual or buccal expansion or perforation (**Figs. 1A to C**).
- Enucleation has been seen to be associated with a recurrence rate of 60–80%. Hence, more aggressive treatment is recommended.

TABLE 1: Classification of jaw tumors.

Odontogenic tumors	Nonodontogenic tumors

• Epithelial tumors
  – *Benign*:
    - Ameloblastoma
    - Calcifying epithelial odontogenic tumor
    - Adenomatoid odontogenic tumor
    - Squamous odontogenic tumor
  – *Malignant*:
    - Malignant ameloblastoma
    - Clear-cell odontogenic carcinoma
    - Odontogenic carcinoma
• Mesenchymal tumors
  – *Benign*:
    - Odontogenic fibroma
    - Cementoblastoma
    - Odontogenic myxoma
    - Cementifying fibroma
  – *Malignant*: Ameloblastic fibrosarcoma
• *Mixed epithelial and mesenchymal tumors (all benign)*:
  – Odontoma
  – Ameloblastic fibroma
  – Ameloblastic fibro-odontoma
	• *Benign*:
	  – Fibro-osseous tumors
	    - Ossifying fibroma
	    - Juvenile ossifying fibroma
	  – Langerhans cell disease:
	    - Chronic localized
	    - Chronic disseminated
	    - Acute disseminated
	  – Lesions-containing multinucleated giant cells:
	    - Central giant cell granuloma
	    - Giant cell tumor
	    - Hyperparathyroidism
	    - Cherubism
	    - Aneurysmal bone cyst
	  – Neurogenic tumors
	    - Schwannoma
	    - Neurofibroma
	  – Osteoid osteoma and osteoblastoma
	  – Osteoma
	  – Chondroma
	  – Desmoplastic fibroma
	• *Malignant*:
	  – Osteosarcoma
	  – Peripheral osteosarcoma
	  – Chondrosarcoma
	  – Mesenchymal chondrosarcoma
	  – Fibrosarcoma of bone
	  – Malignant fibrous histiocytoma
	  – Ewing's sarcoma
	  – Burkitt lymphoma
	  – Multiple myeloma
	  – Solitary plasmacytoma of bone
	  – Malignant peripheral nerve sheath tumor
	  – Postradiation sarcoma of bone
	  – Metastatic carcinoma

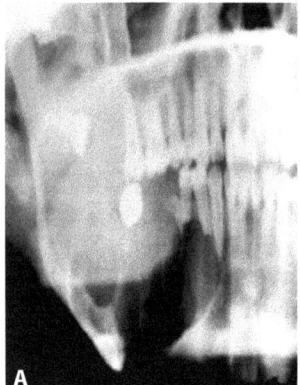 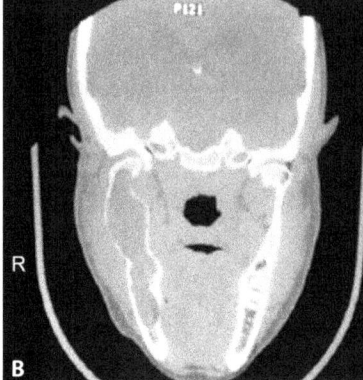 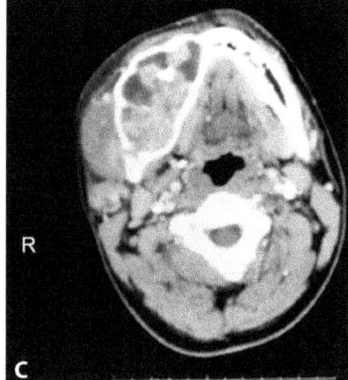

Figs. 1A to C: A large multilocular solid ameloblastoma of the right angle of the mandible and displacing teeth: (A) Panorex; (B) Coronal computed tomography (CT) scan; (C) Axial CT scan.

- Under microscope, cells have been found several millimeters from the radiographical margin of the lesion. This finding has led to a concept that surgery should be performed with 1 cm bony margins around the radiograph limits of the lesion and a single tissue plane clearance should be attempted when there is soft-tissue extension as in a supraperiosteal dissection.
- The inferior alveolar nerve is often sacrificed.

Maxillary ameloblastomas:
- Maxillary ameloblastomas are rare tumors but can be more troublesome than mandibular tumors.
- Histologically, they behave similar but they infiltrate through various pathways.
- Involvement of the maxillary sinus and nasal cavity appears early with spreading through the posterior wall of the maxilla into the pterygomaxillary space. Infiltration into the greater palatine canal reaching the base of the skull is also seen. Resection is preferred with surrounding 1 cm margin guided by CT or magnetic resonance imaging (MRI). It often requires a maxillectomy with an incontinuity resection of the pterygoid plates **(Figs. 2A and B)**.
- Reconstruction is generally done by means of a skin graft and prosthetic obturator or microvascular free flaps.

Cystic Ameloblastomas

This is difficult to diagnosis because many ameloblastomas have cystic areas within them.
- Unicystic ameloblastoma was first described in 1977 by Robinson and Martinez.
- Unicystic ameloblastoma is a less aggressive variant and simple enucleation is the treatment.
- They occur in younger age group (third decade) than the solid variant (fourth decade).
- It is commonly seen in the posterior mandible, followed by the parasymphysis region, anterior maxilla, and posterior mandible
- During the 1988s, unicystic ameloblastomas were classified into three histological

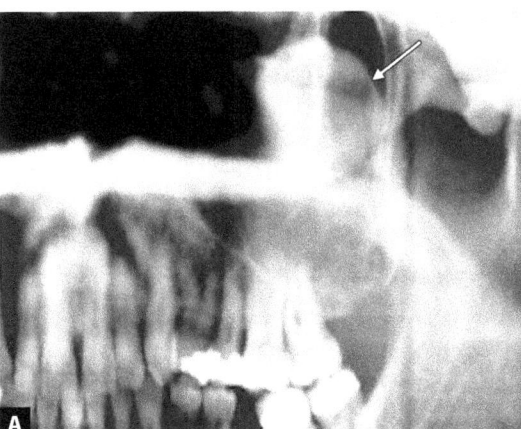 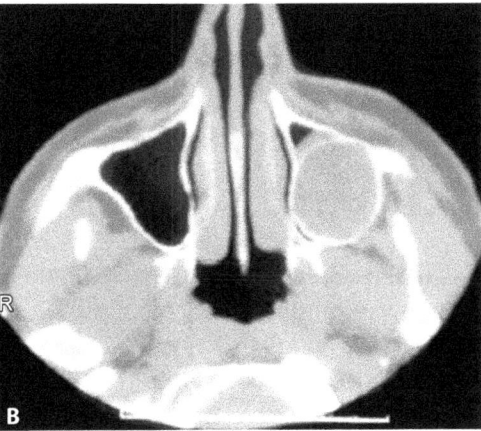

Figs. 2A and B: An ameloblastoma of the posterior maxilla extending to the pterygoid plates. (A) Panorex (lesion arrowed); (B) Axial CT scan.

subtypes, depending on whether they had a:
1. Cystic lining composed of simple odontogenic epithelium.
2. A cystic lesion with intraluminal plexiform proliferation of the epithelial lining.
3. A cystic lesion with epithelial invasion of the supporting connective tissue in either a follicular or plexiform form.

- The first two types are not aggressive and are treated by enucleation. The third type requires aggressive treatment.
- The prognosis of multicystic ameloblastomas is similar to the solid counterpart.
- Treatment is with peripheral ostectomy or liquid nitrogen cryotherapy, or both.

Peripheral Ameloblastoma

The peripheral ameloblastoma is also known as extraosseous ameloblastoma, or the soft-tissue ameloblastoma.

- It is generally seen in the gingiva, but with no bony involvement. Actually the lesions that were earlier called as basal cell carcinoma of the gingiva might have been peripheral ameloblastomas.
- These are painless, sessile, firm, and exophytic growths, mostly smooth or granular. They may sometimes look warty.
- They constitute between 2 and 10% of all diagnosed ameloblastomas.
- They are seen in all age-groups between the ages of 9 and 92 years, with a mean age of 52 years.
- Males are affected more than females, incidence being 1.9–1.
- 70% of peripheral ameloblastomas appear in the mandible, with the body of the mandible anterior to the mental foramen being the most commonly affected site. Histologically, they are similar to intraosseous ameloblastomas though the palisading is not always conspicuous in the stellate reticulum.

Ghost cell formation and clear cells may be found. Peripheral ameloblastomas usually arise directly from the surface epithelium or from residual dental lamina, outside the bone rather than from the ameloblasts. Some studies say they could be hamartomas rather than true neoplasms. They behave like benign tumors and do not recur after simple complete excision.

Calcifying Epithelial Odontogenic Tumors (Pindborg Tumor 1955) (Figs. 3A and B)

- Earlier they were categorized as variants of ameloblastoma.
- This is a rare rumor, and only 200 cases have been reported in the literature.
- The lesion is found in ages ranging from 13 to 80 years in both sexes.
- Most of the cases occur in the mandible with a ratio of approximately 3:1.
- The mandibular premolar molar area is the most common site.
- These are slow growing and asymptomatic.
- Radiographically, they are classically seen as well-defined, mixed areas of radiolucent/radiopaque lesions.

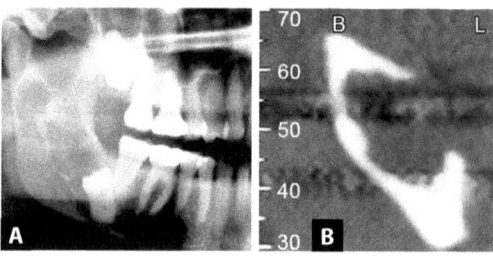

Figs. 3A and B: Imaging studies of a calcifying epithelial odontogenic tumor. (A) Panoral radiograph of a lesion of the posterior right mandible; (B) Coronal CT scan of lesion showing lingual perforation by the lesion.

- They may be unilocular or multilocular.
- Histologically, the calcifying epithelial odontogenic tumor (CEOT) is characterized by sheets of large eosinophilic staining epithelial cells. The stroma consists of a hyaline-like homogeneous material that has been identified as amyloid.
- The amyloid areas may contain Liesegang rings as areas of calcifications in concentric shapes. These areas account for the radiopacities seen radiographically. The lesion is believed to arise from the stratum intermedium of the developing enamel organ.
- The CEOT is locally aggressive with recurrence rates of 14–20%.
- Malignant variants (odontogenic carcinoma) are rare.
- A prominent clear cell component when seen in 8% of lesions, may be associated with increased aggressiveness and perforation of the cortex. In general, the CEOT appears to be less aggressive than the solid ameloblastoma.
- Treatment is wide local excision with margins of 5–10 mm. In the mandible, it may require a marginal resection or even segmental resection with subsequent reconstruction.

Adenomatoid Odontogenic Tumors (Figs. 4A to C)

Adenomatoid odontogenic tumor contains structures similar to enamel formation. It is believed to be originating from odontogenic cells, as it occurs only in the jaws.

- Immunohistochemical and ultrastructural findings show that the eosinophilic deposits are positive for amelogenin in limited areas and probably represent a form of enamel matrix.
- This tumor is more common in females than males (1.9:1).
- It constitutes about 3% of all odontogenic tumors and seen in the ages of 5–30 years.
- The most common site is the anterior maxilla, and is often associated with impacted teeth.
- Different varieties such as intraosseous follicular (70%), extrafollicular (26%), and peripheral (4%) have been described, but they are all histologically same.
- A subvariant of the extrafollicular type of adenomatoid odontogenic tumor may mimic periapical disease radiographically.
- The classic look is of pear-shaped radiolucency with speckled opaque foci of calcification distributed throughout the lesion radiographically.

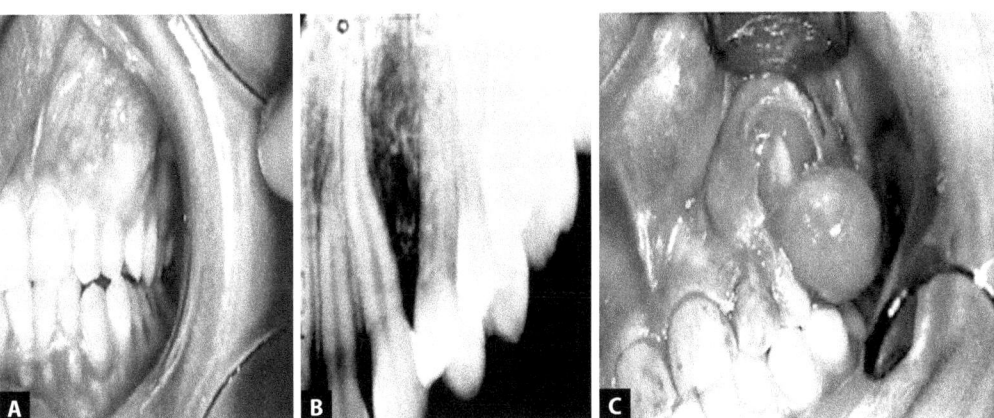

Figs. 4A to C: Adenomatoid odontogenic tumor: (A) A firm swelling over the upper left canine and first premolar; (B) X-ray shows a pear-shaped lesion with speckled opaque foci; (C) Clinical appearance of enucleated lesion.

- They are generally discovered incidentally on X-rays.
- Treatment is simple enucleation. Recurrences have been noted, but generally due to incomplete primary excision. They behave more like hamartoma.

Squamous Odontogenic Tumors

- It generally involves the alveolar process and arise from the rests of Malassez in the periodontium.
- They are asymptomatic but sometimes may cause pain and loose tooth.
- It arises from the mandible and maxilla equally. When in the maxilla, it is more frequently in the anterior maxilla. In the mandible, it occupies the posterior mandible.
- Multiple lesions have also been reported.
- *Age*: Second to the seventh decade, mean age around 40 years.
- There is no gender predilection.
- The radiographic characteristic is a triangular or semilunar radiolucency associated with the roots of erupted or erupting teeth.
- Histologically, the tumor is characterized by variably sized nests and cores of uniform benign-looking squamous epithelium with occasional vacuolization and keratinization. Treatment is curative, by conservative surgical excision, though recurrences have been seen.

MALIGNANT EPITHELIAL ODONTOGENIC TUMORS

Malignant odontogenic tumors are rare and comprise only about 4% of all odontogenic tumors.

Malignant Variants of Ameloblastoma

- *Malignant ameloblastoma* is diagnosed when a histologically benign-looking ameloblastoma produces a metastasis. It is well differentiated and has the characteristic histological features of an ameloblastoma.
- *Ameloblastic carcinoma*: This term is reserved for lesions that demonstrate a malignant morphological appearance, regardless of presence or absence of metastasis present at the presentation.

Malignant Ameloblastoma

- These are diagnosed retrospectively with a metastasis. These metastases are isolated pulmonary metastases that can mostly be treated surgically. They generally arise only after many surgical attempts of the original lesion.
- Lymph-node metastases also occur.

Ameloblastic Carcinoma

- The primary or the metastatic lesion shows less microscopic differentiation showing cytologic atypia and mitotic figures.
- The lesion has a spindle-cell appearance, and are epithelial in origin, being positive for cytokeratin and negative for vimentin.
- Metastasis is seen locally to the lymph nodes, and distant metastases to the lungs and bone.
- Treatment of the primary site is surgical and often along with a lymph node dissection of the neck.
- Radiation therapy has not found to be effective. Chemotherapy with paclitaxel and carboplatin and oral cyclophosphamide has been used with some benefit.
- Most ameloblastic carcinomas are thought to arise de novo. They may also change from a normal well-differentiated ameloblastoma into an ameloblastic carcinoma.

- Death from ameloblastic carcinoma is often due to extensive local recurrence at the base of the skull and cranial cavity.

Clear-cell Odontogenic Carcinoma

- This is a rare neoplasm, of unknown etiology, described in both the mandible and maxilla. It is probably of odontogenic origin.
- It occurs commonly in females, older than 60.
- It is locally aggressive and poorly circumscribed.
- Histologically, it consists of clear cells, positive for cytokeratin and negative for vimentin and for mucicarmine. This differentiates it from other clear cell tumors like mucoepidermoid carcinoma and renal carcinoma and CEOT.
- Metastases to the lungs and neck may occur, necessitating a thorough metastatic workup.

Odontogenic Carcinoma

- This is a central lesion seen most often in the mandible arising from remnants of the dental lamina or enamel epithelium.
- Histologically, it has appearances of a well-differentiated squamous cell carcinoma.
- Its odontogenic origin can only be assumed when there is no connection to the epithelium, as it cannot be differentiated from any other squamous-cell carcinoma histologically.
- Treatment involves a metastatic workup followed by primary surgery, which can often involve a neck dissection followed by radiation therapy depending on the adequacy of the surgical margins, their histological appearance, and metastatic spread.

BENIGN MESENCHYMAL ODONTOGENIC TUMORS OF THE JAW

Odontogenic Fibroma

- The central odontogenic fibroma, found in both the mandible and maxilla is a rare lesion seen equally in both males and females and across all age groups.
- Radiographically, the lesion looks radiolucent, often multilocular causing cortical expansion. It has similarity to other odontogenic lesions.
- The lesions are well demarcated and noncapsulated.
- Treatment consists of enucleation or excision. Recurrence is rare.

Cementoblastoma

- The cementoblastoma, also known as a true cementoma, is a rare odontogenic tumor. It constitutes <1% of all odontogenic tumors.
- It is common in the second and third decades and affects the lower molar area.
- It is intimately associated with the root of a tooth, usually lower molar tooth including the third molar, being formed from the cementum. The tooth may remain vital, and symptoms produced are cortical expansion and a mild intermittent pain.
- Radiographically, the lesion looks radiopaque attached to and encasing the root of a tooth. Typically, a radiolucent ring representing the periodontal ligament space surrounds the tumor.
- Treatment is enucleation of the lesion and the associated tooth. Thorough curettage is mandatory. Recurrence is uncommon.

Odontogenic Myxoma (Fig. 5)

- Odontogenic myxoma comprises 15–20% of all odontogenic tumors.

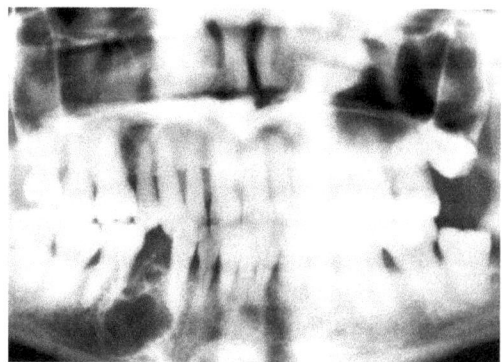

Fig. 5: An odontogenic myxoma of the right mandible, with well-defined multilocular radiolucency.

- It is the second most common odontogenic tumor with an incidence of 0.07 new cases/million people/year.
- It is seen around the second and fourth decades, more commonly in females, male-to-female ratio being 1:1.5. Approximately two-thirds of the cases appear in the mandible and one-third in the maxilla.
- The tumor usually presents as a swelling in the affected jaw or sometimes as an asymptomatic incidental radiographic finding.
- More than 50% of these tumors are multilocular on radiographs. Less than 50% are unilocular with well-defined edges. Larger ones are likely to be multilocular.
- Histologically, the lesion is bland looking with loose mesenchymal fibrous tissue without any atypia. Odontogenic epithelium may not be found within the lesion.
- The odontogenic myxoma is believed to arise from primitive dental pulp or dental papilla.
- The odontogenic myxoma is benign but aggressive locally, but slightly less aggressive than the solid ameloblastoma.
- Treatment suggested is enucleation and radical curettage or peripheral ostectomy.
- For those large lesions or those perforating the buccal or lingual plate, segmental resection of the mandible or maxillectomy could be performed.
- Other treatment adjuncts such as liquid nitrogen cryotherapy or Carnoy's solution have also been practiced along with enucleation.
- Recurrence rate is between 15 and 20%.

Cementifying Fibroma

- This tumor is the odontogenic equivalent of the ossifying fibroma. They are similar clinically and histologically, but not identical.
- Lesions in the jaws with cementum and calcified spherules are believed to be cementifying fibromas. They are common in the mandible, and are classified as benign fibro-osseous lesions.
- Although histologically similar, there are differences on immunohistochemical staining from ossifying fibromas as the latter does not produce immunoreactivity for keratin sulfate or chondroitin 4-sulfate unlike the former.
- Although cementifying fibromas are generally believed to be benign and they respond well to enucleation, recurrences have been described necessitating local resection.

MALIGNANT MESENCHYMAL ODONTOGENIC TUMORS

Ameloblastic Fibrosarcoma

- Malignant odontogenic are rare tumors representing about 4% of odontogenic tumors.
- The ameloblastic fibrosarcoma is a rare variant, only about 80 cases noted in literature.

- Two-thirds arise de novo, and only about one-third appear in pre-existing benign odontogenic lesions.
- Malignant transformation has been seen from benign ameloblastic fibroma.
- These tumors are commonly located in the posterior part of the mandible.
- The average age of onset is 22.9.
- The lesion is locally aggressive.
- The prognosis is good.
- Wide surgical excision is the standard of care. Adjuvant radiation therapy and chemotherapy given whenever necessary.

MIXED EPITHELIAL AND MESENCHYMAL ODONTOGENIC TUMORS

Odontoma

- The odontoma, or odontome, is the most common odontogenic tumor, constituting 22% of all such tumors. They contain fully differentiated, irregularly arranged, mature dental tissues.
- Odontomas are mixed benign tumors, having both epithelial and mesenchymal elements.
- They are found in younger age group and are thought to be developmental abnormalities detected on routine radiographs. Sometimes they may appear as a swelling or associated with an infected lesion, when they erupt. Since these tumors contain mature dental tissue, they are often found in place of a missing tooth.
- They are most commonly seen in the molar area of the mandible. There are two types of odontomas that have been described having similar prognosis and treatment. The difference is only on radiographs and histology.
    - The compound odontome is found in the anterior part of the mouth (**Fig. 6**).
    - The complex odontome is found in the posterior part of the mouth (**Fig. 7**).
- Radiographically, these tumors are well-circumscribed and radiopaque, often surrounded by a small, clear margin representing a periodontal ligament.
- Odontomes have limited growth. They reach to a certain size and then stop growing.
- The curative treatment is enucleation and recurrences uncommon.

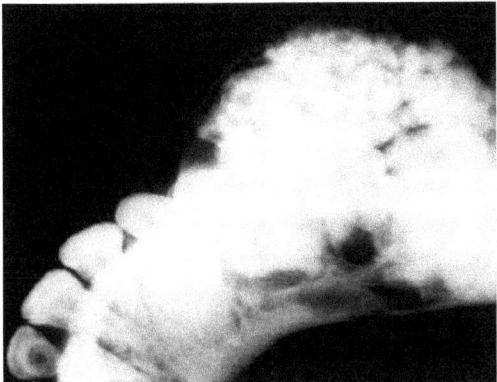

Fig. 6: A compound odontome, occlusal radiograph shows discrete and separate denticles.

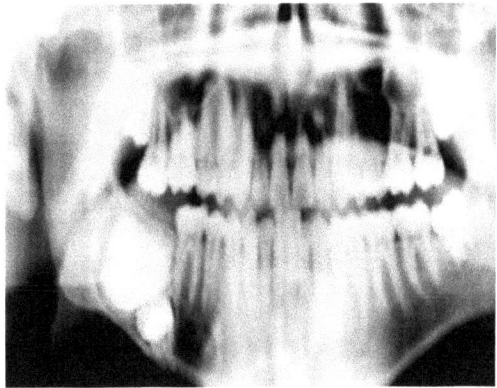

Fig. 7: A complex odontome. Amorphous mass of enamel and dentin, a radiolucent border, and an embedded tooth.

Ameloblastic Fibroma

- This is a true mixed odontogenic tumor with both epithelial and mesenchymal neoplastic elements.
- It is generally associated with an impacted tooth. It appears as a radiolucent area associated with the crown or with the root of an impacted tooth.
- The lesion is encapsulated, and treatment consists of enucleation.
- Recurrences are not common.

Ameloblastic Fibro-odontoma

- These tumors are combination of an ameloblastic fibroma and an odontoma.
- The age, gender predilection, and treatment remain the same as ameloblastic fibroma.

BENIGN NONODONTOGENIC TUMORS OF THE JAW

Fibro-osseous Tumors

Ossifying Fibroma (Cemento-ossifying Fibroma) (Fig. 8)

Ossifying fibroma (cemento-ossifying fibroma) are benign tumors. The normal bone is replaced by a fibrous tissue and amounts of newly formed bone or cementum-like material, or with both.

- Ossifying fibroma, fibrous dysplasia, and cemento-osseous dysplasia are classified together as benign fibro-osseous lesions because of histological similarities.
- Chromosomal abnormalities have been detected in these tumors; the molecular mechanisms underlying the origin of this tumor is unknown.
- An ossifying fibroma clinically presents as a painless, slow-growing, expansile swelling.
- Most occur in the third and fourth decades of life. Females are more commonly affected.
- Ossifying fibromas are confined to the jaws and the craniofacial complex. The mandible, especially the premolar-molar region, is most commonly involved.
- Multicentric or familial ossifying fibromas have been reported rarely.
- The radiographic appearance is of a well-defined radiolucent lesion with internal calcification. The borders may appear sclerotic. Larger lesions in the mandible produce bowing of the inferior border.
- The treatment recommended for ossifying fibromas is complete surgical excision. Characteristically they can shell out from the bone with ease.
- Reported rates of recurrence are <1 to 63%.
- Ossifying fibromas do not infiltrate into bone and therefore require smaller margins than 1 cm.

Juvenile Ossifying Fibroma (Juvenile Aggressive Ossifying Fibroma; Juvenile Active Ossifying Fibroma)

- There is a tendency to affect children and adolescents. They are more aggressive.

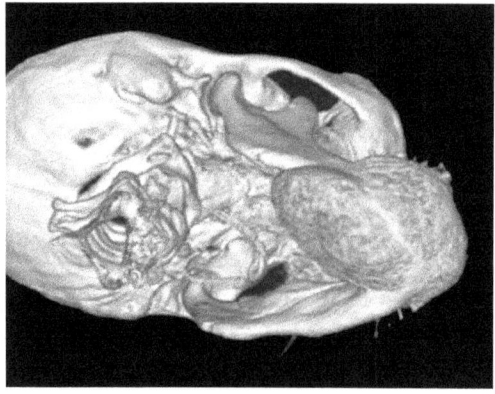

Fig. 8: Ossifying fibroma: Submental 3D reconstructed CT scan showing the expansion of the mandible.

- Two variants have been described:
  1. *Trabecular variant*: Seen in childhood with a slight maxillary predilection
  2. *Psammomatoid variant*: Seen over a wider age group range than the trabecular variant and usually affects the orbit or paranasal sinuses
- Conservative excision is the treatment.
- Lesions of the craniofacial bones need more extensive surgery.
- Recurrence rates of 20–58% have been seen. They could be managed by local excision, and malignant transformation have not been seen.

Langerhans Cell Disease

- Langerhans cell disease was known as histiocytosis X earlier and also as a set of three separate diseases: (1) Eosinophilic granuloma, (2) Hand-Schüller-Christian disease, and (3) Letterer–Siwe disease
- The etiology and pathogenesis of this disease are not known. The pathogenesis may be from neoplastic process, viral etiology, and an overwhelming allergenic challenge.
- Langerhans cell disease is commonly seen in children and young adults.
- The common presentation include bone lesions, either solitary or multiple. They frequently involve the skull, mandible, ribs, and vertebrae, although any bone may be involved. Jaw lesions may be painful and tender, tooth mobility, and expansion.
- Lesions generally involve the bone of the alveolus, producing the classic "floating teeth" appearance.
- Accessible bone lesions are usually treated with aggressive local curettage or resection with 5 mm margins wherever possible.
- Less accessible lesions are treated with low-dose radiation therapy. Intralesional steroids have also been used and cases of spontaneous regression are common.

Lesions-containing Multinucleated Giant Cells

Central Giant Cell Granuloma

- The central giant cell granuloma is a benign proliferation of fibroblasts and multinucleated giant cells.
- They are most commonly found in children and young adults, 75% of them occurring before the age of 30 years.
- Females are twice as frequently affected as males.
- The lesion frequently occurs anterior to the first permanent molar tooth. The mandible is involved three times more than the maxilla.
- Surgical curettage is associated with a recurrence rate of 15–20%.

Giant Cell Tumor

- The giant cell tumor is frequently seen in the long bones and is an aggressive type of lesion.
- The recurrence rate of giant cell tumors in long bones after curettage is higher than for central giant cell granulomas of the jaws **(Fig. 9)**. Hence, many advocate resection.

Hyperparathyroidism

- Increased levels of parathyroid hormone (PTH) stimulate bone resorption mediated by osteoclasts. This produces a focal bone lesion called as a brown tumor of hyperparathyroidism.
- The name of this lesion is derived from the tissue color as seen on surgical exploration, which is due to

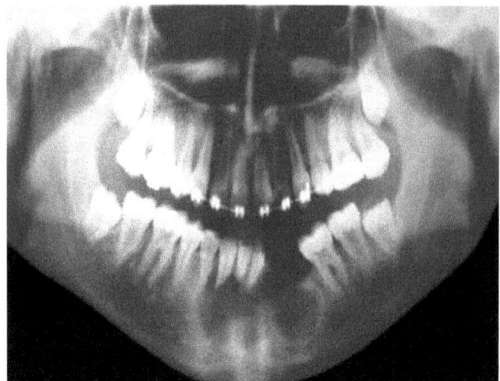

Fig. 9: Central giant cell granuloma: Radiolucency of the anterior mandible seen to cross the midline in a 17-year-old male.

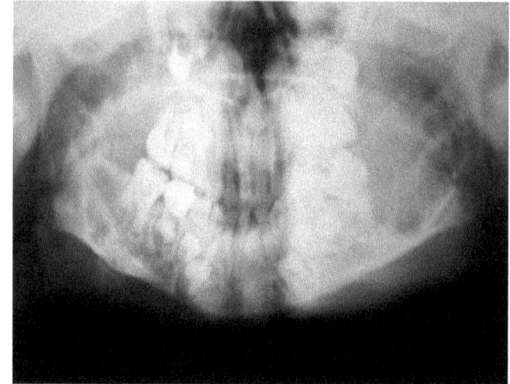

Fig. 10: Cherubism: Multilocular radiolucencies seen in the maxilla and mandible bilaterally. Note the sparing of the mandibular condyles.

the extravasation of erythrocytes and deposition of hemosiderin within the lesion.
- Normal PTH levels are found in central giant cell granulomas. Therefore, hyperparathyroidism must be excluded by getting serum calcium and PTH levels in patients with giant cell lesions.
- If a diagnosis of hyperparathyroidism has been confirmed, then treatment of the cause must be aimed at and the lesions will resolve with no further treatment.

Cherubism (Fig. 10)

- Cherubism is a rare hereditary condition with bilateral, painless, symmetrical expansion of the jaws seen in age group of 2–5 years.
- It has autosomal dominant pattern of inheritance with 100% penetrance in males, 50–75% penetrance in females, and variable expressivity.
- The lesions in cherubism increase in size until puberty, and then they begin to regress.
- Treatment is conservative, allowing natural regression to take place. If surgical recontouring of expanded bone is required, it is preferred to defer it until puberty.

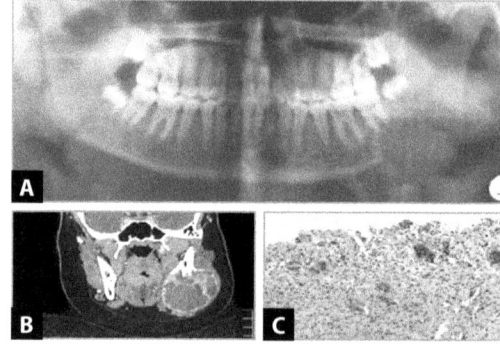

Figs. 11A to C: Aneurysmal bone cyst: (A) A radiolucent lesion seen to produce expansion of the mandibular left angle in a 13-year-old girl; (B) Coronal CT scan demonstrating cortical expansion and thinning; (C) Numerous small sinusoids surrounded by a connective tissue stroma and scattered multinucleated giant cells.

Aneurysmal Bone Cyst (Figs. 11A to C)

- The aneurysmal bone cyst (ABC) is a pseudocyst. It consists of blood-filled spaces within a connective tissue stroma with multinucleated giant cells.
- The lesion most commonly is found in the long bones and vertebrae. Within the craniofacial complex, it is most common in the mandible, followed by the maxilla.
- The etiology and pathogenesis of ABC is not known, though it is generally regarded as reactive.

- The peak incidence is in the second decade of life, with most appearing before the age of 30 years.
- There is a slight female predilection. Mandibular and maxillary lesions are frequently found in the molar regions.
- Radiographically the lesion appears as a multilocular radiolucency, although it may also be unilocular.
- Many authors believe that ABCs are associated with a high recurrence rate. Curettage is the treatment of choice. At the time of surgery, the lesion appears like a "blood-soaked sponge," but significant hemorrhage is usually not found.

Neurogenic Tumors

Schwannoma (Neurilemmoma)

- The schwannoma is a slowly growing, benign tumor arising from the Schwann cells of the nerve sheath (neurilemma). As this encapsulated tumor enlarges, it pushes the involved nerve aside without enveloping it.
- Intraosseous lesions are uncommon. But the mandible is the most common site of origin of the central lesions.
- Intraosseous schwannomas are treated by enucleation and curettage. When the lesion arises from an identifiable nerve such as the inferior alveolar nerve, it can be excised from the nerve while preserving the integrity of the nerve. Recurrences are rare.

Neurofibroma

- They originate from a mixture type of cell including Schwann cells and perineural fibroblasts.
- They occur both as solitary lesions or associated with neurofibromatosis.
- Neurofibromatosis is an autosomal dominant condition 50% of cases resulting from spontaneous mutation. Two types are seen: (1) Neurofibromatosis type 1 (von Recklinghausen's disease) and (2) neurofibromatosis type 2 (**Table 2**). Type 1 is characterized by multiple cutaneous neurofibromas and café-au-lait spots.
- Treatment of solitary lesions is local excision.
- The lesions are vascular, and extensive blood loss have resulted from surgical

TABLE 2: Types of neurofibromatosis.

Neurofibromatosis type 1	Neurofibromatosis type 2
A diagnosis is established when two or more of the following findings are present: 1. Six or more café-au-lait spots >5 mm in diameter in prepubertal patients and >15 mm in postpubertal patients 2. One plexiform neurofibroma or two or more neurofibromas of any type 3. Two or more pigmented iris hamartomas (Lisch nodules) 4. Axillary or inguinal region freckling 5. Optic nerve glioma 6. A distinctive osseous lesion such as dysplasia of the greater wing of the sphenoid or pseudoarthrosis 7. A first-degree relative with neurofibromatosis type 1	*A diagnosis is established when one or more of the following findings are present*: 1. Bilateral cranial nerve VIII masses 2. A first-degree relative with neurofibromatosis type 2 and either a single cranial nerve VIII mass or any of the following findings: • Schwannoma • Neurofibroma • Meningioma • Glioma • Juvenile posterior subcapsular lens opacity

management of mandibular lesions; therefore, some have advocated mandibular resection.
- Neurofibromas that occur with neurofibromatosis type 1 makes complete surgery impractical. In such cases, surgery is reserved for those lesions which are large and symptomatic or compromise function, or both.
- Malignant transformation to neurogenic sarcoma are seen in 5–15% of neurofibromas associated with neurofibromatosis.

Osteoid Osteoma and Osteoblastoma

- The osteoid osteoma and osteoblastoma have similar histological features.
- They are benign neoplasms of unknown etiology.
- Most are seen in the second decade, with 85–90% occurring before the age of 30.
- A 2:1 male predilection exists.
- The osteoid osteoma is <2 cm in diameter, occurring mostly in the femur, tibia, and phalanges. Rarely, it is seen in the jaws.
- An osteoid osteoma characteristically has symptoms of nocturnal pain, i.e., responds to aspirin.
- The osteoblastoma is >2 cm in diameter, occurring most frequently in the vertebrae and long bones of the extremities.
- The craniofacial skeleton is the site of involvement in 15% of osteoblastomas. The mandible is affected more frequently than the maxilla.
- Within the jaws, the posterior tooth-bearing portion is the most commonly involved area.
- Clinically, it grows rapidly, with swelling and pain. In contrast to osteoid osteomas, the pain is not typically nocturnal and it does not respond as well to aspirin.
- These lesions are well-defined with a mixed radiolucent-radiopaque pattern.
- Conservative surgical excision either with curettage or local excision is the treatment of choice.
- Recurrences and malignant transformation are rare.

Osteoma

- Osteomas are benign tumors composed of mature compact or cancellous bone.
- They are distinguished from the common palatal and mandibular tori, as well as buccal exostoses, although they have identical histopathology.
- Tori and buccal exostoses are developmental or reactive in origin and are not true neoplasms.
- Osteomas may arise from the surface of bone (periosteal osteoma), or in the medullary bone (endosteal osteoma).
- Osteomas may also arise in the paranasal sinuses, skull bones, and facial bones including the maxilla and mandible. They are most commonly seen in young adults.
  - *Periosteal osteomas* present as slow growing, painless, discrete bony masses.
  - *Endosteal osteomas*: They are usually asymptomatic and detected on routine radiographs.
- Osteomas are usually solitary, except in cases of Gardner syndrome.
- Osteomas in association with Gardner syndrome are found at the mandibular angles, as well as in other facial bones and long bones. In most cases, the development of osteomas precedes manifestations of the syndrome.
- Osteomas are diagnosed and treated by local excision. Recurrences are uncommon. Small, asymptomatic cases may simply be followed clinically and radiographically.
- Patients with multiple osteomas must be investigated for Gardner syndrome.

Chondroma

- The chondroma is a benign tumor made of mature hyaline cartilage.
- It commonly occurs in the bones of the hands and feet, and rarely in the craniofacial bones.
- Within the maxillofacial region, chondromas occur in the nasal septum and anterior maxilla most often. They have also been seen in the mandibular condyle, coronoid process, body, and symphysis.
- Chondromas present as painless, slowly progressive swelling.
- They are usually seen before 50 years of age. No sex predilection has been seen.
- Radiographically, they are unilocular or multilocular radiolucency, which may have internal foci of calcification.
- To avoid undertreating a malignancy, some authors consider chondromas of the jaws as potentially malignant and manage them accordingly.
- They recommend wide surgical excision with a margin of 1 cm. If the lesion recurs after conservative surgical treatment, the lesion must be considered a low-grade chondrosarcoma and then treated with wide surgical excision.

Desmoplastic Fibroma

- The desmoplastic fibroma is a benign, locally aggressive tumor of bone. They are considered to be the osseous counterpart of soft-tissue fibromatosis.
- The etiology and pathogenesis remain unknown, although genetic, endocrine, and traumatic factors have been suggested.
- The lesion usually found in children and young adults, with most being discovered before the age of 30 years.
- It most commonly affects the long bones and occasionally the jaws.
- Within the jaws, the posterior mandible is the most frequently involved site. Patients present with a painless, slow-growing, firm swelling of the affected jaw.
- Recurrence rates after conservative surgery like curettage and local excision are high, while lesions treated by resection or wide excision do not recur. Thus, despite a benign histology, the desmoplastic fibroma should be treated aggressively. Radiation and chemotherapy have been recommended for lesions involving vital structures and those located in areas where resection would be debilitating.

MALIGNANT NONODONTOGENIC TUMORS OF THE JAWS

Osteosarcoma (Figs. 12A and B)

- Osteosarcoma is a malignant tumor which produces osteoid by a sarcomatous stroma.
- It is the most common primary sarcoma of the bone, second only to plasma cell neoplasms, which is the most common primary tumor of bone.
- It may develop in a previously radiated bone, as well as in pre-existing bone abnormalities such as Paget's disease, fibrous dysplasia, and giant cell tumors.
- Osteosarcomas may be of two types
  1. *Central type*:
     - More common
     - Arises from the medullary portion of the bone.
  2. *Peripheral (juxtacortical) type*:
     - Less common
     - Originates on the surface of the bone and initially grows outward.

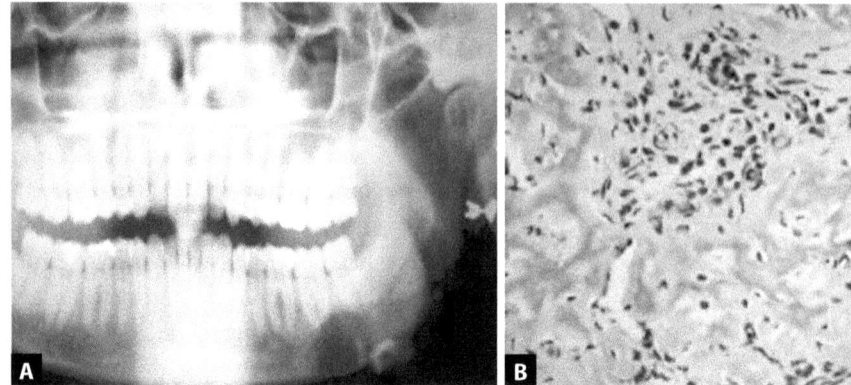

Figs. 12A and B: Osteosarcoma: (A) Poorly-defined radiolucency of the posterior left mandible; (B) Production of osteoid by a sarcomatous stroma.

- The molecular mechanisms in the pathogenesis of osteosarcoma may be related to genetic alterations resulting in inactivation of *tumor suppressor genes* and overexpression of *oncogenes.*
- Osteosarcomas of the jaws constitutes 5–7% of all osteosarcomas and most commonly found in third and fourth decades of life, with a mean age of 35 years. There is a slight male predilection. The mandible is affected more frequently than the maxilla.
- Symmetric widening of the periodontal ligament and extracortical bone producing a "sunburst" appearance are typical radiographic features classically seen in osteosarcoma.
- Cortical destruction and root resorption may be apparent on radiography.
- Lesions are histologically subdivided into osteoblastic, chondroblastic, and fibroblastic subtypes, depending on the relative amounts of osteoid, cartilage, or collagen produced by the stroma. The chondroblastic type is most common in the jaws.
- The prognosis does not depend on the histologic subtype. But patients with high-grade lesions have a poorer prognosis.
- Rare examples of the telangiectatic and small cell variants have been found in the jaws.
- Wide surgical resection with negative margins is the only treatment leading to increased survival. A bone margin of 3 cm from the radiographical margin is recommended.
- Majority of studies indicate that radiation therapy has no beneficial effect on survival. Chemotherapy with surgery has shown better prognosis of osteosarcoma of the long bones. Benefit in the jaws are not established. Overall 5-year survival rate for head and neck osteosarcomas is between 40 and 70%.
- The main cause of death in osteosarcoma of the jaws is local recurrence.
- Metastasis occurs in about 18% of cases, though high rates of 50% have also been reported. The lungs are the most common site of metastasis.
- Because regional lymph node metastasis is rare, neck dissection is not needed.
- Osteosarcomas of the jaws generally metastasize less frequently and have a better prognosis in comparison with lesions of the extremities.

Chondrosarcoma

- This is a malignant tumor characterized by the formation of cartilage by the tumor cells.
- It is next to osteosarcoma as the most common primary sarcoma of bone. Only 1–2% of chondrosarcomas occur in the head and neck region.
- The maxilla is the most common involved site. Maxillary lesions occur most often in the anterior region, and mandibular lesions occur most often in the molar-premolar region.
- This tumor is seen over a wide age range with a peak incidence in the third decade.
- Chondrosarcomas have been classified into grades I, II, and III on the basis of its mitotic rate, cellularity, and nuclear size. This grading system correlates with prognosis. In the head and neck region, grades I and II chondrosarcomas are common.
- Radical ablative surgery is the recommended treatment.
- Radiation therapy has not shown to provide a survival benefit; thus radiation therapy is considered in unresectable, residual, or recurrent tumors.
- Chemotherapy showed no significant therapeutic benefit.
- The overall 5-year survival rate for chondrosarcomas of the jaws ranges from 32–81%.
- Factors influencing the prognosis for chondrosarcomas of the jaws are the site of origin, histological grade, and therapeutic modality.
- Mandibular tumors have a better prognosis than maxillary lesions.
- The lung is the most common site of metastasis, while lymph node metastasis is not common; hence neck dissection is not recommended.
- The most common cause of death for jaw lesions is uncontrolled local recurrence.
- Recurrences may occur even after 10–20 years of surgery; thus long-term follow-up is required.

Mesenchymal Chondrosarcoma

Mesenchymal chondrosarcoma is a rare tumor that is clinically and histologically distinct in comparison with chondrosarcoma.

- One-third of these lesions arise from soft tissue. The maxilla and mandible are the more commonly involved bony sites.
- The tumor occurs commonly between 10 and 30 years of age, with an equal distribution between genders.
- The cartilaginous component distinguishes mesenchymal chondrosarcoma from Ewing sarcoma and hemangiopericytoma, which resemble the undifferentiated small cell component.
- Surgical resection with wide margins is recommended to achieve local control.
- Information regarding the use of both radiation therapy and chemotherapy is limited.
- The 5-year and 10-year survival rates are approximately 50% and 28%, respectively.
- Mesenchymal chondrosarcoma has a predilection for local recurrence and metastasis. The lung being the most commonly seen site of metastasis. Recurrences and distant metastases may take up to 20 years to manifest following treatment of the primary tumor.

Fibrosarcoma of Bone (Figs. 13A and B)

- It commonly affects the long bones, although some occurs in the jaws.
- Jaw lesions present with expansion of the jaw and tooth mobility.
- Surgical resection with wide margins is the recommended treatment.

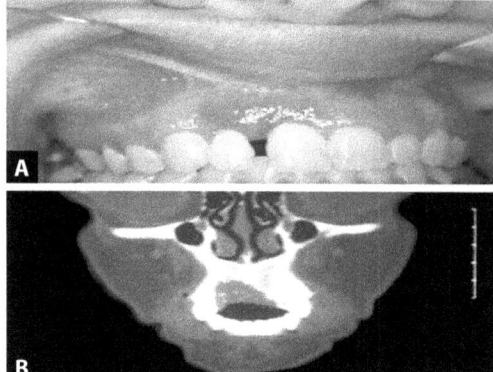

Figs. 13A and B: Fibrosarcoma of bone: (A) Erythematous gingival lesion seen in the anterior right maxilla; (B) Coronal CT image demonstrating the extent of tumor.

- The efficacy chemotherapy or radiation therapy is not established.
- The tumor has minimal metastatic potential.
- Recurrences are common and are best managed with salvage surgery.
- Factors that influence the prognosis negatively are high grade and age more than 40 years.

Malignant Fibrous Histiocytoma

- It occurs in soft tissues and represents 2–6% of all primary bone cancers.
- The long bones, particularly the femur, are the commonly affected osseous sites. Lesions of the jaws are rare. They arise as a primary tumor of bone (70%) and secondary to a preexisting bone condition (30%) including previously irradiated bone, Paget's disease, or bone infarct.
- The tumor appears over a large age range, mostly in older than 40 years of age. A male predilection has been seen.
- Most malignant fibrous histiocytomas are high-grade malignancies.
- Wide surgical resection is advocated for lesions of the jaws.

Ewing's Sarcoma

- Ewing's sarcoma is a family of tumors that include the primitive neuroectodermal tumors, defined as round cell sarcomas that show varying degrees of neuroectodermal origin.
- These tumors are characterized by a recurrent t(11;22)(q24;q12) chromosomal translocation, which is detectable in approximately 85% of cases.
- This family of tumors accounts for 6–8% of primary bone malignancies, although it is second to osteosarcoma as the most common sarcoma in bone and soft tissue in children.
- The bones of the lower extremity and pelvis are most commonly involved. Lesions of the jaws account for <3% of Ewing's sarcomas.
- The posterior mandible is most frequently affected in the jaw, while maxillary lesions are not common.
- Ewing's sarcoma primarily affects children and young adults, with 80% of cases occurring in patients younger than 20 years of age.
- A male predilection is seen, and black individuals are rarely affected.
- The tumor grows rapidly with extensive destruction of bone and a tendency for metastasis, particularly to the lungs and other bones. Clinically apparent metastases are seen in 15% patients of nonpelvic tumors at the time of diagnosis.
- Management consists of involve multiagent chemotherapy with either surgical resection or radiation therapy or a combination of surgery and radiation therapy. Surgery offers slightly better local control compared with radiation therapy alone.
- The incidence of secondary sarcomas after radiation therapy is approximately 6.5%.

- The 5-year survival for nonmetastatic patients presenting is 60%, and for those with metastatic disease the 5-year survival is 30%.
- Patients younger than 15 years tend to have a better prognosis than those older than 15 years of age.
- Ewing's sarcoma of the mandible appears to have a more favorable prognosis than that for other sites of involvement.

Burkitt Lymphoma

- Burkitt lymphoma is a high-grade, non-Hodgkin's B-cell lymphoma.
- Dennis Burkitt in 1958 originally described it as a jaw tumor of African children.
- The endemic (African) and sporadic (American) forms of Burkitt lymphoma are characterized by the activation of the *c-myc oncogene* through reciprocal chromosomal translocations, most commonly t(8:14).
- The endemic form is associated with Epstein–Barr virus (EBV) in >95% of cases, while the sporadic form is mostly EBV negative.
- Another third type of Burkitt lymphoma is found associated with HIV infection in adults.
- The endemic form shows a peak incidence between 3 and 8 years of age.
- Involvement of the jaw is common and age-related, with 90% of patients younger than 3 years of age and 25% of older than 15 years have jaw lesions.
- The maxilla is involved more commonly than the mandible, although all four quadrants may be involved.
- Sporadic form is seen in older age group with a maximum incidence between 10 and 12 years of age; the jaws are affected in 16% of cases at diagnosis; the lesions are more localized, most commonly involving single quadrant; and the mandible is involved more than the maxilla.
- Jaw lesions of Burkitt lymphoma progress rapidly, presenting with facial swelling or exophytic mass. These tumors may be associated with mobility of teeth, pain, and paresthesia.
- If untreated, it results in death within 4–6 months of diagnosis.
- Intensive chemotherapy has resulted in a dramatic improvement in the prognosis.
- Current treatment consists of intensive, short-term, multiagent chemotherapy along with intrathecal drugs for central nervous system prophylaxis.
- For advanced-stage disease, survival rates of between 70 and 87% have been achieved using these regimens.

Multiple Myeloma

- Multiple myeloma is a monoclonal, malignant, neoplastic proliferation of plasma cells with multicentric involvement of bone marrow.
- Extraskeletal sites may also be involved.
- It is the most commonly seen primary malignancy of bone. The bones involved are the vertebrae, ribs, skull, pelvis, femur, clavicle, and scapula. The mandible and maxilla may also be affected.
- The median age at diagnosis is 68 years with 90% of cases seen in older than 40 years of age.
- Signs and symptoms include bone pain, pathological fracture, hypercalcemia, anemia, renal failure, and recurrent bacterial infections.
- Monoclonal light chain (Bence-Jones protein) is found in the urine of approximately 50% of patients. Bence-Jones protein is directly toxic to renal epithelial cells and is a major contributing factor in the development of renal failure in multiple myeloma.

- In 25% of patients, the light chain protein may also accumulates in soft tissues, resulting in the development of amyloidosis, which may manifest in the maxillofacial region as macroglossia.
- Some of multiple myeloma patients do not have an identifiable M component in the serum or urine. This form of the disease is termed nonsecretory myeloma.
- The typical radiographical appearance is that of multiple well-defined, punched-out radiolucencies of bone, which are noncorticated.
- The treatment of multiple myeloma is systemic chemotherapy.
- High-dose chemotherapy with autologous stem cell transplantation has greatly improved complete remission rates, event-free survival, and overall survival as compared with conventional chemotherapeutic regimens.
- Improvements in the treatment of multiple myeloma have caused complete remission rates of 20–59% and median overall survival of 4.4–7.1 years, with a large proportion of patients surviving beyond 10 years.
- Death is generally due to infection, renal failure, or progressive myeloma.
- Bisphosphonates, which inhibit osteoclastic resorption of bone, also have direct antitumor effects. Bisphosphonates are beneficial in preventing pathological vertebral fractures, hypercalcemia, and ameliorating bone pain.
- The use of intravenous pamidronate and zoledronate has been found to be associated with osteonecrosis of the jaws.

Solitary Plasmacytoma of Bone

- A solitary plasmacytoma is a unifocal, monoclonal, neoplastic proliferation of plasma cells. They are commonly seen within bone but may also be found in soft tissue.
- To diagnose this disease, a complete radiological skeletal survey and a bone marrow biopsy away from the solitary lesion mandatorily must demonstrate no evidence of plasmacytosis in other locations.
- The lesion is found at a mean age of 50 years with a male predilection. Although rare in the jaws, the mandible is commonly affected than the maxilla.
- Radiation therapy using 3500–4500 cGy is the treatment of choice for solitary plasmacytomas.
- Approximately 70% of patients with solitary lesions ultimately develop multiple myeloma; however, it is not possible to predict which one would.
- The overall mean survival of patients diagnosed with a solitary plasmacytoma is 10 years.

Malignant Peripheral Nerve Sheath Tumor (Neurofibrosarcoma, Malignant Schwannoma)

- The malignant peripheral nerve sheath tumor (MPNST) is a rare malignancy that may develop within a preexisting neurofibroma, de novo, or as a postradiation sarcoma.
- 52% develop in patients with neurofibromatosis type 1.
- The Schwann cell and possibly other nerve sheath cells may be the cell of origin.
- The lesion occurs most commonly in the soft tissues of the extremities and trunk, with intraosseous lesions being involved rarely.
- The most common site for intraosseous lesions is the mandible.

- Radiographically, tumors of the mandible may produce widening of the inferior alveolar canal or the mental foramen.
- The treatment of choice for intraosseous MPNSTs is surgical resection with wide margins.
- Recurrence is common, and metastasis develops in the hematogenous path. Survival data for intraosseous tumors is limited.
- 5-year survival rate for soft-tissue tumors in patients without neurofibromatosis is 53%, compared with 16% for those with neurofibromatosis

Postradiation Sarcoma of Bone

- Postradiation sarcoma of bone is a sarcoma that develops in a bone within a previous irradiated field.
- Radiation-induced sarcomas are seen more frequently in the soft tissues than in bone.
- They are estimated to occur in 0.02% of irradiated patients.
- Postradiation sarcomas develop a mean of 14 years following the initial radiation therapy. But there are cases developing it in <1 year.
- The risk of development of postradiation sarcoma is related to the dose of radiation received.
- The most common sarcomas that appear in an irradiated area are osteosarcoma, malignant fibrous histiocytoma, and fibrosarcoma.
- Postradiation sarcomas behave more aggressively and are less amenable to treatment.
- Wide surgical resection is the best chance for cure.
- Adjuvant chemotherapy has not shown favorable results.
- 5-year survival rate is approximately 30%.

Metastatic Carcinoma

- Metastatic carcinoma is the most common form of malignancy affecting bone.
- Bones with active marrow such as the vertebrae, ribs, pelvis, and skull are the preferential sites for metastasis. The jaws are relatively uncommon sites of metastasis.
- Approximately 1% of all oral malignancies represent malignancies that have metastasized from elsewhere in the body.
- The most common sites of the primary carcinoma are the breast **(Fig. 14)** and lung, followed by the kidney, prostate, thyroid, colon, and rectum.
- Metastatic spread of carcinoma to the jaws occurs through hematogenous route.
- The majority of patients with metastatic carcinoma to the jaws are in their fifth to seventh decades.
- Within the jaws, approximately 80% of the metastases are to the mandible, 14% to the maxilla, and 5% to both jaws.
- The molar/premolar region is the area within both the mandible and the maxilla that is most frequently affected.
- Management of metastatic carcinoma to the jaws begins with identification of the

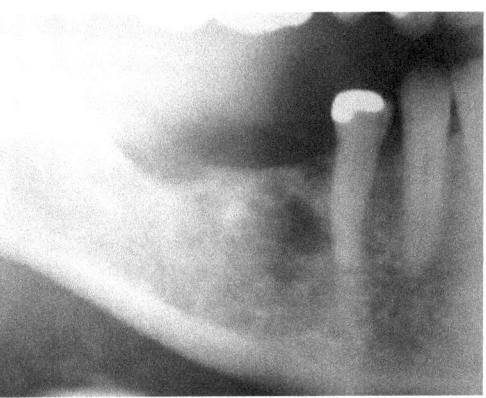

Fig. 14: An irregular radiolucency of the mandibular body: Metastatic from breast cancer.

primary site and determining the extent of metastatic involvement.
- Jaw metastases are usually evidence of widely disseminated disease, and palliative treatment should be aimed at eliminating pain and preserving function.
- If the metastatic lesion of the jaw represents the only site of metastasis, adequate surgical treatment or chemoradiotherapy may improve the prognosis.
- Overall, the prognosis of metastatic carcinoma of the jaws is poor, with a mean survival of 6–7 months.

KEY POINTS

- The pathologist should be given a representative and large enough biopsy specimen along with clinical and radiological information.
- For a lesion of the jaws, there may be debate regarding the order of investigations as to whether biopsy should precede three-dimensional imaging or not. If the biopsy is taken first, it may cause artifact on the three-dimensional imaging. If the imaging is done first, it may prove to have been unnecessary or inadequate once the diagnosis is established.
- Follow-up for aggressive odontogenic tumors (including ameloblastoma, odontogenic myxoma, and calcifying epithelial odontogenic tumor) should be at least 20 years and possibly for life.

CHAPTER 11

Nutrition in Oral Cancer

Ghanashyam Mandal

"Let food be your medicine and not medicine be your food"
—Hippocrates, 337 BC

INTRODUCTION

Nutritional support and timely intervention are an important part of head and neck cancer management. Patients at presentation may be very malnourished and most of these patients will need nutritional support during treatment for head and neck cancer. Early identification of such high-risk patients and timely intervention with nutritional support should be an integral part of their planning and should be discussed when treatment options are being considered.

ETIOLOGY OF MALNUTRITION IN ORAL CANCER PATIENTS

- Tumors may mechanically impede oral intake or cause trismus and odynophagia.
- Surgical therapy can change the anatomy so much that chewing and swallowing may be affected.
- Radiation therapy and chemotherapy also may cause mucositis, dysgeusia, anosmia, xerostomia, trismus, nausea, and vomiting.
- Poor dentition may result in difficulty with mastication. Dental problems induced by radiation such as caries, increased sensitivity further add to the problem.
- Alcohol and tobacco use worsen the problem by suppressing appetite and providing empty calories without essential nutrients. It is also seen that oral cancer patients generally have a lower intake of fresh fruits and vegetables.
- Tumor-induced metabolic dysfunction or cancer cachexia or immune alterations.
- Stored glycogen (exhausted during the first 24 hours) catabolized results in loss of proteins from tissue. Fat is then mobilized to meet the nutritional needs.
- Changes in status of neurotransmitters, immunoregulatory hormones, and also food aversions cause anorexia.
- Tumorigenic and immune-modulating factors [tumor necrosis factor (TNF) and interleukins 1 and 6] give rise to catabolism of muscle and tissue proteins that get converted to glucose in the liver. Without normal immune responses, this available glucose drives replication of cell by cancer cells. Fat is catabolized and elevates the levels of plasma free fatty acids due to hepatic neoketogenesis. This causes relative insulin insensitivity by normal body tissues.
- Deficiency of insulin decreases amino acid uptake in normal tissue and further fuels gluconeogenesis.

IMPACT OF MALNUTRITION (MALNUTRITION-ASSOCIATED MORBIDITY)

- Increased risk of infection
- Delayed wound healing
- Impaired cardiopulmonary function
- Muscle weakness
- Depression
- Poor quality of life (QOL)
- Increased risk of postoperative complications
- Reduced response to chemotherapy and radiotherapy (RT)
- Increased mortality rate

NUTRITIONAL SCREENING AND ASSESSMENT TOOLS

- *Subjective Global Assessment (SGA) tool*: It assesses nutritional status based on history and physical examination.
- Patient-generated Subjective Global Assessment (PGSGA).
- *Malnutrition Screening Tool (MST)*: It compares favorably with the PGSGA.

MONITORING

- Screening weekly for inpatients.
- For outpatients, weight to be recorded at each visit. Any weight loss of 2 kg or more within 2 weeks must be reported to the dietitian.

NUTRITIONAL ASSESSMENT PARAMETERS

- *Clinical observation*:
  - Ability to chew and swallow
  - Clinical signs of weight loss, e.g., fitting clothes
  - Medical history, which may affect nutritional intake, e.g., celiac disease, diabetes
- *Dietary history*: Review of recent intake in last 24 hours.
  - Fluid intake
  - Changes in texture
  - Reports of fullness
  - Length of time and effort taken to eat
  - Changes in appetite
- *Calculation of requirements*:
  - *Energy*: 25–35 kcal/kg/day dependent on activity level
  - *Protein*: 0.8–2.0 g/kg/day
  - *Fluid*: 30–35 mL/kg/day and increases, if infection and excessive fluid losses
  - *Vitamins and minerals*: As per recommended dietary allowance (RDA), unless considered deficient
  - Proposed treatment
  - Disease status and tumor site
  - Nutritional implications of previous and current treatment plan
- *Anthropometry*:
  - Height
  - Weight and percentage weight change
  - Body mass index < 18.5 kg/m^2 suggests undernutrition
  - Triceps skinfold thickness indicates fat stores
  - Mid-arm muscle circumference indicates lean tissue mass
  - Handgrip strength assesses muscle function
- *Personal and social information*:
  - Alcohol intake
  - Smoking
  - Substance misuse
  - Social support
  - Access to food and cooking skills
  - Social and financial circumstances
  - Time taken to eat and drink
  - Patient perception of nutritional status

- *Biochemistry*:
  - Urea and electrolytes—indicate fluid status, although it can be disrupted by disease state and treatment
  - Albumin—not good indicator of nutritional status due to its long half-life (17-20 days) and it is affected by stress and sepsis
  - Prealbumin—shorter half-life 2-3 days, but also affected by infection and stress
  - C-reactive protein—indication of acute phase response
  - Transferrin—affected by inflammation and infection
  - Total lymphocyte count—affected by infection

REFEEDING SYNDROME

- It is defined as potentially fatal shifts in fluids and electrolytes that may occur in malnourished patients receiving artificial refeeding (whether enterally or parenterally).
- It occurs due to hormonal and metabolic changes.
- Hallmark biochemical feature → Hypophosphatemia.
- It is a complex syndrome as a consequence of abnormalities in fluid and sodium balance; changes in metabolism of glucose, protein, and fat; deficiency of thiamine; hypokalemia; and hypomagnesemia.

How does refeeding syndrome develop?

- *Prolonged fasting*:
  - The underlying cause of refeeding syndrome is the rapid refeeding whether enteral or parenteral that causes metabolic and hormonal changes.
  - Early in starvation is the body switches from using carbohydrate to using fat and protein as the main source of energy and the basal metabolic rate decreases by as much as 20-25% causing metabolic and hormonal changes.
  - In prolonged fasting, hormonal and metabolic changes try to prevent protein and muscle breakdown in the body.
  - Muscle and other tissues start using fatty acids as the main source of energy decreasing the use of ketone bodies → The result is an increase in levels of blood ketone bodies and stimulate the brain to change from glucose to ketone bodies as its main source of energy.
  - The liver decreases the rate of gluconeogenesis and, hence, preserves muscle protein.
  - Several intracellular minerals also become severely depleted during the period of prolonged starvation.
  - Since these minerals are located mainly in the intracellular compartment, which contract during starvation, concentration of these minerals (including phosphate) in serum may reflect as normal with a reduction in renal excretion.
- *Refeeding*:
  - With refeeding, glycemia causes increased secretion of insulin and decreased secretion of glucagon.
  - Insulin stimulates synthesis of glycogen, fat, and protein.
  - This requires minerals such as phosphate and magnesium and cofactors such as thiamine.
  - Insulin stimulates potassium absorption into the cells through

- the sodium-potassium ATPase symporter, which also transports glucose into the cells.
- Magnesium and phosphate are also absorbed into the cells.
- Water followed by osmosis.
- They result in a further reduction in the already depleted serum phosphate levels, potassium, and magnesium.
- Clinical findings of refeeding syndrome appear due to the functional deficits of all the electrolytes and the rapid alteration in basal metabolic rate.

Criteria for Determining People at Moderate or High Risk of Developing Refeeding Syndrome

- *Patient has one or more of the following*:
  - Body mass index < 16 kg/m^2
  - Unintentional weight loss > 15% in last 3–6 minutes
  - Little or no nutritional intake for >10 days
  - Low levels of K^+, PO_4^{2-}, and Mg^{2+} prior to feeding
- *Patient has two or more of the following*:
  - Body mass index < 18.5 kg/m^2
  - Unintentional weight loss > 10% within last 3–6 minutes
  - Little or no nutritional intake for >5 days
  - History of alcohol abuse or drugs such as insulin, CT, or diuretics

Approach to Refeeding Syndrome

The approach to refeeding syndrome is given in **Flowchart 1**.

AIMS OF NUTRITION SUPPORT

- Improve the subjective QOL
- Enhance antitumor treatment effects
- Reduce the adverse effects of antitumor therapies
- Prevent and treat undernutrition

METHODS OF NUTRITION SUPPORT

- *Oral*:
  - Traditional food fortification is first-line advice
  - Early use of oral nutrition support, e.g., nutritionally complete supplements
- *Parenteral*
- *Enteral*: When, where, and which tube is to be used depends on the tumor site, expected duration of dysphagia, and interference with further treatment.
- *Types of feeding tubes* (**Fig. 1**):
  - Nasogastric tube
  - Nasojejunal tube
  - Gastrostomy tube
  - Jejunostomy tube
- Nasogastric and nasojejunal tubes are all recommended for short-term use (<4 weeks).
- The National Institute for Health and Care Excellence (NICE) guidelines on enteral feeding suggest that if enteral feeding is expected to be required for >4 weeks, then gastrostomy tube insertion is recommended.
- *Immune-enhanced nutrition*:
  - Feeds containing amino acids, nucleotides, and lipids.
  - There are no additional benefits to immunonutrition preoperatively over standard nutrition support.
- In the perioperative period, omega-3 enriched nutrition support may improve nutritional outcomes including weight, lean body mass and fat mass, reduce postoperative infections, and reduce hospital stay.

Flowchart 1: Approach to refeeding syndrome.

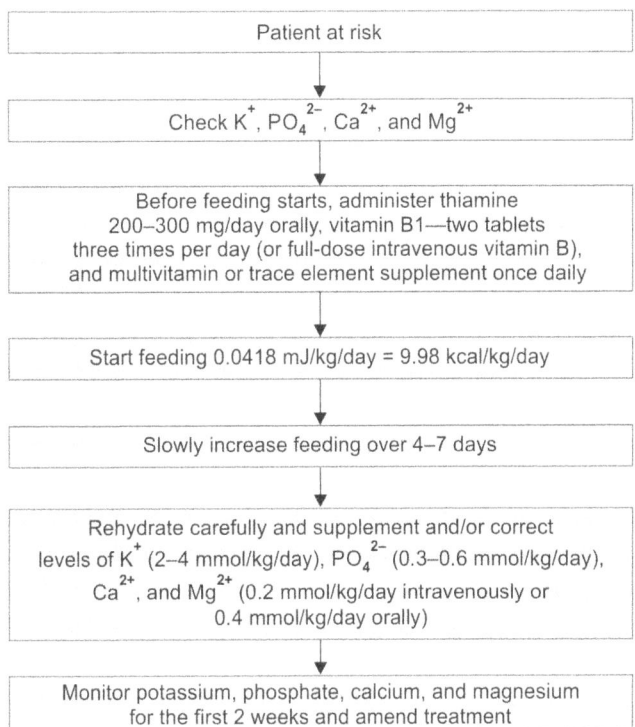

Patient at risk
↓
Check K^+, PO_4^{2-}, Ca^{2+}, and Mg^{2+}
↓
Before feeding starts, administer thiamine 200–300 mg/day orally, vitamin B1—two tablets three times per day (or full-dose intravenous vitamin B), and multivitamin or trace element supplement once daily
↓
Start feeding 0.0418 mJ/kg/day = 9.98 kcal/kg/day
↓
Slowly increase feeding over 4–7 days
↓
Rehydrate carefully and supplement and/or correct levels of K^+ (2–4 mmol/kg/day), PO_4^{2-} (0.3–0.6 mmol/kg/day), Ca^{2+}, and Mg^{2+} (0.2 mmol/kg/day intravenously or 0.4 mmol/kg/day orally)
↓
Monitor potassium, phosphate, calcium, and magnesium for the first 2 weeks and amend treatment

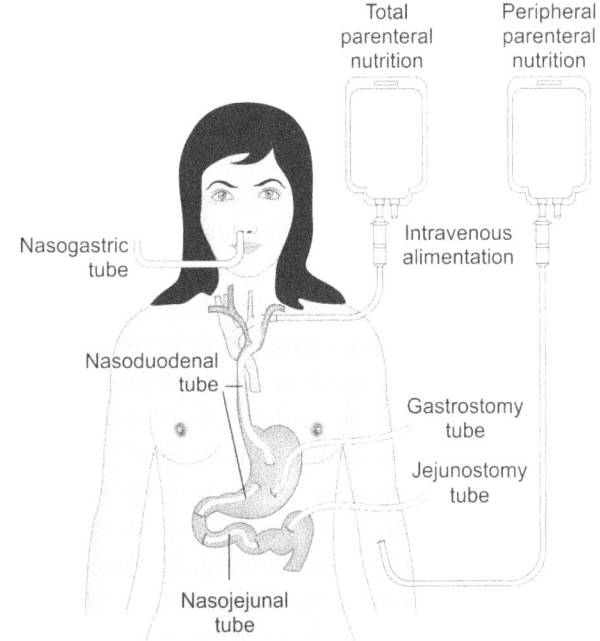

Fig. 1: Types of feeding tubes.

ESTIMATING NUTRITIONAL REQUIREMENTS

- Mildly hypermetabolic with an excess energy expenditure of between 138 and 289 kcal/day.
- Total energy expenditure and protein requirements for nonobese ambulatory patients using their actual body weight can be estimated as follows:
  - *Energy*: 30–35 kcal/kg/day
  - *Protein*: 1.2 g/kg/day
- As energy requirements may be elevated postoperatively, monitor weight and adjust intake.
- During RT/CTRT, the target is same.

NUTRITION CONSIDERATIONS DURING SURGICAL TREATMENT

- *Criteria for initiating preoperative nutritional support*:
  - Indications:
    - Weight loss > 10–15% in 6 months
    - Body mass index < 18.5 kg/m^2
    - Subjective Global Assessment grade C
    - Serum albumin < 30 g/L
    - Unable to maintain intake above 60% of recommended intake for >10 days
    - Patients with severe nutritional risk should receive nutrition support for 10–14 days prior to major surgery
    - Carbohydrate loading is standard practice
- *Postoperative nutrition*:
  - Early postoperative tube feeding (within 24 hours)
  - Nutrition support, especially enteral nutrition, reduces morbidity Postoperatively, standard polymeric enteral feeds are advised with very limited evidence currently to support the use of immunonutrition.
- *Postoperative nutrition with chyle leak*:
  - Nutritional intervention with fat-free or medium-chain triglyceride nutritional supplements either orally or through a feeding tube to be commenced.
  - Parenteral nutrition may be considered in severe cases when drainage volume is consistently high.
  - Medium-chain triglyceride is recommended because it is directly absorbed into the portal system resulting in less chyle production.

NUTRITIONAL CONSIDERATIONS DURING CURATIVE RADIOTHERAPY ± CHEMOTHERAPY

- Patients may develop toxicities from these combined modality treatments which affect adequate nutrition or they need dietary intervention to support their QOL.
- Prophylactic tube feeding has shown reduced weight loss in the short term, compared to oral intake alone, and may decrease unplanned hospital admissions and improve QOL during and after treatment.
- Nutrition of patients receiving biological agents such as cetuximab along with RT needs similar management as those receiving chemoradiotherapy.
- Percutaneous endoscopic gastrostomy (PEG) may be a better option in nutrition management of such patients receiving RT or chemoradiotherapy.
- More than 10% weight loss during and directly after RT has a significant impact on social eating, social contact, and QOL in head and neck cancer patients.

NATIONAL COMPREHENSIVE CANCER NETWORK GUIDELINES: HEAD AND NECK CANCER

- Pre- and post-treatment functional evaluation of nutritional status should be undertaken using subjective and objective assessment tools.
- All patients should receive dietary counseling with the initiation of treatment.
- Regular follow-up with dietitian until patient has achieved a nutritionally stable baseline following treatment.
- It does not recommend prophylactic nasogastric (NG)/PEG tube placement, if good performance score is present.
- Prophylactic tube placement:
  - *Severe weight loss prior to treatment*: >5% over 1 minute and >10% over 6 minutes
  - Ongoing dehydration, dysphagia, anorexia, and pain interfering with swallowing/chewing
  - Comorbidities that may be aggravated by dysphagia
  - Aspiration
  - For whom long-term swallowing disorders are expected

LOOKING INTO THE FUTURE

- To prevent cancers by changes made in diet—an exciting and new oncologic concept.
- Risk of developing head and neck cancer has been found to be more in patients who have food deficient in cryptoxanthin, lycopene, and vitamins C and E. It has been postulated that these substances act as free radical scavengers and, thus, protect deoxyribonucleic acid (DNA) from mutation.
- Recently, research has found that omega-3 polyunsaturated fatty acids derived from fish oils have beneficial effects in immunocompromised patients.
- Special enteral formulas containing arginine, dietary nucleotides, and omega-3 fatty acids are available in market.
- Nutrigenetics studies have also shown the positive effects of nutrition at the gene level, whereas nutrigenomics studies the effect of nutrients on genome and transcriptome patterns.

KEY POINTS

- Malnutrition in oral cancer patients may be not only due to disease per se, but also due to its treatment such as surgery and RT/CT.
- Nutritional assessment and monitoring of weight form an integral part of follow-up.
- *Target*: Energy: 25–35 kcal/kg/day, protein: 0.8–2.0 g/kg/day, and fluid: 30–35 ml/kg/day increases, if infection and excessive fluid losses.
- Nasogastric and nasojejunal tubes are recommended for short-term use *(<4 weeks)*.
- If enteral feeding is expected to be required for *>4 weeks*, then gastrostomy tube insertion is recommended.
- More than 10% weight loss during and directly after RT has a significant impact on social eating, social contact, and QOL in head and neck cancer patients.

Anesthesia in Oral Cancer Surgery

CHAPTER 12

Shagun Bhatia Shah

"Eternal vigilance is the price of safety"
"Anesthesia is a science, but practiced as an art"
— **Ralph Milton Waters**

INTRODUCTION

Oral cancer surgery presents unique challenges such as difficult airway, shared airway, patients with poor nutritional status, postchemotherapy, and postradiotherapy status. The anesthetic and surgical teams require a clear mutual understanding regarding their respective responsibilities in managing the "shared airway" according to the type of procedure and the requirement of the anesthetist to avoid compromise of the airway by way of gas exchange or soiling.

PREANESTHETIC CHECKUP

Airway Assessment

Airway assessment is the cornerstone of preanesthetic checkup in oral oncosurgery patients. Various airway assessment parameters including composite multivariate indices and imaging are employed for this purpose. Nine core airway considerations are tabulated here:

1. Any history suggestive of airway difficulties?
2. Any altered cardiorespiratory physiology?
3. Any impact of surgery on the airway?
4. Any anticipated bag-mask ventilation difficulty?
5. Any anticipated supraglottic airway device (SAD) placement difficulty?
6. Any anticipated intubation difficulty?
7. Any anticipated infraglottic airway difficulty?
8. Any risk of aspiration?
9. How easy will it be to extubate safely?

In nutshell, the "10 commandments" for airway assessment are checking for:

1. Previous anesthesia issues
2. Gastric reflux
3. Obstructive sleep apnea
4. Body mass index
5. Mouth opening
6. Modified Mallampati score
7. Dental status
8. Thyromental distance
9. Jaw protrusion
10. Cervical spine movement

Among the multivariate indices of airway assessment, the El-Ganzouri's index is described in **Table 1**.

Despite careful preoperative evaluation, some patients with difficult airway remain undetected.

The patients have to be explained about overnight retention of endotracheal tube (ETT) (postsurgery) and consequent inability to phonate till such time the tube is removed.

Patients with anticipated difficult airway in whom an awake fiberoptic bronchoscopic/awake videolaryngoscopic intubation has

TABLE 1: Airway assessment: El-Ganzouri's index.		
El-Ganzouri's index		Score
Mouth opening	>4 cm	0
	4 cm	1
	<4 cm	2
Thyromental distance	>6.5 cm	0
	6–6.5 cm	1
	<6 cm	2
Mallampati grade	0/1/2	0
	3	1
	4	2
Neck movement	>90°	0
	80–90°	1
	<80°	2
Jaw protrusion	Yes	0
	No	1
Body weight	<90 kg	0
	90–110 kg	1
	>110 kg	2
History of difficult intubation	None	0
	Questionable	1
	Definite	2

0–3: Standard Macintosh laryngoscope
>3: Videolaryngoscope
>7: Awake fiberoptic bronchoscopy (FOB)

Minimum score: 0
Maximum score: 1–3

been planned need special counseling regarding nerve blocks and detailed explanation about the steps of the procedure and the need to perform it with the patient awake to ensure adequate patient cooperation.

Routine investigations for all oncosurgical patients include a complete blood count, renal function test including serum electrolytes, hepatic function tests including serum proteins, coagulation profile, viral markers, chest radiograph, and an electrocardiogram and echocardiogram.

Airway Plan

Fiberoptic bronchoscopy (FOB), though the gold standard, is not a blanket solution for all difficult airways.

Anticipated difficult airway is not a race against time. So, *pause, plan, prepare, and then proceed*.

With distorted nasal anatomy/reduced nasal patency, nasal FOB is not an option. With grossly distorted, edematous larynx, exposed oropharyngeal structures, and requirement of prolonged postoperative ventilation, preoperative elective tracheostomy is the preferred technique.

When blood and secretions rule out use of FOB as in friable tumors, C-MAC® D-blade videolaryngoscopy with adequate use of Yankauer's suction catheter comes to the rescue. In difficult airways with greater than "one finger" mouth opening, D blade can be used keeping the patient awake/spontaneously breathing.

INTRAOPERATIVE MANAGEMENT

Presence of a difficult airway cart should mandatorily be set before surgery including ensuring availability of fiberoptic bronchoscope, videolaryngoscope, cricothyroidotomy, and tracheostomy sets. Selecting the more roomy nostril or the nostril contralateral to the tumor, if both the nostrils are equally patent, must begin by asking the patient directly or digital palpation with a gloved lubricated little finger or examining the radiographic images (CT/MRI) when available or by point of care ultrasound of the nasal cavity. Adequate nasal preparation, i.e., xylometazoline drops and packing with ribbon gauze soaked in 4% lignocaine should be performed and the nostril which is more patent selected for nasotracheal intubation following preoxygenation.

An armored (flexometallic) ETT helps prevent kinking of the tube caused by the pressure from the robotic arms or patient-side surgeon. The C-MAC™ videolaryngoscope, especially the D blade, is a very good tool for securing the airway under vision with the added advantage of visualizing the cancerous lesion as well. A gauze pad may be used to pack any gap between upper incisors to prevent lodgment of laryngoscope blade in the gap causing trauma.

In patients with a difficult airway, spontaneous respiration has to be maintained preferably till the insertion of a definitive airway is done and a muscle relaxant should be given only after correct tube placement is confirmed. Awake FOB-guided nasal intubation may be used in those patients who have limited mouth opening and trismus. Local anesthetic airway blocks are needed (bilateral superior laryngeal nerve block with 2 mL 2% lignocaine, transtracheal block with 3 mL 4% lignocaine, and glossopharyngeal nerve block with viscous lignocaine gargles) as well as cooperation from patient. "SAYGO" (spray as-you-go) technique can also be used during insertion of the fiberoptic bronchoscope for airway anesthetization. In certain situations, posterior pharyngeal wall tumors could need insertion of orotracheal tube, which may be difficult because the tumor may obstruct the tube entry. Patients scheduled for maxillectomy also require orotracheal intubation. Some patients require a tracheostomy preoperatively and its patency needs to be ensured before induction with anesthesia.

Hemodynamic Stability

Intraoperative hemodynamic stability can be maintained with one or more of the following agents: Esmolol boluses or infusion (0.5–1 mg/kg bolus or 50–100 µg/kg/min infusion), nitroglycerin (NTG) infusion (5–10 µg/min infusion), labetalol bolus (5–20 mg) or infusion (1–2 mg/min infusion), intermittent opioid boluses (20–30 µg fentanyl or 8–25 µg/kg sufentanil), and continuous remifentanil infusion (0.25–0.5–1 µg/kg/min). Esmolol hydrochloride is an ultrashort-acting beta-blocker. NTG is a direct-acting vasodilator. Labetalol is a combined alpha- and beta-blocker. Remifentanil is a unique, ultrashort-acting opioid with a rapid onset (1.3 min) and offset of action (half-time = 3–5 min) with fast and predictable titration of effect and unaltered pharmacokinetics in patients with obesity, renal, or hepatic dysfunction.

Causes of Sudden Rise in Airway Pressure

- Tube kinking
- *Shared airway*: Surgeon leaning on ETT
- Blockage of ETT by secretions, mucus, blood, or tumor/tissue debris

POSTOPERATIVE MANAGEMENT

Postoperatively, the patients are reversed, but not extubated generally, anticipating any edema of the airway after intraoral surgery. Flexometallic tube can be changed to portex (PVC) cuffed ETT with a tube exchanger device before the neuromuscular blockade is reversed. Each patient should be monitored preferably in a dedicated oncosurgical intensive care unit keeping the nasotracheal tube in situ. Humidified oxygen may be given through a T-piece set, which is connected to the distal end of the retained ETT.

Patients admitted to postoperative care units with tracheal tubes in situ must be monitored with continuous capnography. It is the responsibility of the anesthesiologist to remove the tracheal tube.

Anesthesiologist should formally hand over care to an adequately trained physician in the postoperative and intensive care unit. Intensive care unit staff looking after postoperative tracheostomies must understand about those patients who are not suitable for bag-mask ventilation or oral intubation in case of any emergencies.

The patient may be extubated after 24–48 hours over an airway exchange catheter/bougie with supplemental esmolol boluses to prevent sympathetic stimulation and dexamethasone injected 30 minutes before extubation. Remifentanil infusion may be utilized, if available, since it helps clear-headed recovery, rapid extubation, and effective postoperative management of pain. Moreover, the patient must be kept warm. Monitoring has to be continued in the postoperative period to identify any untoward events.

Pre-existing comorbidities such as hypertension, diabetes, coronary artery disease, or thyroid disorders also have to be treated appropriately.

Patients who have reactive airway disease could present with other problems such as bronchospasm during both intubation and extubation. Perioperative steroid and beta-2 agonist nebulization and aerosol inhaler can be used through the ETT for immediate relief. Beta-blockers are avoided in this subgroup of patients and opioids in adequate doses should be used early in surgery to control the heart rate.

Elderly patients, especially those with concurrent cardiac ailments, are very prone to develop arrhythmias during the postoperative periextubation period. This needs prompt detection and treatment.

Both deep vein thrombosis (DVT) and postoperative nausea and vomiting (PONV) prophylaxis must be given to all patients.

POSTOPERATIVE ANALGESIA

Successive stages of cancer surgery may result in several angiogenic factors as described here:
- Malpositioning on the operating table
- Infiltration, ulceration, or pressure of tissue due to tumor
- Intraoperative nerve and muscle damage
- Pain related to extensive tissue resection
- Psychosocial dimension of pain due to cosmetic disfigurement
- Radiotherapy- and chemotherapy-induced oral mucositis
- Infection or coexisting morbidity

Nociceptive pain results from tissue infiltration by neoplastic cells whereas neuropathic pain can be due to nerve compression or invasion by the tumor mass.

Preventive and curative measures to manage acute postoperative pain include:
- Avoiding hyperextension of head and neck
- Sparing nerve and muscle structures during surgery as far as possible to curb painful sequelae

- Patient-controlled analgesia using infusion pumps to deliver morphine for early postoperative pain at tumor resection and flap harvesting sites
- Physical therapy after flap harvesting to minimize painful sequelae
- Proper nutrition, adequate sleep, and physical activity

Multimodal analgesia and a holistic approach are the mainstay of postoperative pain relief.

The World Health Organization (WHO) recommends usage of the oral route, unless contraindicated. Head and neck cancer patients can be administered drugs enterally by nasogastric or gastrostomy tubes or rectal administration. When this is not possible, subcutaneous/intravenous (IV) route or transdermal patches may be employed. The WHO three-step ladder for cancer pain management is useful **(Fig. 1)**.

Postoperative analgesia is multimodality treatment with IV paracetamol, nonsteroidal anti-inflammatory drugs (NSAIDs), and fentanyl infusion (30–40 µg/h) for the first 12–24 hours. Intravenous patient-controlled analgesia (IVPCA) with opioids (fentanyl or sufentanil) can alternatively be utilized for patient comfort.

Ultrasound-guided mental block and superficial cervical plexus block may be supplemented in patients with extensive

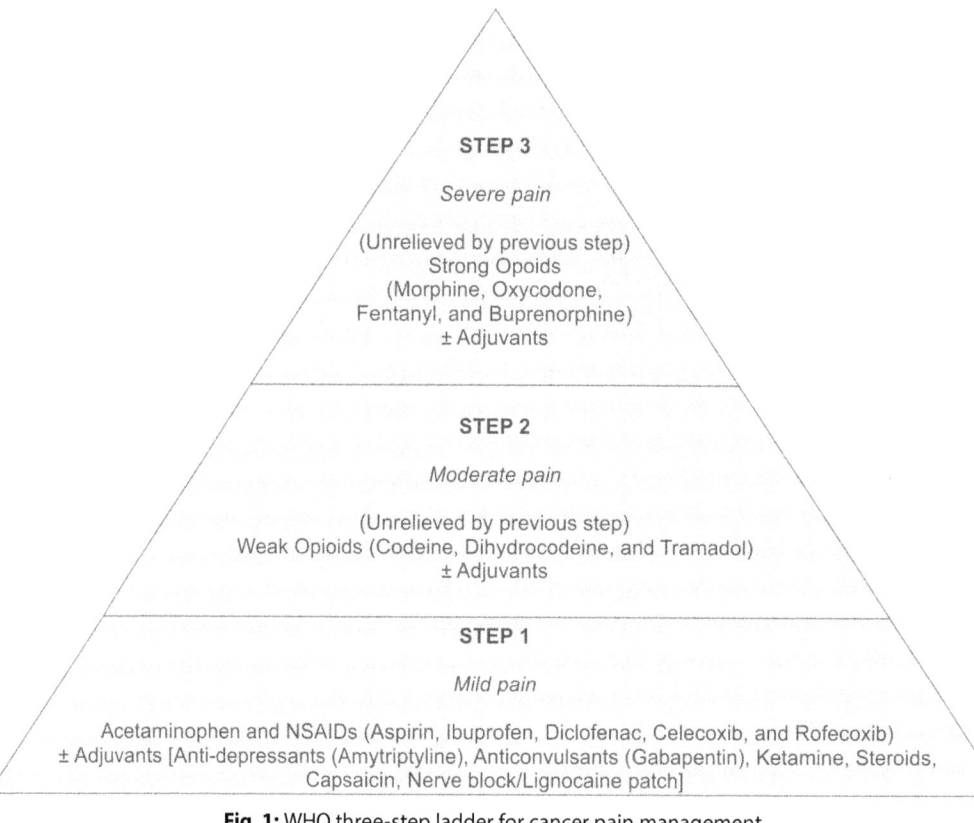

Fig. 1: WHO three-step ladder for cancer pain management.
(NSAIDs: nonsteroidal anti-inflammatory drugs; WHO: World Health Organization)

neck dissections. In patients on oral morphine for cancer pain before surgery, the total 24-hour dosage requires recalculation and supplementation with equivalent (oral morphine dose is approximately three times the IV dose) IV morphine postoperatively.

Interventional Therapy

Regional nerve blocks employed include:
- Trigeminal nerve block
- Glossopharyngeal nerve block
- Cervical plexus block

These nerve blocks may be diagnostic, prognostic, or therapeutic. Therapeutic blocks may be nondestructive or neurolytic. The former employs bupivacaine 2.5%, while the latter administers alcohol or phenol. In the patient with head and neck cancer, interventional therapy for cancer pain is no more the preferred pain management. Single nerve blocks are ineffective because sensory innervation to the head and neck area originates from multiple cranial/cervical nerves.

SPECIAL SITUATIONS

Post-chemotherapy Patients

Securing an IV line may become a mammoth task in some patients who have undergone chemotherapy due to widespread thrombophlebitis of peripheral veins owing to repeated injection of irritant chemotherapeutic agents. Chemoport/peripherally inserted central catheter (PICC) line insertion prior to chemotherapy is a good preventive measure. Two chemotherapeutic agents of utmost importance to anesthetists are adriamycin and bleomycin. The former being cardiotoxic that reduces the left ventricular ejection fraction requiring major changes in anesthesia plan such as use of etomidate instead of the commonly used induction agent propofol, securing an arterial line for advanced hemodynamic monitoring (cardiac output and systemic vascular resistance) to titrate anesthetic drug doses, vasopressors and ionotropes, and keeping the defibrillator as a backup. Bleomycin is no longer used in oral cancer now and is known to cause pulmonary fibrosis.

Post-radiotherapy Patients

Radiotherapy to the anterior aspect of neck renders the neck stiff with inadequate extension resulting in difficulty in alignment of the oropharyngolaryngeal axis for endotracheal intubation. The dermal fibrosis also renders surgical airway/tracheostomy difficult. The thyroid gland too may be affected leading to hypothyroidism and, hence, extra caution with administering opioids and sedatives.

Post-oncosurgery Patients

These patients may have external deformities, contractures, and limited neck extension. Rigidity and distortion of the oropharyngeal tissues also may interfere with facemask ventilation and conventional laryngoscopy. Tracheal deviation, distorted anatomy, and laryngeal edema may result in a difficult airway.

RECONSTRUCTIVE SURGERY IN PATIENTS

The decision regarding the necessity and type of reconstructive surgery (locoregional/myocutaneous/free flap) is taken only after resection is complete by gauging the extent of defect produced. But, the anesthetist has to be prepared for any of the free flaps and accordingly spare the left upper limb (radial artery free flap) and left lower limb (anterolateral thigh flap) and contralateral lower limb (free fibular flap) for the plastic surgeon. IV cannulation, arterial lines, and cubital central venous access are prohibited in these areas leaving just the right upper limb for cannulation. Doppler probes help to monitor vascular flow in perforators during free flap harvest and occasionally to view anastomotic vessel, but they are expensive and of restricted use to inaccessible sites, composite flaps (where skin color may not reflect the deeper layer viability), continued arterial spasm risk, and patients with previous radiation. Prompt return to the OR in case of compromise may allow the blood flow to be restored and flap to be salvaged.

EQUIPMENT

Nasotracheal Tube

The most commonly used PVC tubes (Portex) are replaced by flexometallic armored tubes in head and neck surgery to prevent the rise in airway pressures due to kinking/compression under the surgical assistants elbow/drapes. It should be ensured that fastening tapes are secured in such a way as to avoid columellar necrosis.

Difficult Airway Armamentarium

The C-MAC D-blade (Karl Storz, Tuttlingen, Germany) videolaryngoscope is a new promising tool in the difficult airway armamentarium. D stands for Volker Doerges (anesthesiologist in Kiel, Germany) as coinventor of the D blade and may also denote "difficult." In C-MAC-guided orotracheal intubation, bringing just the pharyngeal and laryngeal axes (and not the oral axis) in the same plane is adequate to view the glottis. This is useful in patients with limited neck extension (cervical spine rigidity/stereotactic localization frame in situ).

The tongue is not to be shifted to the right side as with conventional Macintosh laryngoscope instead the tongue remains in the midline. Essentials for secure videolaryngoscopy are that the three Ts: namely the tip (of the D blade), target (glottis), and the tube are visualized on the monitor. A styleted tracheal tube is prepared with a curvature matching the D blade. A hockey stick-shaped stylet (or S guide with its soft orange distal tip, three oxygen outlets, and proximal malleable part) may be beneficial in obese patients.

LASER SURGERY

The risk of airway fires due to laser is low, if careful precautions and laser-safe tubes are utilized. The concentric outer and inner cuffs of the laser tube should be filled with methylene blue dye and saline, respectively. A polyvinyl chloride (PVC) tube may be wrapped with an aluminum ribbon and its cuff filled with saline, if a commercially-produced laser tube is not available. Postoperative hemorrhage and edema are known risk factors after extensive laser surgery.

TRANSORAL ROBOTIC SURGERY

Transoral robotic surgery (TORS) is a promising, minimally invasive procedure for deep-seated lesions situated in inaccessible nooks and corners of the oropharynx/oral cavity. It works around corners and avoids certain line-of-sight limitations.

The da Vinci Robotic Surgical System (Intuitive Surgical, Sunnyvale, California, USA) enjoys a monopoly for radical surgery of cancers of head and neck. Its purported advantages include reduced blood loss, better cosmesis (no mutilating scars), 15-fold magnified view of difficult-to-reach lesions, lesser pain, and earlier recovery postoperatively. The indications have been increased to radical tonsillectomy, partial laryngectomy, and other complex intraoral lesion excision. The wristed robotic arms (EndoWrist technology) improve dexterity and filter any tremors of the hand of the operating surgeon. Surgical precision can be obtained by optimal port placement with noncollision of the robotic arms. Drawbacks of robotic surgery include the expenses, lack of tactile feedback, and overdependence on the patient-side surgeon. Widespread adoption by high-volume centers worldwide will mitigate costs.

Perioperative anesthetic concerns include positioning of the surgical robotic cart, operating theater (OT) table, anesthesia workstation, surgeon, anesthetist, and nursing staff with instruments trolley relative to each other. Breathing circuit modifications, control of sympathetic stimulation after the insertion of mouth gag or robotic arms, judicious use of fluid, cautious patient positioning with protective padding for eyes, postoperative ETT retention, and meticulous management of difficult airway are among other challenges.

In contrast to open radical head and neck oncosurgeries, the nasogastric tube (for gastric decompression and postoperative nutrition) has to be inserted only after complete excision of the tumor and clearance of the margins on frozen section in patients undergoing TORS. The C-MAC videolaryngoscope is of enormous benefit in helping difficult insertion of Ryle's tube and in visualizing any residual tumor.

The nasogastric tube and oro-/nasopharyngeal temperature probe are not placed immediately after endotracheal intubation. The former is placed after the end of surgery before reversing anesthesia, while the latter may be placed rectally.

Positioning

The patient is laid supine. A sandbag is placed beneath the shoulder blades to provide extension of the head and folded surgical sheets are placed below the donut-shaped gel headrest to provide support. The arms are kept adducted and an oral retractor inserted. Enough space ensured for the patient cart to roll in at an angle of 30° to the OT table from the right side. Traditionally, the anesthesia workstation is at the foot end of the table and, therefore, the breathing circuit needs to be longer. The resultant increase in dead space is regulated by adjusting the ventilatory parameters. The detection of end-tidal carbon dioxide ($ETCO_2$) via a conventional side stream carbon dioxide analyzer may also be delayed. This is of significant importance for detecting intraoperative air embolism (especially when in sitting position) or circuit disconnections. Extension lines have to be connected to IV catheter lines, since the patients' hands would be inaccessible to the anesthesiologist. Placing the anesthesia workstation on the left side of the lower half of the OT table at an angle of 45° diminishes the need for long breathing circuits with their accompanying problems. The breathing circuit tubes are safely secured adjacent and parallel to the long axis of the patient on the left side.

ROBOT-ASSISTED RADICAL NECK DISSECTION

The patient is in supine position with the head turned to the side opposite to that of operating side. An extra-long breathing circuit should be improvised beforehand by joining together end-to-end two standard circuits and extension attached to IV lines after tucking the arms at patient's sides.

ANESTHESIA IN HIV-POSITIVE PATIENTS

Risk of transmission to staff increases during invasive procedures, and this is reduced, if universal precautions are universally followed. Needlestick injury carries a 0.03–0.3% risk of transmission depending on the type (hypodermic) of needle, depth of puncture, and quantity of blood inoculated. Disposable equipment and linen, hydrophobic filter-fitted circuits, visors, double gloves, and protective footwear must be utilized to avoid contact with blood, body fluids, and tissues. Sweat, tears, saliva, sputum, urine, and stool are all considered noninfectious, unless contaminated by above. Robotic endoscopic equipment tray is gas plasma sterilized (STERRAD 100S) before reuse.

EMERGENCY IN ORAL CANCER SURGERY

Flap necrosis and arterial/venous/capillary bleeder with resultant hematoma formation and/or hemodynamic instability are the most frequent causes of emergency in oral oncosurgery. Major neck vessels may get eroded. This sort of hemorrhage can arise suddenly and with little warning. Everyone involved should be aware of what is needed as immediate measures (e.g., pressing on the neck in the event of a "carotid blowout" or removing the skin clips in the event of a rapid expanding hematoma) *versus* the need to reach the theater to manage the issue directly. Proximity to the OT and availability of emergency kit in the ward are important considerations.

Transnasal humidified rapid insufflation ventilatory exchange (THRIVE) combines apneic oxygenation, continuous positive airway pressure, and flow-dependent dead space flushing and can change the nature of difficult intubations from a hurried stop–start process to a more controlled event with an extended apneic window and reduced iatrogenic trauma. THRIVE delivered through a nasal high-flow oxygen delivery system that has shown to increase the apnea time in head and neck patients including those with stridor to an average of 17 minutes.

Do emergency tracheostomy (percutaneous) rather than attempting difficult intubation.

Vortex Approach

The vortex approach is an emergency airway cognitive tool. It allows maximum three attempts for a nonsurgical airway technique out of which at least one attempt must be by the most experienced available clinician. This sequential spiral approach is described here:

A: Intubation: Three categories of manipulations available include:
1. Head and neck (remove head ring and neck extension)
2. Larynx [backward, upward and rightward pressure (BURP) maneuver: BURP externally on larynx and applied digitally by an assistant]
3. Devices (smaller ETT, stylet, bougie, McCoy blade direct laryngoscope, and C-MAC® D-blade videolaryngoscope)

B: SAD: Supraglottic airway device (second generation)

C: Facemask (two-person technique and oral/nasal airway)

D: Cannot intubate and cannot oxygenate situation

A needle or surgical cricothyroidotomy needs to be performed.

ENHANCED RECOVERY AFTER SURGERY PROTOCOL

Extrapolation of enhanced recovery after surgery (ERAS) concepts to patients with oral cancer undergoing major procedures and free-flap surgery could help in improving the outcomes. Relevant preoperative steps consist of carbohydrate loading (maltodextrin drink 2 hours before surgery), while intraoperative measures are those such as goal-directed fluid therapy using cardiac output monitoring to optimize fluid management, maintenance of normothermia, chemical thromboprophylaxis, and tight glycemic control. Early enteral feeding is advocated postsurgery.

TABLE 2: Anesthetic concerns for oral cancer surgery.

Diagnosis	Radical surgical resection	Reconstructive surgery	Anesthesia concerns
Carcinoma of buccal mucosa	• Commando + Radical neck dissection (RND) • Marginal/Segmental mandibulectomy	Radial artery free-flap (RAFF)/Anterolateral thigh free-flap (ALT-FF)/Free fibula	• Nasotracheal intubation • IV line and radial artery on right side/dorsalis pedis in RAFF • In ALT-FF, spare right lower limb for surgeon
Carcinoma of tongue	• Partial glossectomy + Supraomohyoid neck dissection • Tongue Commando		• Nasal PVC tube (may kink) • Nasal flexometallic tube
Carcinoma of maxilla	Commando	• PMMC • Nasolabial • RAFF	• Nasal tube may get damaged • Oral flexometallic tube • Oral south pole and tracheostomy
Carcinoma of mandible/alveolus	• Segmental mandibulectomy • Hemi-mandibulectomy	• PMMC flap • Free fibular flap	• Nasal PVC tube (may kink) • North pole tube • Nasal flexometallic tube • In free fibula, spare the lower limb opposite to the side of head and neck lesion for plastic surgery
Tracheostomy			• *Positioning*: Already desaturated, uncooperative, and unable to lie flat • Heliox mixture and resuscitation
RND/MND	Neck dissection for occult primary		Oral tube

(MND: modified neck dissection; PMMC: pectoralis major myocutaneous; PVC: polyvinyl chloride)

KEY POINTS

- Communicate to the patient about overnight retention of ETT postsurgery and consequent inability to phonate till such time the tube is removed.
- Special counseling regarding nerve blocks and detailed explanation about the steps of the procedure for awake intubation.
- Fiberoptic bronchoscopy, though the gold standard, is not a blanket solution for all difficult airways. So, pause, plan, prepare, and then proceed.
- Selecting the more-roomy nostril or the nostril contralateral to the tumor, if both the nostrils are equally patent, must begin by asking the patient directly, digital palpation with a gloved lubricated little finger, examining the radiographic images (CT/MRI) when available, or by point-of-care ultrasound of the nasal cavity.
- The C-MAC videolaryngoscope, especially the D blade, serves as an excellent tool for securing the airway under vision with the added advantage of visualizing the cancerous lesion as well.
- In difficult airways, spontaneous respiration should preferably be maintained till the insertion of a definitive airway and muscle relaxant must be given only after confirming correct tube placement.
- On encountering intraoperative sudden rise in airway pressure, suspect tube kinking, blockage of ETT by secretions, mucus, blood or tumor/tissue debris, or even the surgeon leaning on the ETT.
- Nociceptive pain results from tissue infiltration by neoplastic cells, whereas neuropathic pain can be due to nerve compression or invasion by the tumor mass.
- Multimodal analgesia and a holistic approach are the mainstay of postoperative pain relief in these patients.
- Perform emergency tracheostomy (percutaneous) rather than attempting heroic difficult intubation: Follow the vortex approach.
- Extrapolation of ERAS concepts to patients with oral cancer undergoing major resections and free-flap surgery may help in improving outcomes.

CHAPTER 13

Preoperative, Peroperative, and Postoperative Nursing Care

Rajan Arora, Ghanashyam Mandal

INTRODUCTION

Malignancies of the head and neck may frequently require complex, labor intensive surgery such as composite oral cavity resections. Surgeries such as free-flap reconstruction for extensive defects add to the length and complexity of these surgeries. Hence, they need a coordinated multidisciplinary team to deliver adequate care before, during, and after surgery.

"The ultimate measure of a man is not where he stands in moments of comfort and convenience, but where he stands at times of challenge and controversy."

—Martin Luther King Jr

PREOPERATIVE NURSING CARE

Definition

Preoperative care is the preparation and management of a patient prior to surgery.
- The preoperative phase begins with patient or someone on his behalf is informed of the need for surgery and he decides to undergo the procedure. It ends with the patient being transferred to operating room (OR) bed.
- This period of time is utilized to prepare the patient physically and psychologically for the surgery.
- The length of the preoperative period is not constant. For elective surgery, this period may be long, whereas for patients who need emergency surgery, this period is shorter.
- During this period, diagnostic tests and medical regimens are begun.
- Information from preoperative assessment tests are used to prepare a plan to care for the patient.
- Nursing activities are aimed for patient support, teaching, and preparation for the procedure according to the orders of the surgeon.

Preoperative Phase

Assessment by Nurses

Regarding past and present illness, patient's drug history, diet, allergies (latex), personal habits, occupation, finances, family support, knowledge about surgery, and attitude.
- Their duty is to send investigations, e.g., complete blood count (CBC), electrolytes, creatinine, urinalysis, X-ray examinations, electrocardiogram (EKG), blood type, partial thromboplastin time (PTT), prothrombin time (PT), platelets, liver function test (LFT), viral markers, radiological investigations.
- Blood donations

Final Surgical Preparation on the Day of Surgery

- Complete preoperative checklist sheet in medical record
- Informed consent
- Start intravenous (IV) fluids

- Removal of prosthetics, hair pins, contact lenses and glasses, dentures, hearing aids, nail polish, and jewelry
- Bowel and bladder preparation, ID band, and preoperative medications
- Hygiene—skin scrub and hospital gown are provided
- Record vital signs
- Height/Weight
- Insert tubes, if required, and preoperative medications
- Promote comfort—antianxiety medicines
- Marking of surgical site

INTRAOPERATIVE NURSING CARE

This period begins with the patient being transferred to the preoperative area or holding area and ends with transfer to the recovery room. Nursing activities in this period center around patient safety, facilitation of procedure, prevention of any infection, and surgical intervention.

Better term is *perioperative nursing care*.

Perioperative nursing is a nursing specialized team that works for patients who are planned for operative or any invasive procedures. Perioperative nurses work closely with surgeons, anesthesiologists, and operation theater (OT) technologists. They deliver preoperative, intraoperative, and postoperative care primarily in the OT.

Preoperative Care in OT

Patient is kept in *preoperative holding area*, where nursing staff identifies and assesses the patient before transferring him or her to the OR.

Here nurses verify all relevant documentation such as history and clinical examination and signed consent form. Any requirement of blood products, implants, devices, and special equipment is made available. All the results of the diagnostic and radiology tests such as X-rays and biopsy reports are labeled and displayed.

When everything is up-to-date, patient is transferred to operation room bed. Nurses help in transferring the patient to and from OR, maintaining proper body alignment.

Intraoperative Care in OR

During this phase, the operation room is prepared for the patient.

Patient is monitored, anesthetized, prepped, and draped and the procedure is performed.

Experienced nursing teams trained with the equipment of each surgical team are very important for performing a smooth surgery and for reducing the risks of complications. Patient safety is the vital concern. Therefore, an intimate coordination between surgical and nursing teams and the anesthesiologists is required.

Responsibilities of OR Nurses

Responsibilities of the OR are shared by the scrub nurse and the circulating nurse.

The *scrub nurse* scrubs before the operation, sets up the sterile table, prepares sutures and special equipment, and helps the surgeon and his assistants throughout the surgery.

The *circulating nurse* manages the OR and monitors cleanliness, humidity, lighting, and safety of equipment. She is also responsible for coordinating the activities of OR personnel and monitoring the aseptic practices.

Other responsibilities during the intraoperative period are positioning of the patient, preparing the incision site, draping the patient, and documenting information such as surgical team information, assessment, the care and handling of specimens, and the count sheet.

Time Out for Safety (Surgical Safety Checklist)

The *"World Health Organization (WHO) Surgical Safety Checklist"* aims to decrease errors and adverse events and increase teamwork and communication in surgery **(Fig. 1)**. This includes three steps:

1. *Before induction of anesthesia*—the entire operative team performs a final verification of the correct patient, procedure to be carried out, and the surgical site.
2. *Before incision* is given—introduction of all the team members, confirmation of patient's name, procedure, antibiotic prophylaxis, and any anticipated critical events.
3. *After completion of surgery* and before shifting out the patient from OR—completion of instrument, sponge and needle count, and specimen labeling.

Two teams of nursing staff are important in microvascular free-flap surgeries, since two simultaneous procedures are performed and two surgical setups are planned. One team (*resection team*) focuses on the head and neck portion of the case in which all instruments are expected to be contaminated with cancer cells. A second team (*the harvest team*) with plastic and microvascular instruments is to be used to obtain the flap, which will fill the defect. Both teams work simultaneously, ensuring not to cross-contaminate the two

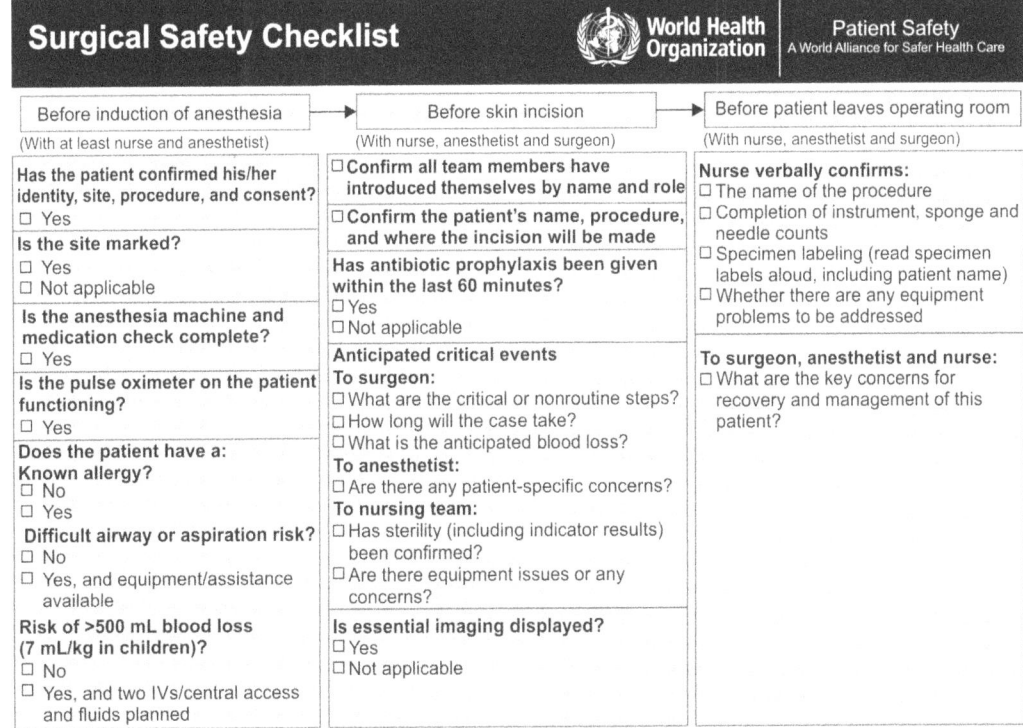

Fig. 1: World Health Organization (WHO) Surgical Safety Checklist.

surgical regions. The circulating nurse has to focus on maintaining the sterile technique throughout the OR and of each team member. It is his primary responsibility to inform each member of the team whenever there is a breach in sterile procedure and to immediately advise correction. At any point of time, the circulating nurse would manage 8-10 people in the sterile area, including surgeons from each team, fellows, residents, and scrub personnel.

Once the surgery is over, nurse secures dressing, drains, tubes, wipes blood off patient, position is corrected, if needed, patient is redressed, covered up, warm blankets given, patient transferred to stretcher, team members are needed to safely move patient to postoperative area, or recovery room on stretcher.

POSTOPERATIVE NURSING CARE IN OPERATION THEATER

The postoperative phase begins with the patient being transferred to the recovery room and ends with the resolution of the surgical outcome.

Here postanesthesia care, nurses assume responsibility for the patients. In this phase, nursing activities center on supporting care of the physiologic system of the patient.
- Cardiovascular—regular, strong heart rate and stable blood pressure (BP), peripheral pulses, and vital signs
- Neurological—level of consciousness, orientation, and sensation
- Fluid and electrolyte and acid-base balance
- Care of drains and tubes
- Medications as advised

Postoperative Nursing Care

It starts when patient is shifted from recovery room and ends once patient is discharged. Postoperatively, these patients will typically stay in the intensive care unit (ICU) for 2–3 days followed by a few more days in the ward.

Recovery may be difficult and patients are kept in bed rest with little mobilization for the first 2 days. They are not allowed to eat or drink for a minimum of 5 days after surgery and are often put on a ventilator from which they would be gradually weaned.

There are many different tubes and drains to be managed as well as pain. Mobilization of patient is begun 2 days after surgery but in few patients of free fibula, the period of immobilization is extended to 5 days.

Throughout postoperative period, the nurse will continuously monitor response of the patient to treatment, prevent complications, patient education, and promote optimum well-being.

The major risks in this type of surgeries are bleeding, infection, pain, problems with blood flow, loss of flap, leakage of saliva, and problems in wound healing.

As with any surgery, a patient who undergoes anesthesia and surgery faces the risks of stroke, heart attack, blood clots, and death.

It is the duty of nurse to timely inform the surgeon in case patient develops any complications in postoperative period.

Discharge plans: Nurses educate patient/family regarding dressing care and comfort, care of drains and tubes, diet, medicines regimen, i.e., antibiotics, analgesics, how to take care of oral hygiene, and fix next visit in follow-up period.

Positioning of patient:
- 30° head up
- Tilt to either side or neutral position as advised by treating surgeon
- Use gel-based head ring

Care of endotracheal tube:
- Fixing with dynaplast and support to be given while shifting to bed
- *Assessment for patency:*
  - Check air blast on dorsal aspect of hand
  - SpO_2
  - Excessive sweating/tachycardia
  - Abnormal breath sounds such as 'whistling'
  - Irregular breathing pattern
- Suctioning to be done as and when needed.
- Cuff of the tube to be kept inflated and pressure of cuff maintained at 15–25 cmH_2O.
- Humidified O_2 to be administered.
- Ventilator support as and when required.

Care of tracheostomy tube:
- Ensure fixing sutures are intact.
- Trachi-hold or nylon tapes which accompany tube packing should be used to keep it fixed to neck.
- Support tube during shifting of beds and changing of bedsheets/pillow/head ring or turning the patient for cleaning.
- *Suctioning* should be done based on the patient's respiratory status, the consistency of secretions and ability to cough/clear secretions from airway.
- *Use multiple-eyed catheters* because it causes less damage to the tracheal mucosa than the single-eyed catheter by dissipating the focus of suction pressure.
- *Size of catheters:* Tracheostomy size (inner diameter) × 1.5 = FG of suction catheter

- *Suctioning pressure:* Between 100 and 120 mm Hg.
- *Suctioning duration:* Less than 15 seconds.
- *Humidification:* Humidify the inspired air using
  - Humidifier system—heated or non-heated
  - Heat moisture exchanger (HME) filter
  - Simple gauze piece in a single/double layer soaked wet in normal saline/clean water
  - Laryngeal bib wet over the area covering the opening of tube
- *Cuff pressure:*
  - Check eight-hourly.
  - Maintain the cuff pressure between 15 and 25 cmH_2O
- Inflate cuff of tracheostomy tube only if indicated (e.g., on ventilator support or on high risk for aspiration).
- Inspect the inner cannula at least 6-hourly to ensure patency.
- *Stoma care:*
  - Ensure dressing to be dry, change stoma dressing and tapes daily and/or whenever soiled.
  - *Signs and symptoms of stoma infection:*
    - Excessive leakage of secretions
    - Foul smelling discharge
    - Erosions/ulceration around stoma site
- Nebulization with normal saline every 6 hourly
- *Assess for airway patency:*
  - Check air blast on dorsal aspect of hand
  - SpO_2
- *Signs of tube blockage:*
  - Excessive sweating/tachycardia
  - Abnormal breath sounds such as "whistling"

- Irregular breathing pattern
- Increase in coughing
- Inability to cough
- Cyanosis/deterioration in oxygen saturation
- *Signs of tube displacement*:
  - All signs of tube blockage
  - Obstruction to passage of a suction catheter/bougie
- *Tube dislodgement/displacement*:
  - Partial—when tube comes out of the trachea into the soft tissue of the neck
  - Complete—when tube comes out of the stoma
  How to manage?
  - Ensure cuffed tube is deflated and provide patient with supplemental oxygen via facemask.
  - Call for help
  - Proper light source must be arranged. Reinsertion of tracheostomy tube done using tracheal dilator and rail roading technique over a bougie.
  - A flexible fiber-optic laryngoscope may be used for identifying trachea and rail-roading tube over it. This additionally helps in tracheobronchial toileting if required.
  - Emergency oral intubation may be done if reinsertion of tracheostomy tube fails.
- *Tube obstruction*:
  How to manage?
  - Ask the patient to cough
  - Remove inner cannula and change it
  - Apply suctioning to remove the secretions
  - Ventilate the patient (and secure airway patency)
  - Deflate the cuff tube bag and mask ventilate patient
  - Call for medical help
  - Prepare for change of tracheostomy tube or oral intubation.

- *Weaning criteria*:
  - Reversal of the medical condition that originally necessitated the procedure
  - Adequate ventilatory reserve
  - Patent upper airway
  - Adequate nutritional state
  - Ability to cough and clear airway secretions
  - Absence of respiratory infection
  - Observe for any signs of increased respiratory distress such as noisy breathing, and hypoxia during the weaning procedure and thereafter.
  - If signs of respiratory distress or aspiration noted then reinsertion of tracheostomy tube is done.

Ryles tube care:
- *Feeding tube selection*:
  - Size 14/16 Fr
  - Polyurethane or silicone tubes for long-term feeding (4–8 weeks)
  - Polyvinylchloride tubes for short-term feeding (<3 weeks), decompression and lavage
- Fixing with adhesives to dorsum of nose
- *Feeding tube placement*:
  - A positive air insufflations test combined with aspiration of gastric contents is a reliable predictor of successful placement.
  - X-ray is the most accurate method of checking tube placement.
  - Regular assessment of feeding tube placement is important because a tube can be partially pulled out during movement. Tube malposition may be caused by faulty initial placement or upward dislocation after bouts of coughing or vomiting.
- *Maintaining tube patency*:
  - Flush feeding tubes with 30 mL of water before and after intermittent feeding, every 4-hourly during continuous feeding and after checking for gastric residue.

- Residue, containing gastric aspirate with an average pH of 4.6 or less interacts with protein formula to form clots. Formula residue that adheres to the tube lumen may cause tube clogging. Thus flushing the tube with water will maintain the patency by eliminating acid precipitation of formula in the feeding tube.
- *Preparation of formula feeds and delivery system*:
  - Wash hands before preparing and handling delivery sets.
  - Use pre-prepared feeds for enteral feeding.
  - Gravity feeding bags may be used for feeding.
- *Feeding position*: The patient should be placed at a semi-recumbent position or elevated to an angle of at least 30° during and after feeding for at least 1 hour.
- *Quantity*: We generally start RT feed on postoperative day 1 @ 250 mL every 3 hourly and supplement IV fluids. On postoperative day 2 we stop IV fluids and give RT feeds @ 300 mL every 2 hourly.
- *Continuous feeding*: Use feeding pump for administration of continuous feeds. Start with an initial slow rate of 10–40 mL/hour. Advance to the goal rate by increasing the rate by 10–20 mL/hour every 8–12 hours as tolerated.
- *Administration of medications*:
  - Enteric-coated and sustained release medications should not be crushed.
  - Medications administered through nasogastric tube should preferably be in liquid form.
  - Flushing the feeding tube prior to drug administration removes any enteral feeds that remain in the tube to prevent drug nutrient interaction.
  - Medications should not be added directly to the enteral formula or into the enteral feeding bag.
- *Management of feeding intolerance*: When patient shows signs of feeding intolerance such as nausea, vomiting, abdominal distension and pain, feeds may be stopped for few hours and restarted with hourly slow feeding.
- *Declogging*: Use warm water to declog obstructed feeding tubes. If unsuccessful, pancreatic enzyme with sodium bicarbonate may be used.
- *Treatment of diarrhea*:
  - Do not dilute enteral feeds.
  - Use enteral feeds with soluble fiber
- *Aspiration pneumonia*: Signs/symptoms
  - Unexplained fever spikes
  - Changes in sputum color or consistency
  - Changes in breath sounds
  - Worsening oxygenation and setbacks in ventilator weaning.

Drain care:
- Tubing should remain free of kinks, debris and clots so as to enhance free drainage.
- The drain should be secured well so as to avoid falling off or its migration into the cavity or erosion of surrounding tissue. Ensure that the drain is fixed to the skin and not to gown of patient.
- Drain should be lower than the incision at all times.
- Skin care and aseptic technique must be observed during application and change of dressing over drains.
- Gauze pieces are used around and over drainage tubes, to protect the tube, absorb some amount of drainage, assist with the stabilization of the tube and help to protect from external contamination.
- Measurement and record keeping of drainage output and color must be ensured.

Oral hygiene: We advice povidone iodine and hydrogen peroxide mouth wash to be used alternately @ 2 hourly.

KEY POINTS

- Free-flap reconstruction for extensive defects due to malignant composite oral cavity resections requires a coordinated multidisciplinary team to deliver care before, during, and after surgery.
- Preoperative care is the preparation and management of a patient prior to surgery.
- In this phase, patient is explained, planned, and prepared for the surgery by the nurses as per the order of the surgeon incharge.
- Intraoperative nursing care begins when the patient is transferred to the preoperative area or holding area and ends with transfer to the recovery room.
- Nursing activities in this period center on patient safety, facilitation of procedure, prevention of infection, and satisfactory surgical intervention.
- Better term is perioperative nursing care.
- Postoperative nursing care starts when patient is shifted from recovery room and ends once patient is discharged.
- Throughout postoperative period, the nurse will always—monitor patient's response to therapeutic regimen, prevent complications, patient education, and promote optimum well-being.

CHAPTER 14

The Lip

Hemant T Bhoye

FUNCTIONS OF LIPS

- Contain and prevent spillage of oral secretions and food bolus
- Help in deglutition
- Speech coordination
- Facial expression of emotions

ANATOMY

- Area between both nasolabial folds from under the nose till upper gingivobuccal sulcus and from chin till lower gingivobuccal sulcus **(Fig. 1)**.
- *Muscle*: Orbicularis oris (circular muscle) forms bulk and other synergistic group of levators and depressors arranged radially.
- *Blood supply*: From both sides, the superior and inferior labial vessels which are branches of facial artery **(Figs. 2A and B)**.

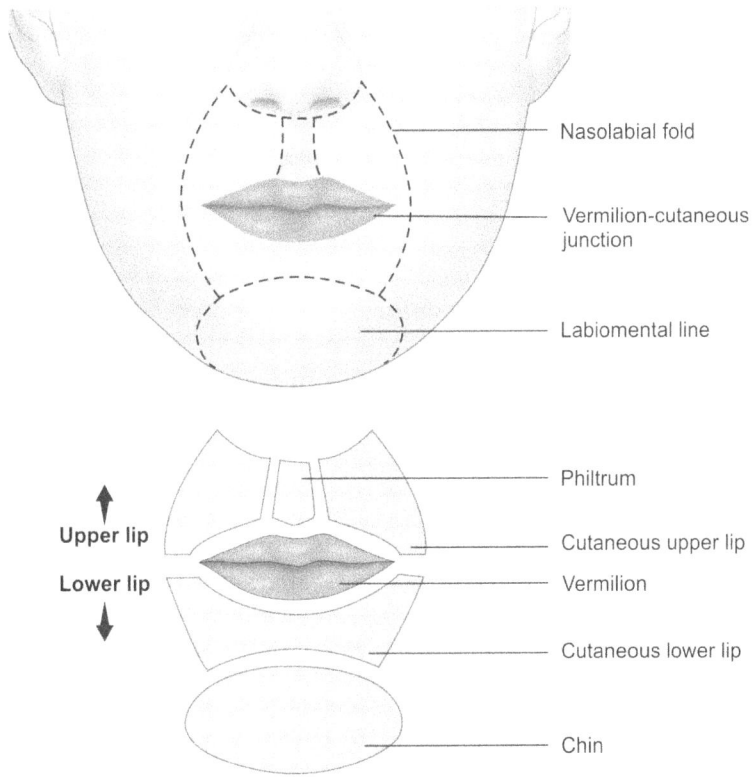

Fig. 1: Lip landmarks.

The Lip

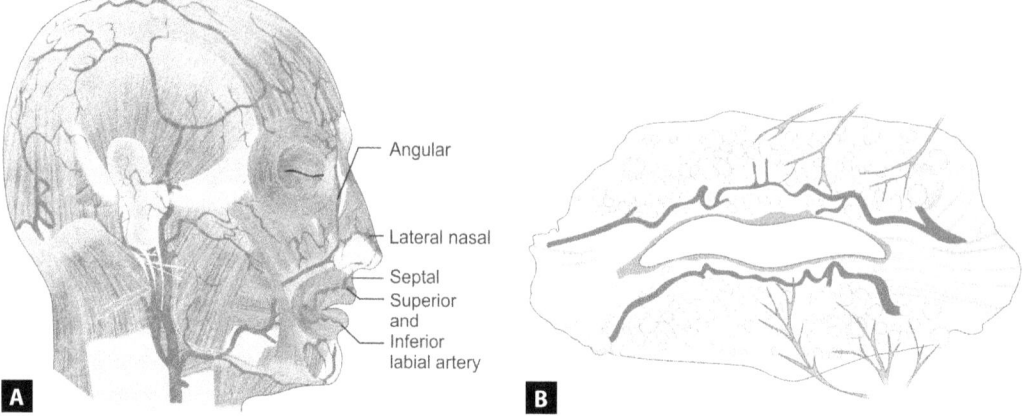

Figs. 2A and B: Vascular anatomy of lip.

- *Lymphatic drainage*: To submental and submandibular lymph nodes.
- *Nerve supply*:
  - *Motor—Facial nerve*:
    - Buccal branch—elevator
    - Marginal mandibular—depressor
  - *Sensory—Trigeminal nerve*:
    - Maxillay—infraorbital—upper lip
    - Mandibular—inferior alveolar—lower lip

COMMON MALIGNANCIES ON LIPS

- *Upper lip*: Cutaneous part—basal cell carcinoma
- *Lower lip*: Squamous cell carcinoma

PRINCIPLES OF CANCER RESECTION IN LIP

- Cancer cure should prioritize over reconstruction and esthetic aspect.
- Tissue conservation is also important and can be achieved by tumor extirpation using Mohs micrographic surgery.
- Borders of subunits of lips give good camouflage after resection, if the resection margins can be placed along it.

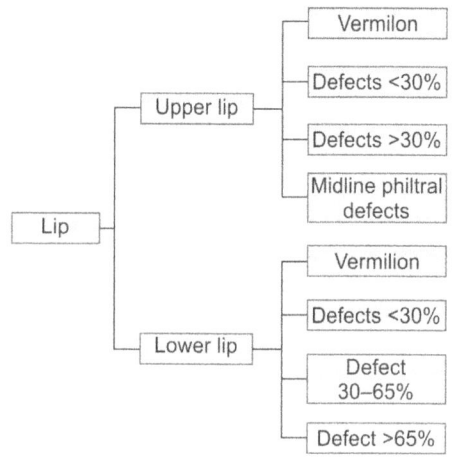

Flowchart 1: Full-thickness lip defects.

LIP DEFECTS

Classification

Depending upon the tissue component resected:
- Full-thickness defects
- Partial-thickness defects

Full-thickness defects can be further classified **(Flowchart 1)**.

GOALS OF LIP RECONSTRUCTION

- Maintain oral competence
- Restore sensation of lip

- Maintain continuity of vermilion border (white roll)
- Provide adequate size of mouth opening
- Restore esthetic appearance of lip

GENERAL RULES OF LIP RECONSTRUCTION

- Defects up to 30% of upper or lower lip can be closed primarily with minimal microstomia, which is due to excellent elasticity of lip tissue.
- Defects >30% of the lip need to be reconstructed by addition of tissue from opposite lip or adjacent area.
- Defects >60% of lip require either combination of two or more adjacent sites or distant tissue.
- In general, for upper lip defects, lower lip tissue can be used as flap but vice versa should be avoided.
- Good orbicularis muscle approximation is necessary to restore competence. If the muscle cannot be restored in its continuity, dynamic slings such as palmaris longus tendon or strip of deep fascia should be placed in the defect.
- Vermilion border (white roll) continuity restoration alone can give esthetically pleasing lip appearance.

RECONSTRUCTIVE STRATEGIES FOR LIP DEFECTS

Partial-thickness Lip Defects

- *Secondary healing*:
  - Small raw area around the subunit borders can be left to heal by secondary intention. It should not be wider than 0.5 cm in maximum dimensions.
  - Mucosal raw areas (wet vermilion) can be left to heal by secondary intention.
  - Chances of infection and hypertrophic scarring

- *Primary suturing*:
  - Superficial defects up to 1.5–2 cm can be closed by primary suturing.
  - Local tissue advancement, "Z" plasty, "M" plasty, or "W" plasty suturing technique can be incorporated to achieve esthetically pleasing outcomes.
  - Underlying muscle layer is freed from skin by dissection while advancing the skin flap.
- *Skin graft*:
  - Both split-thickness skin graft and full-thickness skin graft can be used.
  - The upper lip skin defects can be better covered with full-thickness graft harvested from hair-bearing portion of neck or scalp in male patients to achieve hair growth to replace mustaches.
  - Defects in central region of upper lip (area between philtral column) and near the Cupid's bow can be covered with concave skin perichondral graft harvested from the ear.

Full-thickness Lip Defects

- Full-thickness lip defects involving lip vermilion, orbicularis muscle, and skin require restoration in layers.
- Restoration of continuity of orbicularis oris muscle is most essential for oral competence.
- If large segment of lower lip (>50%) is lost due to resection, orbicularis oris muscle continuity may not be possible to restore. In such cases, a deep fascia or tendon (palmaris longus) is used to restore continuity. Orbicularis muscle medially and tendon can be used as adynamic laterally sling sutured across the lip defect.
- The sling is fixed to periosteum of zygomatic bone and care is taken to maintain

appropriate tension in the sling, so that the lip seal is restored.

Vermilion Defects

The vermilion defects must be closed with "like" tissue to achieve good cosmetic outcomes.

- *Primary closure*: Deliberate V-shaped resection of primary lesion of vermilion allows primary closure by simple advancement owing to its elasticity (**Figs. 3A and B**).
- *Myomucosal advancement*: The buccal part of lip mucosa can be used as local flap along with underlying muscle to cover vermilion defect (**Figs. 4A to C**).
- *Transverse vermilion advancement*: Vermilion defects up to 35% can be closed by transverse vermilion advancement (**Figs. 5A and B**).
- *Lower lip vermilion flap*: For upper lip vermilion defects, lower lip vermilion flap can be raised since lower lip has larger vermilion. The opposite, however, is not recommended (**Figs. 6A to C**).

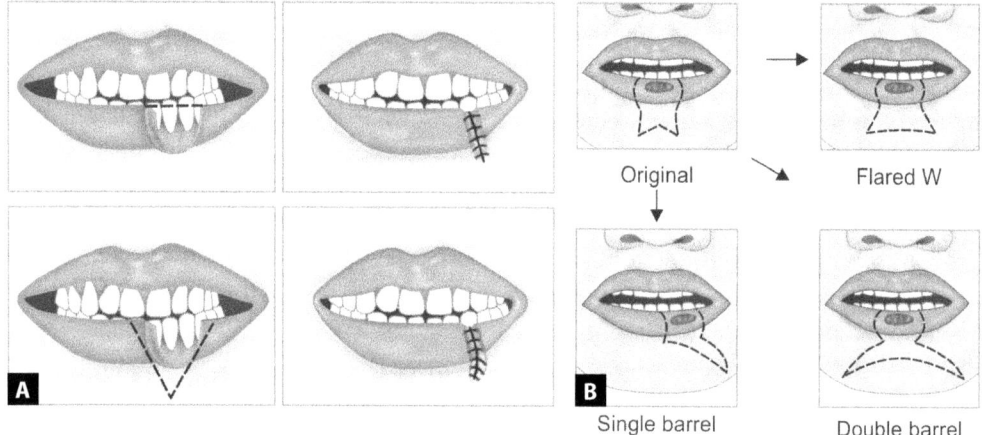

Figs. 3A and B: Primary repair of lip.

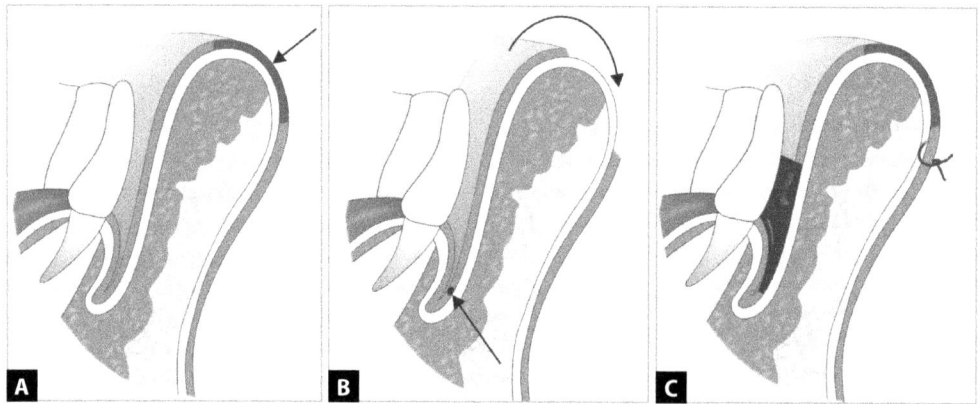

Figs. 4A to C: Buccoalveolar groove of myomucosal advancement for vermilion defect.

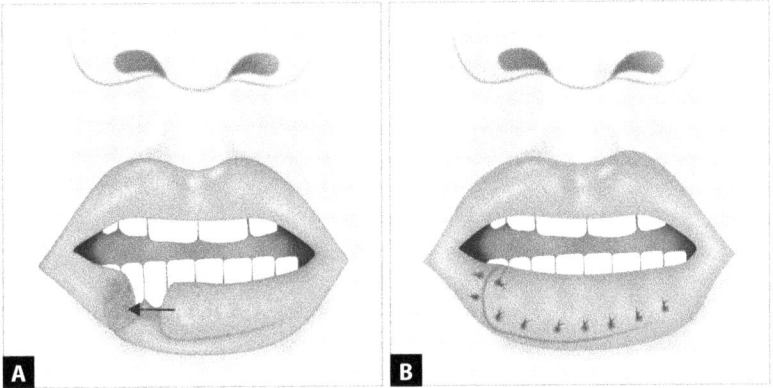

Figs. 5A and B: Transverse myomucosal advancement.

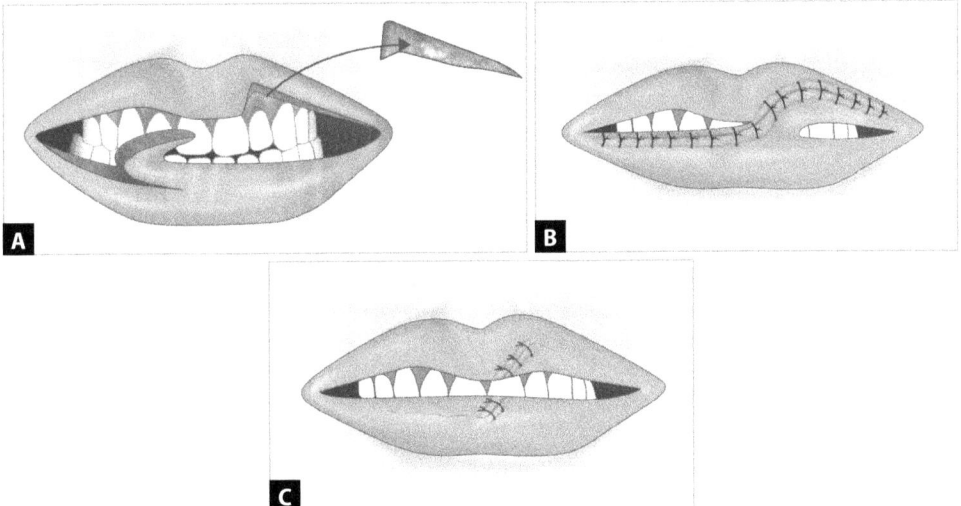

Figs. 6A to C: Cross vermilion flap.

- *Tongue flap for vermilion defect*: Flap can be raised from ventral tongue to cover the defect over lower lip vermilion in staged manner **(Figs. 7A to D)**.
- *Buccal myomucosal flap*:
  - Buccal mucosal flap along with submucosal muscle based on branches of facial vessels and the flap is rotated to fill the ipsilateral vermilion defect providing it identical mucosal lining. This is especially useful for commissural defects **(Figs. 8 and 9)**.
  - Absolute essential prerequisite criteria for buccal myomucosal flap are normal and healthy mucosa.

Upper Lip Defects

- Full-thickness defects of upper lip should be very carefully restored to its near original form, as it is most noticeable part of lip esthetic unit.
- There is paucity of tissue thickness and more defined landmarks such as lip roll, philtral columns, and Cupid's bow.

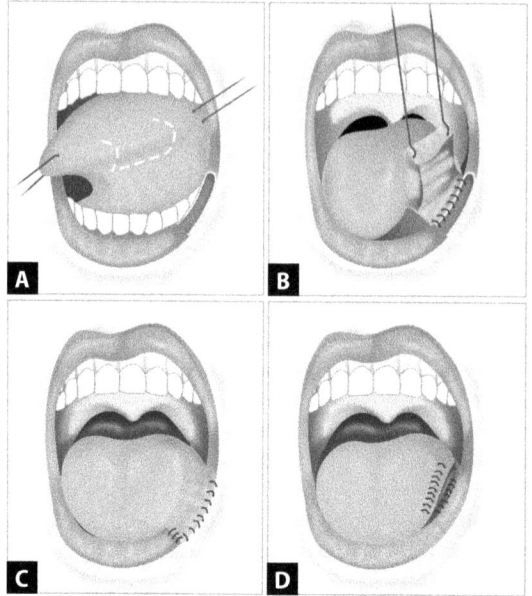

Figs. 7A to D: Tongue flap for vermilion defects.

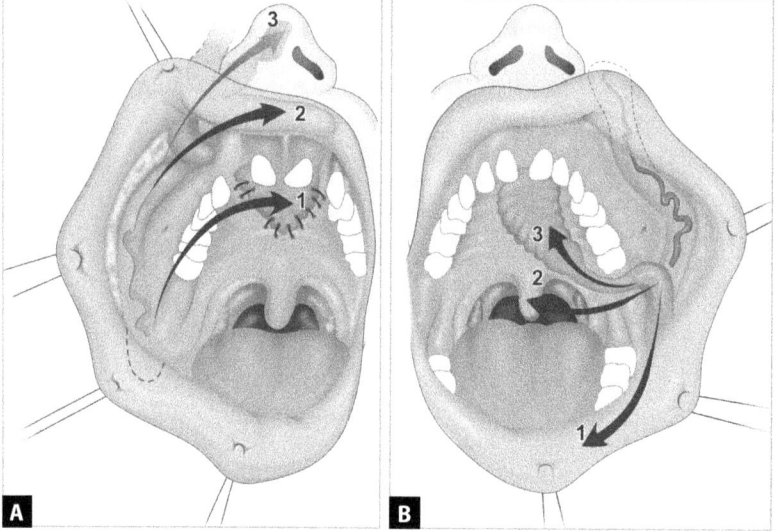

Figs. 8A and B: Buccal myomucosal flap and its utility.

- Most important principle of reconstruction of upper lip defects is placement of the suture lines along the boundaries of the esthetic units.
- Upper lip defects are divided into central and lateral esthetic subunits.
- The two lateral subunits lie between the nasolabial fold and the philtral column on either side.
- A small full-thickness defect measuring up to 0.5–1.5 cm (up to approximately one-third of lip) can be sutured primarily.

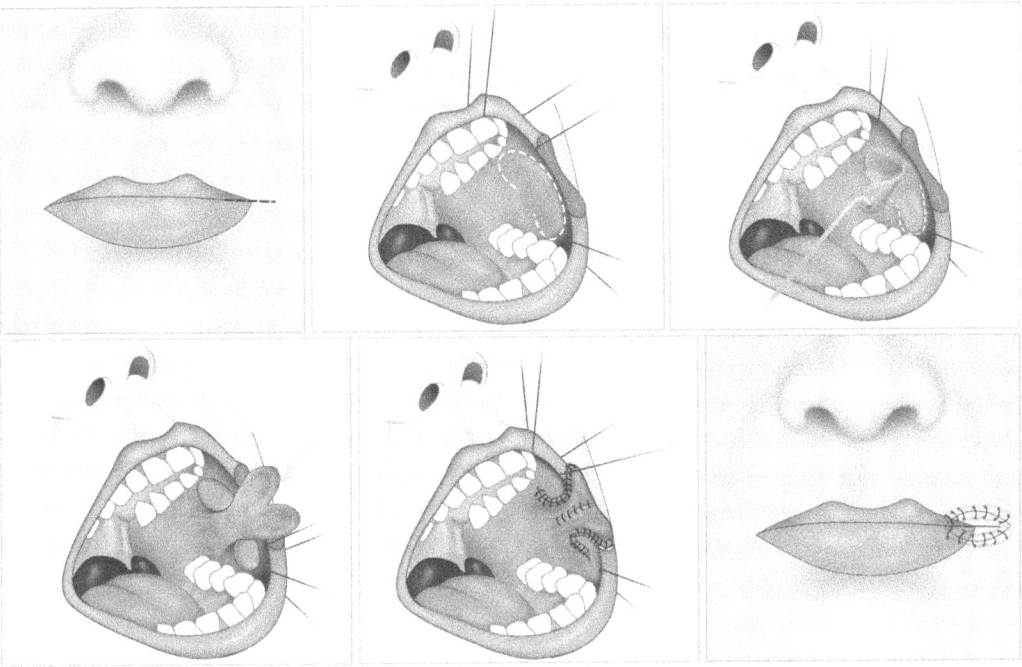

Fig. 9: Commissural reconstruction with buccal myomucosal flap.

- Defect of larger than 1.5 cm or more than one-third of lip needs reconstruction by local flap.
- *Abbe flap*:
  - The flap is based on labial vessels, which run submucosally in vermilion of lip.
  - The flap is harvested from the lower lip and done in staged manner.
  - The size of the flap is always half of what the actual upper lip defect is and the rest of the defect is easily closed due to elasticity of the lip itself.
  - Both central and lateral lip defects can be reconstructed using the Abbe flap technique **(Figs. 10A and B)**.
  - The flap for central upper lip defect needs division after 14 days, while lateral lip defect (involving commissure) is single-stage procedure.
  - Defects between 30 and 50% can be reconstructed.

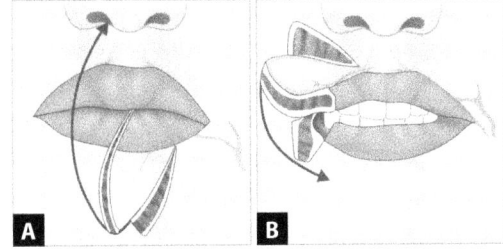

Figs. 10A and B: Abbe flap for central lip defect (A) and lateral lip defect (B).

- *Gillies fan flap* **(Figs. 11A to D)**:
  - It is a modification of the Estlander flap which is used for lower lip reconstruction.
  - It is based on nasolabial flap principle.
- *Bernard's burrow or alar crescent excision* **(Figs. 12A and B)**:
  - It essentially gains length in remnant upper lip tissue after excision of the tumor.

- Crescents of tissue or burrow adjacent to the nasal alae is excised and the lateral lip is advanced to center for lip reconstruction.
- The vermilion, if deficient, can be reconstructed with buccal myomucosal flap or lower vermilion flap.
- *Reverse Karapandzic flap (Fig. 13)*:
  - Flap is based on lower labial vessel
  - The commissure is recreated
- Microstomia is a disadvantage
- Both unilateral and bilateral flap can be used depending on the size of the flap.
- *Kazanjian and Converse reverse cheek flap (Fig. 14)*: Now rarely done due to its poor esthetic outcomes and chances of marginal necrosis.
- *Combination of flaps (Figs. 15A to C)*: Two local flaps can be combined to reconstruct entire upper lip.
- *Microvascular free flap*:
  - In some cases, where there is total upper lip excision along with buccal mucosa, microvascular free flap is required for the reconstruction of such large defect.
  - Free flap need to have qualities such as thin, supple skin paddle and long vascular pedicle that can reach the neck easily for anastomosis.
  - Radial artery forearm flap (Fig. 16) and anterolateral thigh flap (especially in thin individuals) are flaps of choice in upper lip reconstruction.

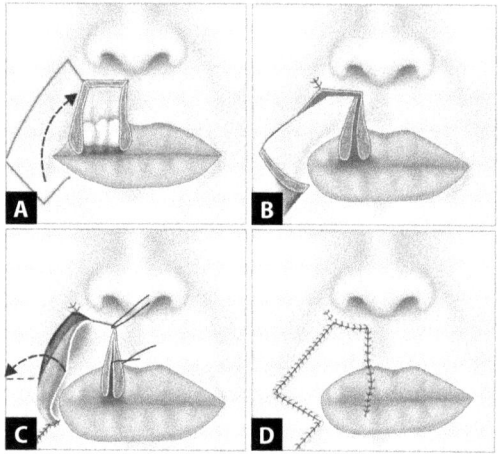

Figs. 11A to D: Gillies fan flap for upper lip.

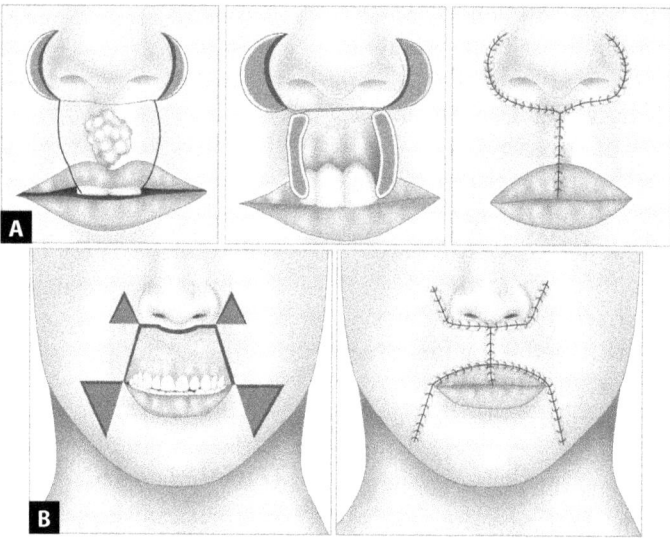

Figs. 12A and B: Perialar excision advancement flap. (A) Perialar crescent excision; (B) Perialar burrow triangle excision (Bernard).

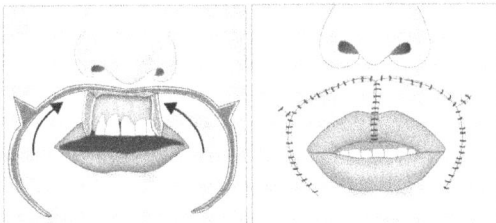

Fig. 13: Bilateral Karapandzic flap.

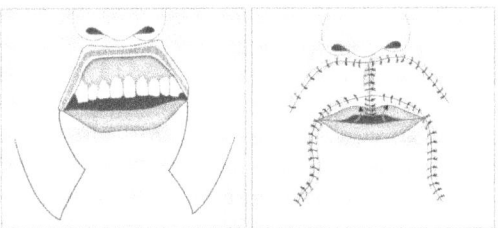

Fig. 14: Kazanjian flap: Kazanjian and converse technique of superiorly-based lower cheek flaps.

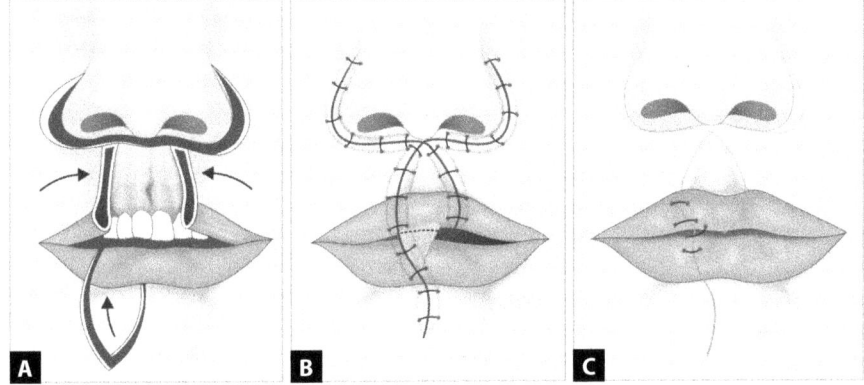

Figs. 15A to C: Celsus method: Lateral lip units by perialar crescent and central with Abbe flap.

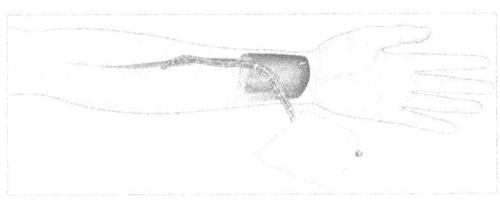

Fig. 16: Outline of radial artery forearm flap.

Lower Lip Defects

- Lower lip has ample of expansile tissue including more tortuous course of labial vessels and thicker musculature.
- The esthetic boundaries are less conspicuous as compared to the upper lip.
- This enables us to utilize the lower lip tissue as flap for upper lip reconstruction.
- It is much easier to plan a primary reconstruction of lower lip defects.
- For any local flap reconstruction in lower lip defects, very important prerequisite is to have intact facial artery (which may have to be ligated during the neck lymph node dissection).
- *Defects < 30% of the lip*:
  - Primary repair is almost always done.
  - The incision is planned to have esthetically pleasing suture line and the scar.
  - A "V" or "W"-shaped incision or its modification is best suited for the primary closure **(Fig. 17)**.
- *Defects 30–65% of the lip*:
  - For defects in lateral lip region and commissural region:
    - *Estlander flap* **(Fig. 18)**:
      - Commissure is shifted.
      - The upper lip adjacent to the commissure now becomes part of lower lip.

- *Nasolabial flap (Fig. 19)*:
  - More common flap to restore lateral third defects of lower lip.
  - Full-thickness flap with little extra mucosa is taken, which is used for vermilion recreation.
- *Karapandzic flap*:
  - Unilateral Karapandzic flap can be used **(Fig. 20)**.
  - Microstomia is common.
- *Johanson's step ladder advancement* **(Figs. 21A to C)**
- *Unilateral Gillies fan flap* **(Figs. 22A and B)**: It distorts the commissure and microstomia can occur.
- *McGregor or Nakajima flap* **(Figs. 23A and B)**:
  - Similar to Gillies flap.
  - Major differences are both preserve the neurovascular pedicle and microstomia is not created as both methods are rotation flap not simple advancement.
- Defects > 65%:
  - Subtotal to total lip defects.
  - Require local flap from both sides.
  - Both facial arteries should be intact for local flap reconstruction.
  - *Bilteral Karapandzic flap* **(Fig. 24)**: Though the neurovascualr bundle is preserved, microstomia is severe.

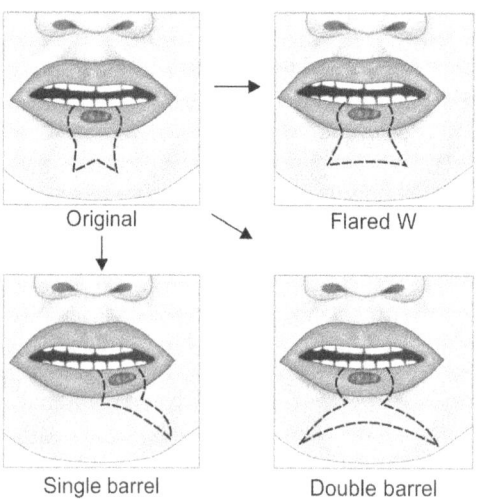

Fig. 17: Incision planning for primary closure of the lower lip defects.

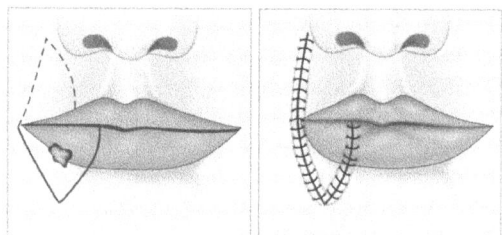

Fig. 18: Estlander flap.

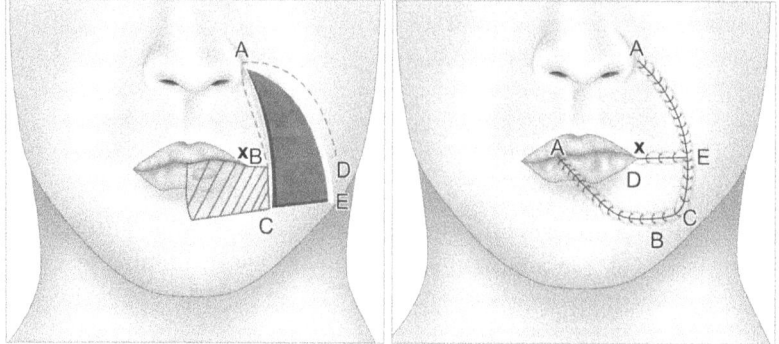

Fig. 19: Fugimori type unilateral nasolabial flap (dotted line represents mucosal incision).

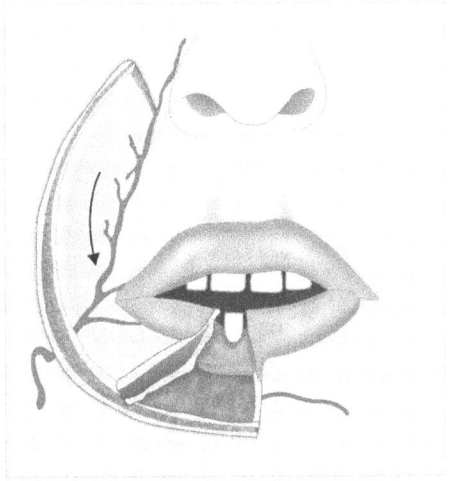

Fig. 20: Unilateral Karapandzic flap.

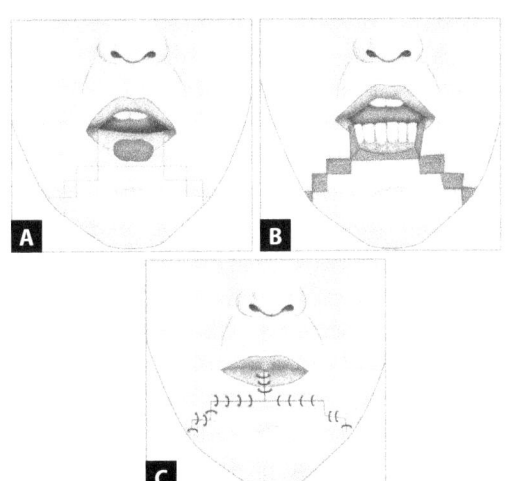

Figs. 21A to C: Johanson's step ladder flap.

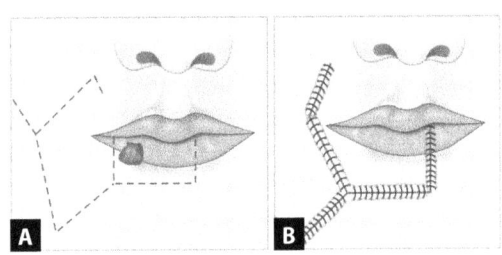

Figs. 22A and B: Gillies fan flap.

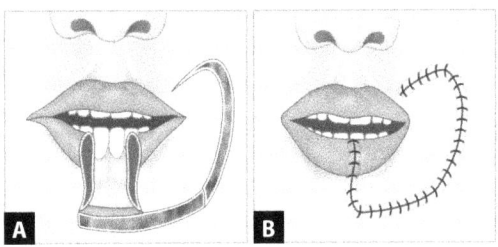

Figs. 23A and B: McGregor flap.

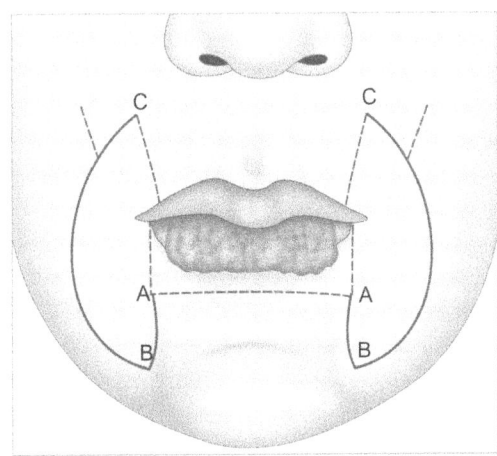

Fig. 24: Bilateral Karapandzic flap.

- *Bilateral Fujimori gate flap* (**Figs. 25A and B**)
- *Von Brown bilateral nasolabial advancement flap* (**Fig. 26**)
- *Bernard, Grimm, and Fries flap* (**Fig. 27**):
  - After Burrow's triangles of skin are cut, the underlying orbicularis oris muscle for upper lip is resected and rerouted toward lower lip via tunnel and, thus, elongates the vermilion.
  - Care is taken not to damage the neurovascular bundle supplying the muscle.

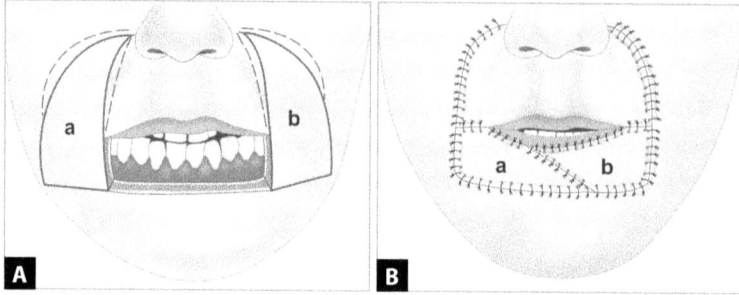

Figs. 25A and B: Bilateral Fujimori gate flap.

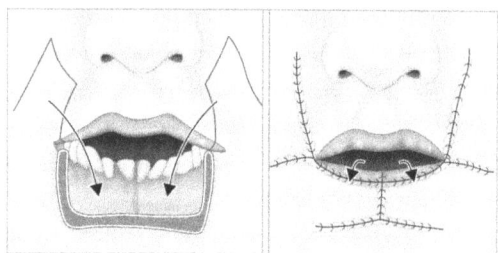

Fig. 26: Bilateral nasolabial flaps.

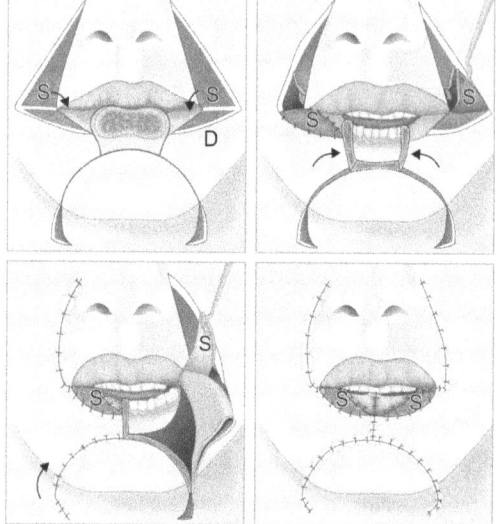

Fig. 27: Bernard, Grimm, and Fries flap.

- *Platysma (submental) flap (Figs. 28A to D)*: Bilobed flap design is used to reconstruct the lower lip defect.
- *Free microvascular flap*: Radial forearm flap, medial sural artery perforator flap, anterolateral thigh flap, and lateral arm flap are the options for lip reconstruction.

Advantages

- Free flap provides ample amount of tissue that is required for lip defects of any size.
- There is no restriction of flap mobility, arc of rotation, and limitation of flap size.
- Vascularity of flap is not dependent of the local tissue vascularity such as locoregional flaps.
- Microstomia does not occur with free-flap reconstruction, which is common with local flaps.

Disadvantages

- Vascular anastomosis needs expertise and has steep learning curve.
- The free-flap surgery demands specialized operative setup and instruments, especially microinstruments and operative microscope.
- The operative procedure involves two teams: (1) Oncosurgery and (2) Reconstructive surgery.
- Despite the expertise in anastomosis, the flap suffers risk of anastomotic complications because of various factors such as pedicle length, vessel quality, blood hypercoagulation, external compression, hematoma, and pre-existing radiation status.
- No matter how much tissue free-flap can provide for lip reconstruction, it is difficult

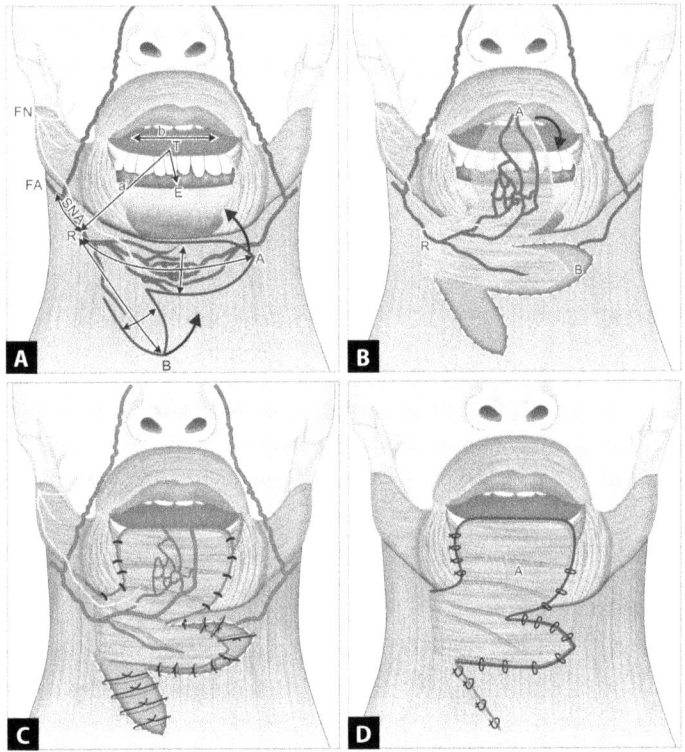

Figs. 28A to D: Platysma flap.

to reconstruct esthetic subunits such as vermilion, white roll, Cupid's bow, and philtral column.
- The lip patency can be a problem if a static sling of palmaris longus tendon or deep fascia is not placed under adequate tension across the lip defect, while doing free-flap reconstruction resulting in spillage of oral contents and difficulty in speech.

KEY POINTS

- Cancer cure should prioritize over reconstruction and esthetic aspect.
- *Goals of lip reconstruction* include maintenance of oral competence, restoration of sensation of lip, maintaining continuity of vermilion border (white roll), providing adequate-sized mouth opening, and restoration of esthetic appearance of lip.
- Defects up to 30% of upper or lower lip can be closed primarily with minimal microstomia, which is due to excellent elasticity of lip tissue.
- Defects > 30% of the lip need to be reconstructed by addition of tissue from opposite lip or adjacent area.
- Full-thickness lip defects involving lip vermilion, orbicularis muscle, and skin require restoration in layers.
- The size of the flap is always half of what the actual upper lip defect is and the rest of the defect is easily closed due to elasticity of the lip itself.
- Both central and lateral lip defects can be reconstructed using the Abbe flap technique.
- A variety of flaps such as *Abbe flap, Gillies fan flap, Bernard's burrow or alar crescent excision, reverse Karapandzic flap, Kazanjian and Converse reverse cheek flap, and microvascular free flap* can be used for upper lip reconstruction.
- Flaps for lower lip reconstruction include *Estlander flap, nasolabial flap, Karapandzic flap, Johanson's step ladder advancement, unilateral Gillies fan flap, McGregor or Nakajima flap, bilateral Fugimori's flap, platysma (submental) flap, and free microvascular flap.*

Management of Buccal Mucosa and Retromolar Trigone Cancer

Vishal Yadav

INTRODUCTION

- Buccal mucosa (BM) cancer constitutes 10% of all head and neck cancers and 41% of all oral cavity cancers. This is in contrast to the site wise incidence of oral cancers seen in the West, where cancers of the anterior tongue and floor of the mouth form the bulk of oral cancers.
- Majority of BM cancers encountered (80%) are in stages III and IV at presentation.
- The reported 5-year survival rates for BM cancers in India range from 80% for stage I disease to 5–15% for locally advanced disease.

SURGICAL ANATOMY (FIG. 1)

- The BM includes the pliable inner lining of cheek extending from the maxillary alveolus superiorly to the mandibular alveolus inferiorly. Posteriorly, the BM is contiguous with retromolar trigone (RMT).
- The layers of the buccal region are BM, submucosa, buccinator muscle, subcutaneous fat, and cheek skin. Once a lesion is deep enough to invade the buccinator muscle, the overlying cheek skin is potentially involved. Resection frequently results in through-and-through defect requiring flap coverage.
- Deep posterior invasion from both buccal and RMT tumors extends toward the masseteric space. Meticulous attention to this potential direction of spread is required to avoid local recurrence.
- The RMT mucosa provides reasonably thin cover over ascending ramus of

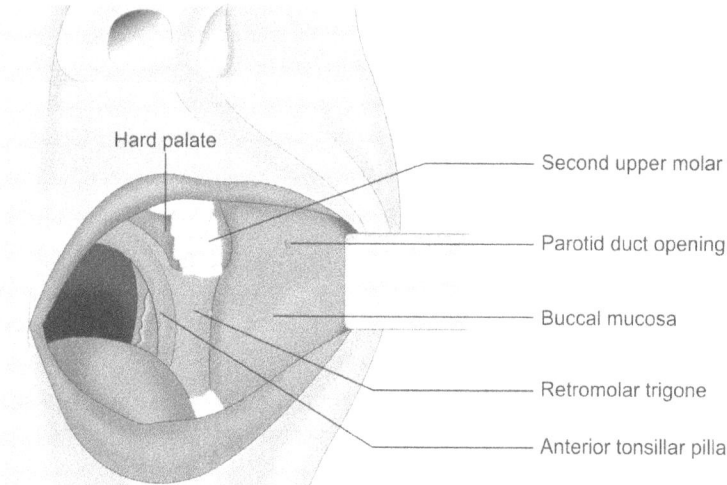

Fig. 1: Anatomy of buccal mucosa.

mandible. Larger tumors quickly invade the bone and continue into masticator space.
- Retromolar trigone tumors often extend posteriorly into the oropharynx. Many clinicians consider the biological behavior to be more consistent with oropharyngeal carcinoma than oral cavity carcinoma.
- Stenson's duct opens in the BM adjacent to the second upper molar tooth after crossing the masseter muscle and passing through the buccinator muscle. Duct stenting should be done to prevent the risk of salivary leak.
- *Arterial supply*: The BM is supplied by the facial and buccal arteries. The buccal artery originates from the pterygoid branch of the maxillary artery. The inferior alveolar artery is a branch of the mandibular branch of the maxillary artery and enters the mandibular canal to supply the inferior alveolus. The superior alveolus is supplied by the posterior superior alveolar artery, a branch of the pterygopalatine segment of the maxillary artery.
- *Venous drainage*: The pterygoid plexus drains into the facial vein, which eventually drains into the internal jugular vein.
- *Lymphatics*: The BM drains into the deep cervical nodes. Level IB (submandibular nodes) is the first echelon of lymphatic spread of tumor.
- *Innervation*: Sensory supply is via the maxillary and mandibular divisions of the trigeminal nerve. Motor supply to the muscles of mastication is by the mandibular nerve; the buccinator muscle is innervated by the buccal branch of the facial nerve.

CLINICAL RELEVANCE

- Involvement of masticator space (MS) is considered to be locally very advanced disease, i.e., T4b stage.
- Infratemporal fossa (ITF) involvement can be either "high" or "low." Tumors involving the high ITF (involving lateral pterygoid and temporalis muscles) are considered unresectable because tumor can escape through the pterygomaxillary and inferior orbital fissures making the possibility of complete (R0) resection unlikely.

STAGING

The stage of cancers of the BM is based on the size of the primary tumor along with involvement of surrounding structures, depth of invasion, cervical lymph node status, and distant metastases [2018 American Joint Committee on Cancer (AJCC) revised cancer stage groupings for oral cavity squamous cell carcinoma (SCC)] **(Box 1)**.

Box 1: Salient features.

Changes in new American Joint Committee on Cancer (AJCC) staging, 8th edition:
- *Inclusion of depth of invasion in T staging*:
  - 5 mm = T1
  - 5–10 mm = T2
  - >10 mm = T3
- Including depth of invasion in oral cavity will better discriminate the higher-risk small cancers as demonstrated by deeply invasive tumors from those with less invasive cancers that have an excellent prognosis **(Fig. 2)**
- *Inclusion of clinical and pathological extranodal extension (ENE)*:
  - Clinical ENE upgrade stage to cN3b
  - Pathological ENE in single node < 3 cm = pN2a
  - Pathological ENE in single node > 3 cm or multiple ipsilateral or bilateral node = pN3b

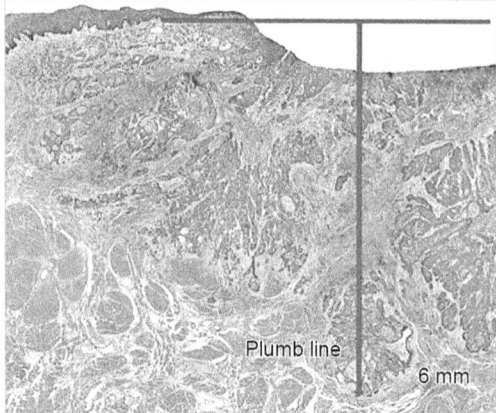

Fig. 2: Depth of invasion in an ulcerated carcinoma. Note how "tumor thickness" would be deceptively thinner than depth of invasion.

PREOPERATIVE EVALUATION

A combination of clinical assessment (under anesthesia, if indicated) and imaging is required to evaluate buccal lesions and to assess resectability and to plan the extent of resection.

UNRESECTABLE CANCERS

- Extension into IFT up to the lateral pterygoid and temporalis muscles (evaluated on imaging as lesion extending superior to sigmoid notch)
- Skull base involvement and intracranial extension
- Perineural invasion along V3 to foramen ovale or to trigeminal ganglion
- Significant oropharyngeal involvement with encasement of great vessels
- Unresectable nodal disease, encasement of great vessels, and prevertebral fascia involvement

Factors to be considered when planning a resection:
- Incisions to approach the tumor
- Management of mandible and maxilla
- Paramandibular disease
- Deep soft-tissue infiltration

IMAGING OF BUCCAL MUCOSAL CANCERS

- Tumor abutting mandible to determine presence of bone invasion
- Tumors involving RMT to assess involvement of IFT
- Deep-seated buccal mucosal lesion to assess involvement of the MS
- Severe trismus that precludes proper clinical assessment

Imaging

- *Orthopantomogram (OPG)*: Requires a loss of up to 30% of bony cortex to detect mandibular invasion (poor sensitivity)
- *Magnetic resonance imaging (MRI)*:
  - Superior soft-tissue delineation compared to computed tomography (CT)
  - To assess involvement of the buccal space and IFT
  - To determine involvement of marrow and inferior alveolar nerve and perineural invasion along V3
  - Inferior to CT to assess cortical erosion
- *CT scan*:
  - Multidetector CT scan with sagittal reformatting can detect mandibular involvement with an accuracy of up to 90%.
  - Soft-tissue delineation is poor.

SURGICAL PRINCIPLES (TABLE 1)

- Adequately expose all tumor margins before approaching the tumor.
- A cheek flap may be required to avoid compromising margins, even for small tumors that are located posteriorly **(Figs. 3 and 4)**.

TABLE 1: Surgical approaches.

Surgical approaches	Indications	Benefits
Peroral	Small anterior lesion of buccal mucosa	No external scar
Cheek flap:		
Midline lip split	When a lesion is located away from the oral commissure	Better oral competence
Lateral lip split	• When the lesion approaches close to the commissure • When adjacent skin excision is required	Avoids devascularization of the lip segment between the commissure and the midline

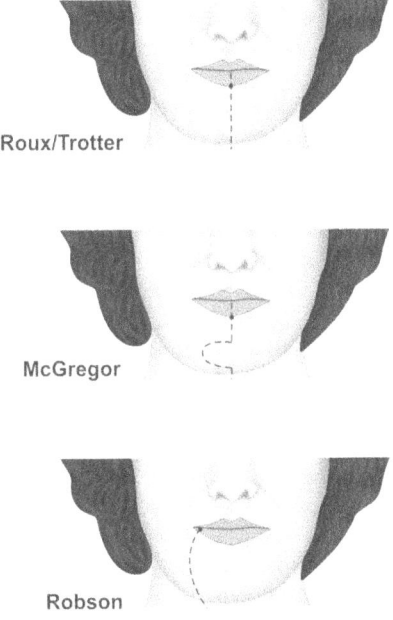

Fig. 3: Lower lip split incisions.

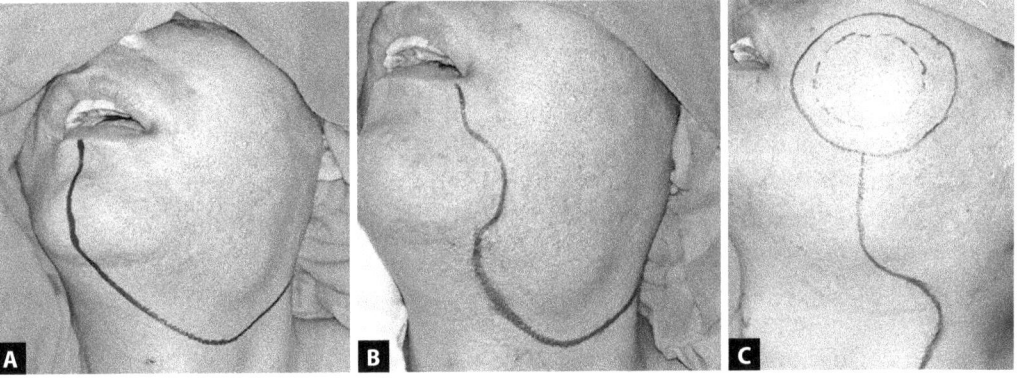

Figs. 4A to C: Intraoral approaches: (A) Midline lip split; (B) Lateral lip split; and (C) Lip sparing.

- Mucosal, soft tissue, and bone margins of >5 mm
- Neck dissection (depending on clinical status, if neck):
    - Suspicious nodes on imaging
    - T3/T4 cancers
    - T1/T2 cancers with:
        - Poor differentiation
        - Tumor thickness > 4 mm (rule of thumb—tumor has palpable thickness)
- Preserve function and avoid trismus with selection of appropriate reconstruction technique
- Avoid obstruction of parotid duct; stent it

SELECTION OF TREATMENT

Role of Surgery

- Surgery is the preferred treatment for early as well as advanced buccal/RMT carcinoma. Patients with advanced disease should receive postoperative radiation or chemoradiation.
- Surgical approach depends on the size of the tumor. Small lesions can usually be treated via transoral wide local excision, whereas advanced lesions usually require excision via a cheek flap.
- Surgically, tumors are excised with a normal margin of 1 cm in all dimensions from the primary tumor. A margin < 5 mm is considered compromised.
- Complete resection of the tumor with negative margins confirmed by frozen section histopathology is the goal.
- Positive margins are associated with increased recurrence and decreased survival rates.
- Early-stage tumors (I/II) are managed with a single treatment modality such as surgery or radiotherapy (RT).

Management of Bone

Periosteum of mandible is a robust barrier to bone invasion. Mandibular invasion from BM/lower gingivobuccal sulcus (GBS) can be through following possible routes:

- From the oral cavity through the upper surface of the mandible (occlusal route)
- Through the mental foramen
- Secondary tumors in the neck through the lower border
- Mandibular foramen
- Cortical bone defects in the edentulous ridge
- Periodontal membrane in the dentate mandible
- Attached gingiva
- MacGregor and MacDonald showed that tumors tended to enter the mandible through small defects in the occlusal part of the edentulous mandible and based this finding on their rim resection, junction-preserving approach to the jaw.
- Later, James S Brown postulates that the route of tumor entry is at the point of tumor abutment (often the junction of the attached and reflected mucosa) rather than entrance into the periodontal membrane at the crest of the ridge in the dentate jaw or the occlusal surface in the edentulous ridge.

Marginal mandibulectomy **(Figs. 5A to C):**
- Involvement of the bone, clinically or radiologically, is a contraindication to marginal mandibulectomy
- Contraindications of marginal mandibulectomy even in case of uninvolved bone are:
    - *Gross paramandibular spread*: Line of resection may inadvertently pass through the infiltrated paramandibular tissues and make marginal mandibulectomy unsound and unsafe.

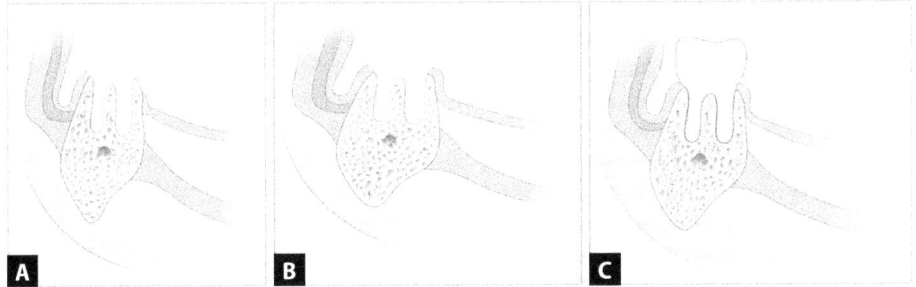

Figs. 5A to C: Marginal mandibulectomy: (A) Vertical marginal; (B) Oblique marginal; (C) Horizontal marginal.

- *Lesions with retromolar extension with masseteric space involvement*: Clearance of the soft tissue in the pterygoid region is possible only, if the ascending ramus of the mandible is resected.
- Irradiated/edentulous bone

Key Points—Marginal Mandibulectomy
- Three types of marginal mandibulectomy—(1) horizontal, (2) vertical, and (3) oblique.
- The edges of the bone should be "canoe shaped" to avoid sharp corners.
- Inferiorly, a bony bridge of >1 cm in height should be retained to avoid a stress fracture.
- With marginal mandibulectomy for RMT cancer, the anterior aspect of the ascending ramus of the mandible is excised in continuity with the coronoid process, as releasing the attachment of the temporalis muscle avoids postoperative trismus.
- *Contraindication*—gross bone erosion/gross paramandibular spread/irradiated/edentulous bone/lesions with retromolar extension with masseteric space involvement.

Surgical steps:
- Neck dissection:
  - Elective neck dissection (levels I-III) at the time of resection of the primary tumor confers an overall survival benefit in patients with early-stage, clinically node-negative oral SCC.
  - In the presence of nodal metastasis, either levels I-IV, or modified neck dissection (levels I-V) is done.
- *Primary resection*:
  - After incising the mucosa around soft tissue using diathermy or a knife, bone cuts are marked adjacent to the soft tissue. The posterior mucosal cut is made according to the extent of tumor. Attention should be paid mainly to the third dimension, i.e., deep resection margin.
  - With lesions deeper, e.g., adhering to skin or causing peau d'orange, the overlying skin is excised to achieve an adequate margin.
  - If the lesion is involving upper GBS, then ITF clearance ± upper alveolectomy is also needed.
- *Infratemporal fossa* (**Fig. 6**):
  - If the lesion does not involve the ITF, then the bone cut is made anterior to the pterygoid plates.
  - If the lesion involves the medial pterygoid muscle, the pterygoid plate is included in the specimen to ensure adequate soft-tissue resection that includes the pterygoid muscles.
  - Infratemporal fossa clearance showed should be done in upper GBS or infrazygomatic lesion. ITF clearance may need zygomatic excision. Dissection of pterygoid plexus may be quite bloody.

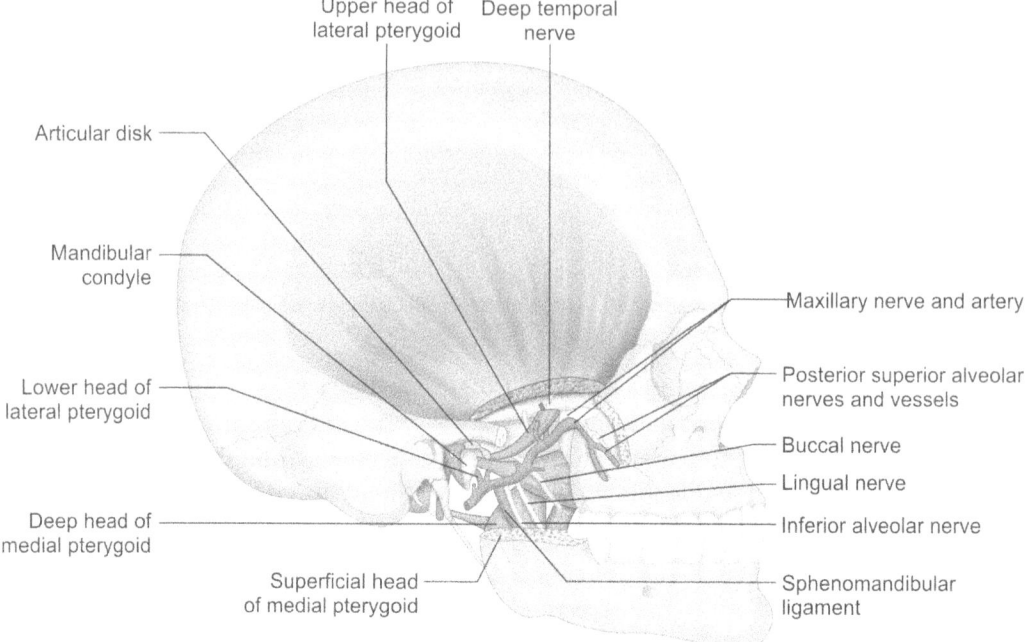

Fig. 6: Contents of infratemporal fossa (ITF).

Role of Radiotherapy

- In early-stage lesions, RT is suitable only for superficial lesions measuring <3 cm away from bony structures and accessible for brachytherapy.
- In locally advanced unresectable BM cancer → chemoradiation followed by salvage surgery may be done.
- Well-differentiated keratinizing SCC involving mandible/maxilla often has less reliable response to RT and chemotherapy.

Role of Chemotherapy

- Chemotherapy by itself is not definitive in the management of BM cancer.
- A Cochrane systematic review on oral cancer analyzed 89 trials related to chemotherapy in the management of oral cavity and oropharyngeal cancer. 11 of these trials had only oral cancer patients. Pooled data of the included 25 trials of induction chemotherapy plus locoregional treatment versus locoregional treatment alone showed no significant benefit for overall survival [hazard ratio (HR): 0.92; 95% confidence interval (CI): 0.84–1.0; $p = 0.06$]. The implications for practice based on this meta-analysis are as follows:
  - Induction chemotherapy is not associated with statistically significant improvement in overall survival compared to locoregional treatment alone.
  - There is evidence that concomitant adjuvant chemoradiotherapy improves overall survival compared to these treatments given sequentially.
  - In patients with unresectable tumors, there is evidence that concomitant chemoradiotherapy leads to improvement in overall survival of 10–20%.

Role of Adjuvant Treatment

- Recommendations for adjuvant RT include multiple pathologically positive lymph nodes in the neck, perineural invasion, angiolymphatic invasion, high-grade histopathology, and advanced T (III or IV) stage.
- Adjuvant concomitant chemoradiation is recommended when surgical pathology shows extracapsular spread in the cervical nodes and positive or close margins (<5 mm) at the primary site.
- In adjuvant RT, the dose and volume for primary and uninvolved cervical nodes are 55–60 Gy/28–30 fractions over 6 weeks using reducing fields, for residual disease and positive margins a 4–10 Gy boost, and for uninvolved cervical nodes 45–50 Gy.

LOCALLY ADVANCED/ BORDERLINE RESECTABLE BUCCAL MUCOSA CANCER

- The AJCC subdivides T4 into T4a and T4b as moderately advanced and very advanced tumors, respectively. The patients with T4a classification disease are considered surgically resectable and are generally offered curative intent treatment. The patients with T4b classification tumors are considered unresectable and usually treated nonsurgically (either chemoradiation or palliative intent treatment).
- The tumors that involve masticator space, pterygoid plates, skull base, or encases internal carotid artery are classified as T4b.
- Certain T4a BM cancer with features such as extensive skin edema up to the zygomatic arch is generally considered unresectable with substantially increased functional and cosmetic morbidity. Patient with brawny induration and satellite nodules on cheek/face should be treated as T4b.
- *Issues of operating locally advanced tumors*:
  - Possibility of getting a positive or close margins much higher in these patients.
  - The bleeding from pterygoid venous plexus also makes surgery technically difficult.
- Induction chemotherapy or chemoradiation can be used to convert potentially unresectable tumors to resectable disease and produce better results.
- The concept of compartment surgery was proposed by Trivedi NP et al. The authors advocate removal of the entire content of MS in en bloc fashion. Their rational of improving margin control with this approach was based on some fundamental issues of operating in MS area.
- Liao et al. evaluated various factors to identify a subgroup of patients with potential for favorable outcome. The study consisted of 45 patients with T4b stage due to MS involvement. The level of mandibular notch in transverse plane served as dividing line between the supranotch and infranotch compartment. A vertical line drawn from middle of ascending ramus divided tumors into anterior and posterior compartments **(Figs. 7A and B)**.

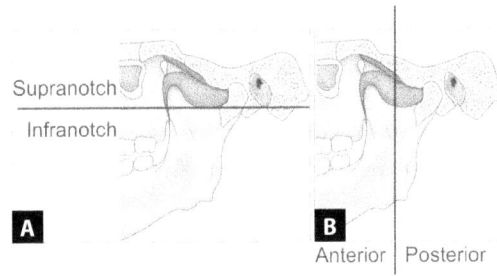

Figs. 7A and B: Supranotch versus infranotch tumors.

He found that infranotch pT4b without nerve invasion had outcomes comparable with those of pT4a tumors.
- Recent studies showed favorable disease outcome in T4b (infranotch) BM cancer patients treated by multimodality treatment of primary surgery and adjuvant RT or concurrent chemoradiotherapy.

TREATMENT FOR RECURRENT AND METASTATIC HEAD AND NECK CANCER

Treatment guidelines and prognostic factors for recurrent oral cancer are explained in **Table 2** and **Box 2**, respectively.

Key Points
- Median survival in most series is 6–15 months
- Choice of systemic regimen is influenced by multiple clinical factors including patient comorbidities, performance status, previous therapy, and pathologic features [i.e., programmed death ligand 1 (PD-L1) expression status].
- *Treatment options include the following*:
  – Administered as single-agent therapy or in combination:
    - Immunotherapy with PD-L1 checkpoint inhibitors (e.g., pembrolizumab, nivolumab)
    - Conventional cytotoxic chemotherapy [e.g., cisplatin, 5-fluorouracil (5-FU), taxanes]
    - Molecularly targeted agents [e.g., epidermal growth factor receptor (EGFR) inhibitors, cetuximab]

TABLE 2: Treatment guidelines.

T1 and T2 tumors	• Surgery or radiotherapy (RT) • *Surgery*: Wide excision ± marginal mandibulectomy with appropriate reconstruction • *Radiotherapy*: Radical RT/Brachytherapy
T3 and T4 tumors	• Surgery + Postoperative RT/chemotherapy (CT)-RT • *Surgery*: Composite resection of the buccal mucosa with mandible or upper alveolus ± ITF clearance • Overlying skin with reconstruction
For locally advanced/borderline resectable cancer	• NACT followed by reassessment • If operable, then surgery followed by adjuvant radiation and concurrent CT • If unresectable, then concurrent chemoradiation
For locally advanced/unresectable cancer (primary or nodal disease)	• Concurrent systemic therapy and RT Or • NACT followed by RT or RT-CT Or • Palliative RT Or • Single-agent systemic therapy Or • Best supportive care (unfit for any active treatment)
Metastatic (M1) disease at initial presentation	• Clinical trial Or • Combination or single-agent systemic therapy Or • Best supportive care

Contd...

Contd...

Recurrent/Metastatic disease	• Salvage surgery (if resectable, locoregional disease) Or • RT ± concurrent CT (if unresectable, locoregional disease/unfit for surgery) Or • Palliative CT • First line—pembrolizumab + Platinum + 5-FU • Better overall survival in programmed death ligand 1 (PD-L1) combined positive score (CPS) of ≥20 and ≥1 (KEYNOTE-048 trial) • Metronomic therapy Or • Best supportive care

(5-FU: 5-fluorouracil; ITF: infratemporal fossa; NACT: neoadjuvant chemotherapy)

Box 2: Prognostic factors for recurrent oral cancer.

- Ambulatory performance status [Eastern Cooperative Oncology Group (ECOG)]
- Prior response to chemotherapy
- Time since completion of definitive therapy
- Human papillomavirus (HPV)-associated oropharyngeal cancers
- Tumor programmed death ligand 1 (PD-L1) expression status (a predictive marker for response to anti-PD-1 therapy)

KEY POINTS

- Treatment for early-stage BM and RMT carcinoma is surgery followed by adjuvant therapy as per histopathology report.
- Advanced-staged tumors will require multimodality treatment, which include surgery followed by adjuvant RT with or without concurrent chemotherapy.
- No definite role of neoadjuvant chemotherapy in BM cancer; however, some recent studies support neoadjuvant chemotherapy in locally advanced borderline resectable disease. Patients who become resectable after chemotherapy had better overall and disease-free survival as compared to patients who managed nonsurgical modality.
- For recurrent disease, the extent of disease and disease-free interval play a significant role in management. Resectable disease should undergo surgery followed by adjuvant therapy.
- For recurrent/metastatic unresectable diseases, palliative chemotherapy with immunotherapy with programmed death-ligand L1 (PD-L1) checkpoint inhibitors (e.g., pembrolizumab, nivolumab) is the first-line therapy.

CHAPTER 16

Carcinoma of Lower Alveolus

Rajeev Kumar

INTRODUCTION

Lower alveolus can be involved by cancers arising from alveolus itself or cancer arising from adjacent areas such as gingivobuccal sulcus and floor of mouth. It can also be involved through inferior alveolar canal. The cancer can involve the mandible and retromandibular area and can extend into infratemporal fossa making its management difficult and there are high chances of local recurrence, if not adequately resected in first go.

The bone of the mandible is close to some soft-tissue structures, which are important for both function and form **(Fig. 1)**. These are anteriorly, the chin, lips, and oral commissures; laterally, the external cheek and intraoral lining; posteriorly, the pharyngeal pillars; and medially, the floor of the mouth and tongue. Resection of tumors in this region can create not only bony defects, but also cause loss of surrounding soft tissues. Mandibular movement is due to largely the four muscles of mastication, which are the masseter, temporalis, medial pterygoid, and lateral pterygoid. These muscles are supplied by the mandibular division of the trigeminal nerve. During the resection, preserving the attachments of these muscles, wherever possible, would prevent an imbalance in the forces resulting in pain and altered mouth opening, more so after radiation therapy.

Dental alveoli (singular *alveolus*) are sockets in the jaws within which the roots of teeth are held in the *alveolar* process with the periodontal ligament. The *gums* or *gingiva*

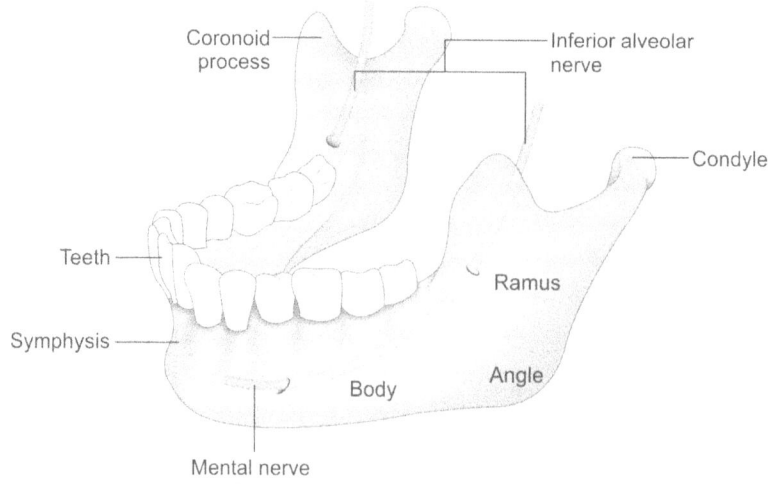

Fig. 1: Bony landmarks of mandible.

(plural: gingivae) consists of the mucosal tissue over the mandible and maxilla from gingivobuccal sulcus laterally to floor of mouth medially.

Squamous cell carcinoma (SCC) may originate within the body of the mandible bone either from the odontogenic epithelium or from the epithelium that is trapped during embryonic development. It is more common in the mandible than in the maxilla and is frequently found in the molar regions. SCC invades the periosteum and the adjacent buccal mucosa and floor of the mouth. Low-grade lesions produce a smooth, saucerized defect before they invade the mandible. Moderate- to high-grade lesions directly invade the bone or through some newly opened dental sockets.

Lymphatic spread is seen in levels I and II. About 18–52% of cases of carcinoma alveolus may show clinically positive nodes.

Magnetic resonance imaging (MRI) is useful to evaluate any malignant infiltration of the marrow cavity, though this is generally a very late finding. A fine-cut/high-resolution computed tomography (HRCT) scan with bone algorithm can show erosion of the cortex of the mandible.

TYPES OF MANDIBULECTOMY (FIGS. 2A AND B)

- *Segmental mandibulectomy*: Different segments of mandible are excised depending on the position of tumor and it may be hemimandibulectomy including the condyle and coronoid process or a segment of mandible leaving two cut ends open. The central arch of the mandible may be excised primarily in the tumors of anterior floor of mouth.
- *Marginal mandibulectomy*:
  - Vertical marginal mandibulectomy—floor of mouth tumors
  - Horizontal marginal mandibulectomy—alveolar ridge tumors

Indications for Segmental Resection of the Mandible

- Invasion of the medullary space of mandible
- Tumor fixation to the occlusal surface of the mandible in edentulous patient
- Invasion of tumor into the mandible through the mandibular or mental foramen
- Tumor fixity to the mandible after prior radiotherapy to the mandible,

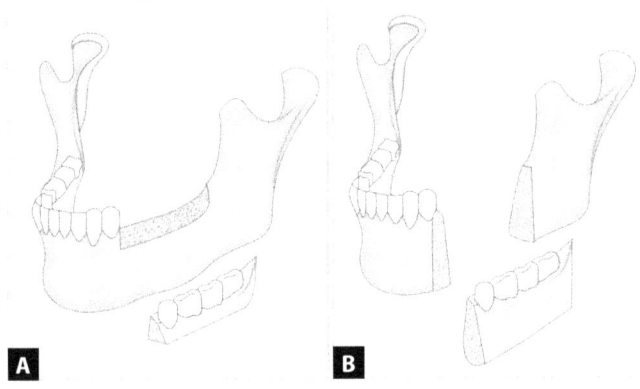

Figs. 2A and B: Types of mandibular resections: (A) Marginal mandibulectomy; (B) Segmental mandibulectomy.

particularly, if the tumor is located on the occlusal surface
- Tumor adjacent to carious teeth with involvement of the periodontal ligament
- Hypoplastic edentulous mandible with significant loss of vertical height precluding safe performance of rim resection
- In selected cases, a segmental resection may be indicated for nononcologic reasons. Previously irradiated patients with trismus may show improvement in jaw opening with a segment removed and newly vascularized soft-tissue interposed

Indications for Rim Resection of the Mandible

- Tumor near but not involving the periosteum of the mandible
- Tumor that involve only mandibular periosteum
- Tumor adjacent to cortical bone of mandible but with no invasion beyond superficial cortex
- Tumor adjacent to dentition with no evidence of involvement of periodontal ligament

Resection margins—gross 1 cm margins are desirable both on soft tissue and bone. Therefore, the resection is performed with a 1 cm minimum margin of what is believed to be healthy mandible on either side of the tumor. Marrow from either side of mandible may be sent for frozen section examination to see the adequacy of resection.

Contraindications for Marginal Mandibulectomy

- Recurrence postradiation therapy with tumor closely associated with the mandible, rim resection is contraindicated.
- Patients with very hypoplastic mandibles where oncologically safe resection of the tumor would leave <1 cm of bone width and height.

COMPLICATIONS

- Orocutaneous fistula
- Bone exposure
- Extrusion of titanium plate
- Loss of graft or flap

KEY POINTS

- *Mandible uninvolved or minimally involved*:
  - *Surgery*: Wide excision with marginal mandibulectomy [avoided in retromolar trigone (RMT) disease, edentulous mandible, paramandibular disease, and postradiotherapy], if required with reconstruction
  - ± Adjuvant treatment [as per histopathological report (HPR)]
- *Mandible grossly involved*:
  - *Surgery*: Wide excision (cheek flap) with segmental/hemimandible resection with reconstruction
  - Postoperative radiotherapy (RT) ± CT

17 Upper Alveolus and Palate

Vikas Arora

SURGICAL ANATOMY (FIGS. 1A AND B)

- The hard palate and upper alveolar ridge comprise the superior boundary of the oral cavity.
- The hard palate has minor salivary glands located in the submucosa, which is responsible for frequent occurrence of salivary gland tumors in this subsite.
- The mucoperiosteum of both alveolar ridge and palate is firmly attached to the underlying bone and it can be stripped cleanly as a single layer to leave a bare bony surface. The alveolar bone with its smoother surface allows steady stripping than the rougher hard palate.
- The hard palate separates the oral cavity from the nasal cavities and maxillary sinuses. Thickness of hard palate varies at different sites. Its overall thickness diminishes in midline as well as toward its posterior border.
- The hard palate contains three major foramina—a single anterior midline incisive foramen that transmits the nasopalatine artery and nerve and two paired posterolateral greater palatine foramen that transmit the greater palatine nerve and artery.

The alveolar ridge lies close to the buccal and upper gingival mucosa. Posteriorly, it is firmly attached to pterygoid plates. During maxillectomy, presence of pterygoid plexus in this region may lead to torrential bleeding which requires careful hemostasis. The alveolar processes of the maxilla along with the overlying mucosa form the upper

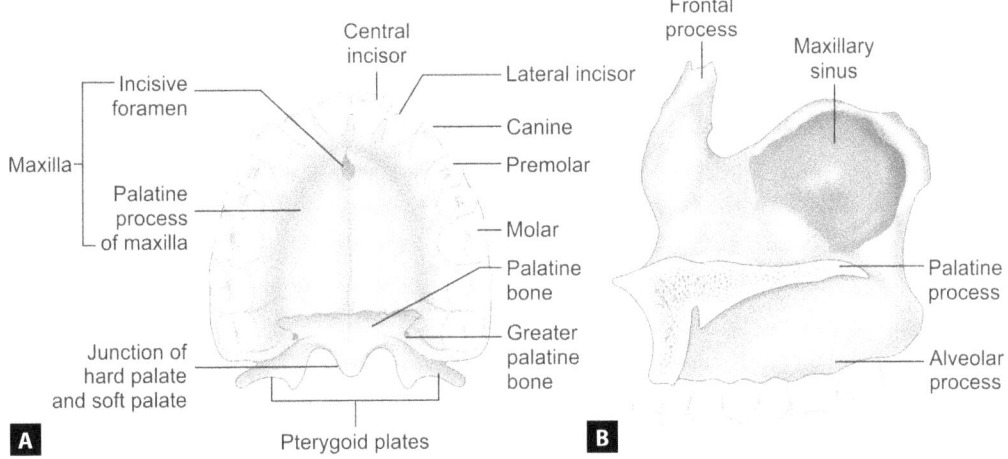

Figs. 1A and B: Bony landmarks of hard palate.

alveolar ridge. The hard palate lies within the horseshoe shape of the maxilla.

- Cancers of the upper alveolus can spread to the upper gingivobuccal sulcus and upper part of the buccal mucosa because of its close proximity and this makes it difficult to identify the exact site of origin of the disease. Tumor of upper alveolar ridge and hard palate, although infrequent, along with upper gingival cancers, constitutes nearly 3.5% of all oral malignancies.
  Upper gingival-buccal cancers (UGBCs) are generally more aggressive biologically than the lower gingivobuccal cancers.
- The aggressive behavior is possibly due to the late presentation of the UGBC and early invasion through the infratemporal fossa (ITF).
- Metastasis to lymph nodes from squamous cell carcinoma (SCC) of upper alveolus is around 34%.

CLINICOPATHOLOGICAL ASPECTS

The cancers of the palate, upper alveolus, and upper gingivobuccal sulcus may have varied histology such as SCC, adenoid cystic carcinoma, mucoepidermoid carcinoma, melanoma, sarcoma, and neuroendocrine tumor of the maxillary region.

- *Squamous cell carcinoma*: More than 85% oral cancers are SCC. The tumors can arise in any part of alveolar-palatal complex, but most frequent site is the alveolar ridge. It may initially present as a "dry socket" after tooth extraction or as an extraction site that produces what may appear to be granulation tissue but does not heal.
  Palatal lesions are usually multifocal. They usually have a warty appearance or sometimes develop into a malignant ulcer.
  In countries where reverse cigar (chutta) smoking is very common, they arise as a single focus at central palate.

Routes of local spread:
- Tumor spread occurs anteriorly and posteriorly along the alveolar ridge toward molar and incisor regions.
- Medially toward center of palate.
- Laterally toward the upper buccal sulcus.
- The spread in lateral direction merely involves the outer surface of alveolus, but further marginal extension brings the tumor round the sulcus onto the ITF and buccal mucosa. Management of such lesions is similar to buccal mucosa tumors.
- Deep spread of tumor involves the bone immediately underlying the mucosal site. This process is quite slow, probably due to mucoperiosteum, its close adherence to the bone, and characteristic of cancellous bone. Once through the bone, tumor involves mucosa of the maxillary antrum or nasal floor.

Other lesions that originate from the lining of the mouth include:
- Carcinoma in situ
- *Multifocal leukoerythroplakia syndrome* **(Fig. 2)**: Leukoerythroplakia of upper and lower mouth usually behaves independently of one another. It needs

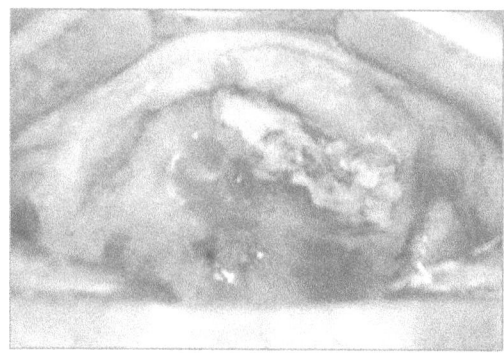

Fig. 2: Erythroleukoplakia hard palate.

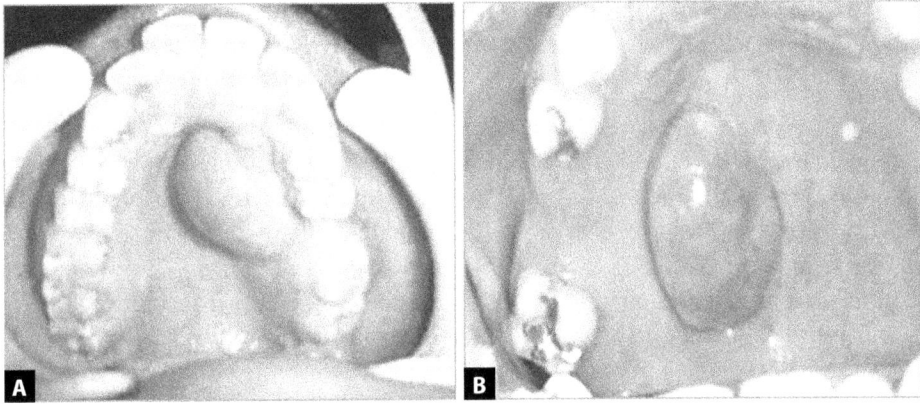

Figs. 3A and B: Adenoid cystic carcinoma of hard palate.

close follow-up after histopathological evaluation.
- *Verrucous carcinoma*: This type of SCC has better prognosis since it is less likely to spread. But, these are treated like any other SCC.
- *Salivary gland cancers*: The lining of the hard palate has many minor salivary glands located underneath. This is why cancers in this region may be glandular malignancies as adenocarcinomas including mucoepidermoid carcinomas and adenoid cystic carcinomas.

  In rare instances, salivary gland cancers may grow inside the bone itself. These tumors are slow-growing tumors and usually get obscured in patients who wear dentures. If the tumor is large and long enough, it may sometimes erode the hard palatal bone.

  Adenoid cystic carcinoma is the most common submucosal malignant salivary tumor **(Figs. 3A and B)**. Silent local infiltration to the skull base and perineural spread are known characteristics of these tumors.
- *Mucosal melanoma*: In this site, the tumor most often takes the form of patchy areas of pigmentation, representing lentiginous

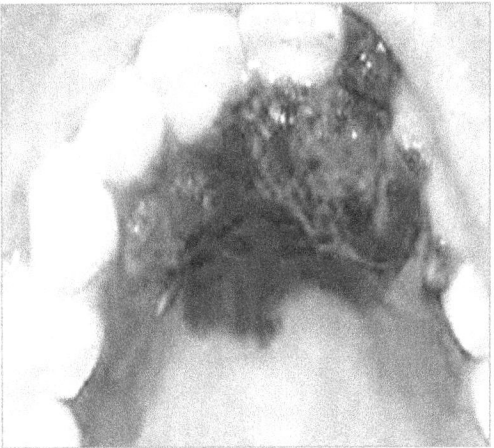

Fig. 4: Malignant melanoma of hard palate.

mucosal spread surrounding a focus of invasive malignant melanoma, presenting as nodule **(Fig. 4)**. Resection should include both focus of invasive melanoma and the surrounding lentigo.
- *Kaposi's sarcoma*: This tumor is usually associated with acquired immunodeficiency syndrome (AIDS). It usually appears on the skin. It may also be seen in the mouth, looking like a purple lesion filled with blood vessels.
- *Osteogenic sarcoma*: Very rarely, it can occur in the jaw.

PREOPERATIVE STAGING AND EVALUATION

For all patients with cancers of the head and neck, a detailed history should be taken with special consideration to:
- Duration of complaints
- Rate of growth
- Any loose dentition
- Ill-fitting dentures, if present
- Palatal and facial numbness
- Velopharyngeal insufficiency
- Presence of any facial swelling
- History of sinusitis
- Evidence of oronasal fistula

The area around the tumor must be mapped with all details including areas of swelling and those suspicious for subepithelial tumor spread.

All loose dentition should be thoroughly examined for the possibility of malignant involvement of the dental sockets and bone.

Any palatal or trigeminal numbness on neurological examination may indicate involvement of the foramina by malignant cells and they may subsequently lead to the skull base.

Nasal endoscopy may be performed to examine the extent of intranasal involvement.

RADIOLOGIC EVALUATION

Chest radiographs are advised for surveillance of any pulmonary metastasis.

CT scan delineates structure of the cortical bones and areas of bony invasion with a great accuracy.

Magnetic resonance imaging (MRI) has the advantage of demonstrating malignancy within the bone marrow and the perineural extension and, therefore, considered as the preferred modality.

Whole-body positron emission tomography computed tomography (PET-CT) is an important tool to evaluate distant metastasis in patients with locally advanced palatal lesions and bulky nodal metastasis.

DENTAL PROSTHETIC EVALUATION

A consultation with the dental prosthetics should be planned presurgery. A prosthodontist will design a temporary surgical prosthesis to be used during surgery to hold the skin graft in place and also to obturate the surgical defect.

Early obturation helps the patient to take orally immediately in the postoperative period. This also helps to avoid a nasogastric tube insertion. Postoperative rehabilitation helps in achieving good cosmesis, nutrition, and speech in most of the cases.

In patients who may need subtotal or complete maxillectomy, process of obturation may be difficult and, hence, free tissue transfer would be necessary.

MANAGEMENT

The management of hard palate and alveolus is described in **Flowcharts 1A to D**.

SURGICAL TECHNIQUE

Common approaches to the surgical management of cancer limited to the hard palate and alveolar ridge include:
- Upper alveolectomy/Partial lateral maxillectomy **(Fig. 5)**
- Infrastructural maxillectomy

Surgical Approach
- Peroral
- Upper cheek flap

Upper Alveolectomy

This surgical approach is customized for smaller tumors of the lateral maxillary alveolar ridge and hard palate.

Flowcharts 1A to D: Management of carcinoma of hard palate and alveolus.

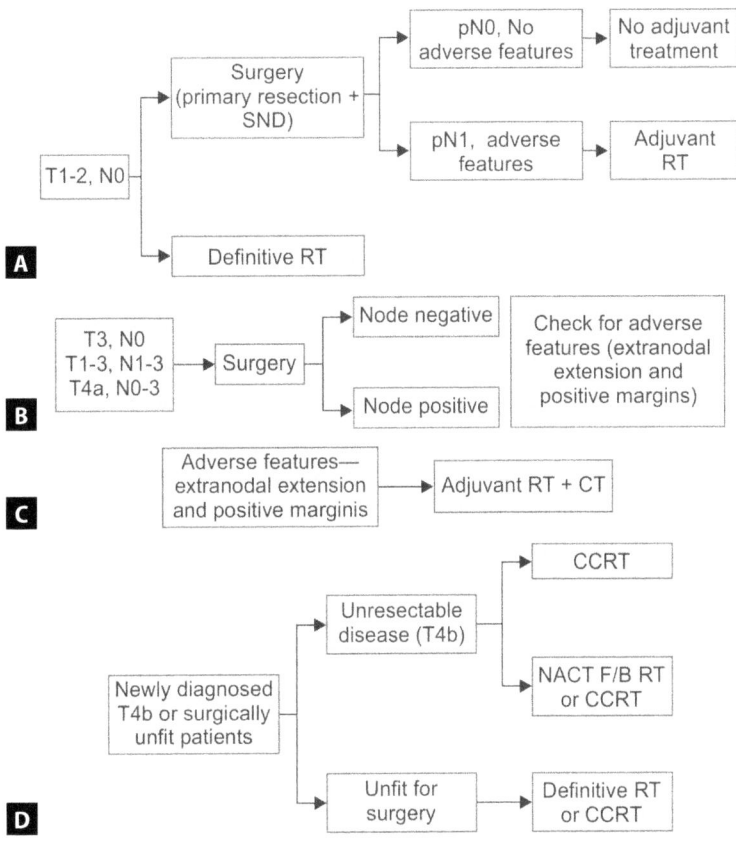

(CCRT: concurrent chemoradiotherapy; NACT: neoadjuvant chemotherapy; SND: selective neck dissection)

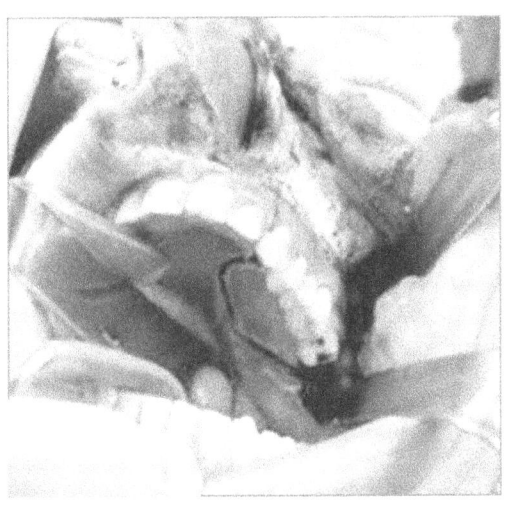

Fig. 5: Partial maxillectomy.

Soft-tissue Dissection/Bony Exposure

- Mucosal incisions should allow for at least 1 cm margin as there is postexcision shrinkage by 30% or more, which creates an artificially close margin.
- Gingivobuccal and palatal incisions are made with scalpel or cautery and taken up to the maxillary bone. Scalpel technique may result in more bleeding, but it gives cleaner surgical margins for pathological analysis.
- The anterior and lateral walls of the maxillary sinus are then exposed with a heavy periosteal elevator.

Bony Resection

- The maxillary sinus is entered with an anterior osteotomy, inferior to the infraorbital rim, provided the sinus is not invaded. Care has to be taken, so as not to disrupt the roots of the tooth with a low osteotomy. An osteotome or sagittal saw may be used in creating the anterior maxillotomy.
- A Kerrison Rongeur too can be used to widen the osteotomy, allowing for direct visualization of the floor of the maxillary sinus.
- The osteotomy is carried through the lateral wall of the maxilla past the area of cancer involvement with a reciprocating or sagittal saw.
- The hard palate is transected lateral to the midline and into the maxillary sinus, thus avoiding the lateral nasal wall and nasal cavity. This is performed with powered instrumentation using the reciprocating or sagittal blades.
- The soft palate is transected, if necessary, with electrocautery, freeing the posterior and inferior portions of the specimen, which include mucosa, palate musculature, and the medial pterygoid muscle.
- The posterior osteotomy is performed with an osteotome, if possible, preserving the posterior wall of the maxillary antrum and avoiding significant blood loss. The posterior osteotomy is reserved for the final step to avoid unnecessary blood loss because bleeding from the pterygomaxillary space can be completely controlled only after removal of the specimen.
- A large osteotome is placed behind the last molar tooth at a 90° angle to the hard palate aiming superomedially. Once the pterygoids are fractured, brisk bleeding will be encountered from the plexus and internal maxillary artery. Often a curved Mayo scissor will facilitate completion of the transection. Bleeding is then controlled with clamp and ligature technique.

Analysis of the frozen-section margins will confirm the efficacy of the obtained margins. Frozen-section margins will be very accurate for soft tissue and muscular margins. The bony surgical margins are left to the discretion of the surgeon.

A split-thickness skin graft is sewn into place to line the exposed bone and soft tissue. Xeroform gauze and a dental obturator are then used to hold the skin graft in place.

Infrastructural Maxillectomy (Figs. 6A and B)

Infrastructural maxillectomy is carried out with tumors limited to the palate and the floor of the maxillary sinus and nasal cavity. It entails resection of the hard palate and may include the walls of the maxillary sinus and nasal floor and inferior turbinate, but spares the orbital floor and ethmoid sinuses.

The operation may be considered in three stages: (1) Soft-tissue dissection/bone exposure, (2) Bone resection, and (3) Closure/reconstruction.

Soft-tissue Dissection/Bone Exposure

It is important to complete the soft-tissue dissection and bone exposure before going ahead with any bone cut to avoid blood loss.

- Infrastructural maxillectomy is done through a sublabial incision or a midfacial degloving approach. Local anesthetic with vasoconstrictor is injected along the planned mucosal or skin incisions.
- The sublabial mucosa is incised along the gingivobuccal sulcus with electrocautery.

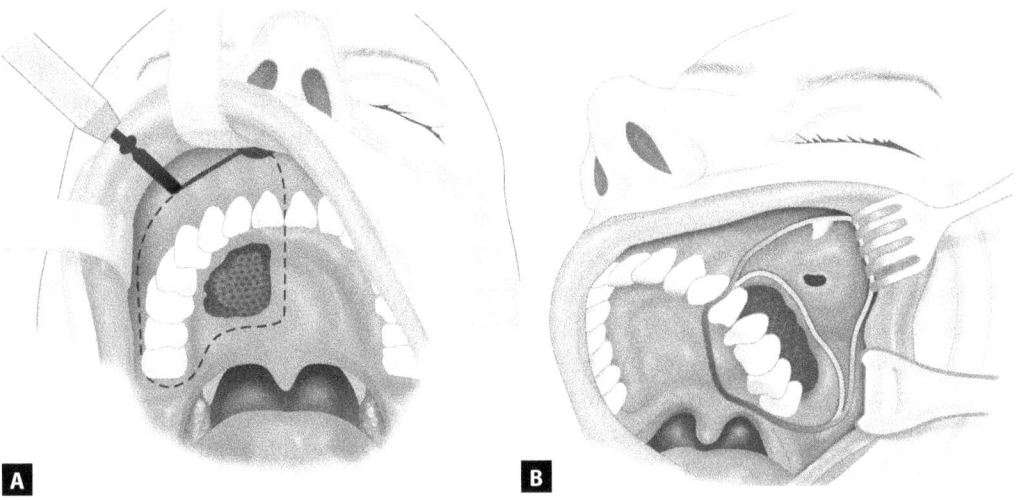

Figs. 6A and B: Infrastructural maxillectomy.

The soft tissues of the face are elevated off the face of the maxilla using cautery or an elevator, remaining hard on bone while doing so.
- Expose the entire face of the maxilla. Stop the dissection superiorly at the infraorbital foramen taking care to preserve the infraorbital nerve and to avoid troublesome bleeding from the infraorbital artery.
- Next, free the soft tissues medially from the bone up to the anterior-free margin of the nasal aperture with diathermy. Retract the nasal ala and incise the lateral wall of the nasal vestibule to expose the ipsilateral nasal cavity and inferior turbinate, taking care not to injure the inferior turbinate or septum to avoid bleeding.
- Using a mouth gag retracted, visualize the hard and soft palate and the tumor. Identify the maxillary tuberosity and the bony spines of the pterygoid plates immediately posterior to the tuberosity.
- Using electrocautery, incise the mucosa of the hard palate along the planned medial resection margin and extend the sublabial incision laterally around the maxillary tuberosity and into the groove between the tuberosity and the pterygoid plates.
- Palpate and define the posterior edge of the hard palate and divide the attachment of the soft palate to the hard palate with electrocautery, thereby entering the nasopharynx.
- Anticipate and coagulate bleeding from branches of the greater and lesser palatine arteries. At this point, the soft tissue dissection is complete.

Bony Resection

- An antrostomy is made in the anterior face of the maxilla with a hammer and gouge or a burr, entering the antrum through the thin bone of the canine fossa.
- A punch or bone nibbler is used to remove enough bone of the anterior wall of the maxillary sinus to evaluate the tumor extent in the antrum, but taking care to leave a margin of bone around the infraorbital foramen, so as to protect the nerve and to avoid bleeding from the infraorbital vessels. Inspect the antrum and determine the extent of the tumor and plan the subsequent bony cuts.

- The infrastructural maxillectomy can now be done using sharp osteotomes and/or a powered saw.
- The extent of the bony resection is tailored to the tumor. The sequence of the osteotomies is planned to reserve troublesome bleeding to the end. The sequence may have to be adjusted depending on the location and extent of the tumor.
- Perform an osteotomy through the lateral wall of the maxillary sinus with an osteotome, bone nibbler, or powered saw up to its junction with the posterior antral wall.
- Perform an osteotomy through the anterior medial wall of the maxillary sinus up to the nasal.
- Free the pterygoid plates with a curved osteotome from the maxillary tuberosity. Perform a palatal osteotomy in a sagittal plane with an osteotome or saw, taking care not to traumatize and cause bleeding from the inferior turbinate and nasal septum when entering the nasal cavity.
- The palatal resection should extend through the floor of the ipsilateral nasal cavity and then the lateral nasal wall needs to be divided parallel to the palate with scissors or an osteotome. Similarly, the nasal septum must be divided, if the resection extends beyond the midline.
- The infrastructural maxillectomy specimen is then leveraged downward, fracturing across the posterior antral wall in the process, and the specimen is removed. Hemostasis is obtained.
- The maxillary artery should be looked for as it might have been transected and gone into spasm and clipped or ligated.
  The specimen is inspected to determine the adequacy of the tumor resection margins.

Closure/Reconstruction

The objectives are to restore palatal integrity to separate the oral cavity from the nose and antrum, to maintain midfacial projection, and to facilitate dental restoration.

This may be achieved in the following ways:
- *Denture*: Retention may be difficult
- Buccinator flap
- Nasolabial flap
- *Temporalis muscle flap*: This is very well suited, but care must be taken not to injure the deep temporal arterial pedicle during maxillectomy
- Radial free forearm flap (± bone)
- Anterolateral thigh free flap
- Free fibula flap (permits dental implants)
- Thoracodorsal artery scapular tip (TDAST) flap

CONTRAINDICATIONS/CAUTIONS

- Distant metastasis (in selected minor salivary gland tumors with pulmonary metastasis, surgery may be done)
- Lack of physical fitness
- Lack of patient cooperation or patient denial
- Patients on anticoagulant therapy should discontinue their medication and go on bridging therapy, so that they can be reversed at the time of surgery.
- Patients with severe comorbidities must have their condition optimized prior to surgery.
- Invasion into the floor of the orbit or invasion of the infraorbital nerve precludes inferior maxillectomy. These patients need more extended resections.
- Invasion of the pterygoid muscle requires a wider exposure than obtainable by

inferior maxillectomy, so that total maxillectomy would be a better surgical option.
- Prosthetic rehabilitation is essential and in those instances where some form of dental rehabilitation is not available to the patients, they should be well aware of nasal regurgitation as well as difficult swallowing and speaking.

Elective neck dissection may be offered to patients with advanced cancer of the hard palate and alveolar ridge who have an N0 neck.

ROLE OF RADIATION THERAPY

Indications for Adjuvant Radiation Therapy Alone

- T3 or T4 (upper alveolus/palatal lesions)
- Close surgical margin, not adequately cleared with additional margins
- Perineural invasion (PNI)
- Lymphovascular invasion (LVI)
- Two or more positive nodes without extracapsular extension (ECE)
- Surgery followed by adjuvant radiotherapy is preferred whenever disease is confined to the infrazygomatic part of ITF.

Indications for Postoperative Radiation Therapy with Concurrent Chemoradiotherapy

- Positive surgical margin
- Extranodal tumor extension (ENE and ECE)

Indications for Primary Radiation Therapy

- Patient unfit or denies for surgery
- Unresectable disease, usually combined with chemotherapy (central palate involvement).
- Advanced disease for patients intolerant of surgery due to poor performance status or comorbidities.
- Whenever the disease is extending into suprazygomatic region of ITF or borderline resectability.

ROLE OF CHEMOTHERAPY

- Primary treatment for advanced disease or unresectable disease in combination with radiotherapy.
- Adjuvant treatment combined with radiotherapy for positive resection margins or extracapsular nodal extension (stage III-IVB lesions).
- Salvage/palliation

REHABILITATION

The main purpose of an obturator is to separate the oral cavity from nasal cavity and forms a pressure resistance seal against the oral mucosa to prevent leakage of air and fluid from nasal cavity, which helps in speech and swallowing functions.

Surgical planning for prosthetic rehabilitation reduces the postsurgical complications and helps in preserving and increasing the supporting areas for the obturator.

The standard treatment protocol for oral rehabilitation of maxillectomy cases are:
- Surgical obturator placed at the time of surgery
- Interim obturator after 7–10 days after surgery
- Definitive obturator is made 3–6 months postsurgery.

An interim obturator supports the soft tissues after surgery and prevents irritation of the mobile, noncicatrized, and bleeding tissues and minimizes the scar contraction and facial disfigurement that helps in mastication and speech.

FOLLOW-UP

- *Complete head and neck examination or fiberoptic examination*:
  - Initial 2 years—every 4 months
  - 3-5 years—every 6 months
  - >5 years—every 12 months
- *Imaging [contrast-enhanced magnetic resonance imaging (CEMRI) or contrast-enhanced computed tomography (CECT)]*:
  - Post-treatment within 6 months
  - Further imaging is based on worrisome symptoms, smoking history, and areas inaccessible to clinical examination.
  - Routine annual imaging with contrast MRI or CT, especially for areas, which are difficult to visualize for examination.
- Serum thyroid-stimulating hormone (TSH) every 6 months, if neck is irradiated
- Dental evaluation for oral cavity or sites exposed to significant intraoral radiation treatment
- Speech and swallowing evaluation and rehabilitation
- Nutritional evaluation and rehabilitation
- Smoking cessation and counseling
- Psychological counseling

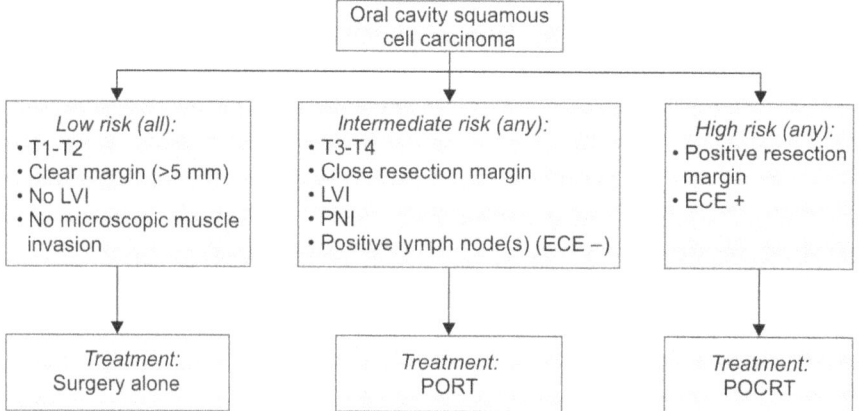

Flowchart 2: Management of oral cavity squamous cell carcinoma.

(ECE: extracapsular extension; LVI: lymphovascular invasion; PNI: perineural invasion; POCRT: postoperative chemoradiotherapy; PORT: postoperative radiotherapy)

KEY POINTS

- Upper alveolus and palatal tumors are uncommon and are diagnosed at advanced stage.
- Adenoid cystic carcinomas have the tendency for silent skull base involvement and PNI. They are the only cancers, which are still resectable in presence of pulmonary metastasis.
- In locally advanced tumors of hard palate and upper alveolar ridge, surgery offers the best form of treatment.
- Upper gingival–buccal cancers behave more aggressively than lower gingival–buccal cancers; therefore, they have poor overall survival.

Management of Tongue and Floor of Mouth Cancer

Ankita Jain, AK Dewan

INTRODUCTION
- *Cancer of the floor of mouth (FOM)* may have devastating outcome. It begins as a small asymptomatic nodular or ulcerative area, which could be overlooked due to its hidden location and being diagnosed in many patients at an advanced stage, when the lesion is painful or causes functional impairment.
- *Cancer of the FOM* constitutes 28–35% of all oral cancers. Although malignant tumors of the FOM develop most commonly after the fifth decade of life, they have been seen in younger persons too.
- *Cancer of the tongue*, on the other hand, may be noticed early by the patient by virtue of its location. However, its location and subsequent surgery have a bearing on the functional outcome. Lesions involving the tip of tongue usually affect the speech in the postoperative period with lesions involving the middle third that affect swallowing function and cause pooling of saliva.

ETIOLOGY
- Tobacco and alcohol together produce additive effects on oral cancer. Tobacco also includes smokeless tobacco derivatives such as snuff and betel nut.
- In India, tobacco is mixed with slaked lime and rolled in a betel nut leaf *(Paan)* to form a quid, which is held against the buccal mucosa for long hours leading to continuous exposure to irritants.
- Consumption of alcohol and smoking has a linear dose-specific relationship with oral cancer.
- Consumption of >40 tobacco cigarettes and 7 or more ounces of alcohol per day increases the incidence of oral cancer by three to five times.
- Continued intake of alcohol or smoking elevates the risk of being diagnosed with a second primary cancer to 15% within 5 years and to 40% thereafter. Additionally, the rate of recurrence also increases and with decreased response to radiotherapy.
- Associated poor oral hygiene and poor dentition may further increase the risk by eight times.

PRESENTATION
Floor of Mouth
- Usually, patients present with a painless inflamed superficial ulcer with well or poorly defined margins **(Fig. 1)**. If asymptomatic, it may be overlooked by the patient for prolonged periods.
- Pre-existent or coincident leukoplakia may also be seen in 20% of cases.
- Coexistent erythroplakia strongly suggests an invasive tumor.
- The patient may present with a neck mass. The incidence of metastases to regional nodal at the time of diagnosis being 30–35%.

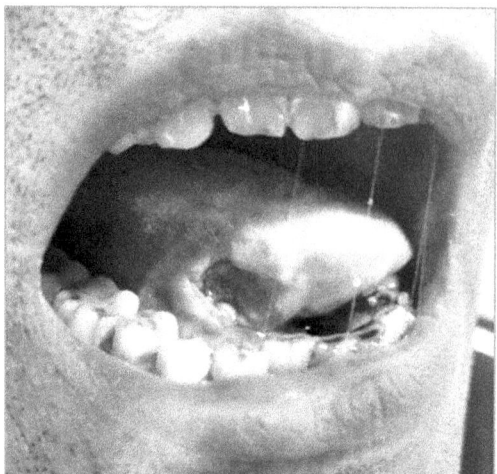

Fig. 1: Ulcerative lesion in the right lateral border of tongue encroaching the floor of mouth (FOM).

- Advanced disease may present with referred pain to the ear, halitosis, evidence of regional lymph node involvement, and bleeding. The base of the tongue and the lingual surface of the alveolus may also become involved.
- A systematic clinical examination includes inspection of the teeth, labial, buccal and gingival mucosae, tongue, and palate. The FOM is carefully examined with a tongue depressor retracting the tongue.
- Bimanual examination helps in the assessment of the extent of the primary tumor and the involvement of the surrounding structures of the submandibular triangle.
- A direct examination of the ears, nose, and oropharynx and palpation of the neck are done to complete the examination of the head and neck.

Tongue

- The lateral border of the tongue is the most common subsite of origin.
- The relative laxity of the tissue planes between the intrinsic muscles of the tongue allows cancer cells to spread easily and the patient becomes symptomatic only when the tumor size is big enough to interfere with mobility of the tongue. Involvement of the root of tongue might lead to ankyloglossia.
- Squamous cell carcinoma of the tongue arises in normal epithelium, in areas of leukoplakia, or in an area of chronic glossitis.
- The patient may have dysfunction of speech and swallowing.
- Pain appears when the tumor involves the lingual nerve and the pain may also be referred to the ear.

SURGICAL ANATOMY

- The FOM is a *horseshoe-shaped area* that is bounded peripherally by the inner surface (lingual surface) of the mandible **(Fig. 2)**.
- It extends posteriorly to the junction of anterior tonsillar pillar and the tonsillolingual sulcus or the insertion of the anterior tonsillar pillar into the tongue and merges medially with the ventral surface of the oral tongue.
- Posterolaterally, the tonsillolingual sulcus separates the tongue from the tonsillar fossa. Posteriorly, the valleculae separate the base of tongue from the lingual surface of the epiglottis.
- Its concavity is important for efficient swallowing of the saliva.
- It is covered with oral mucosa through which the thin-walled veins of sublingual/ranine area are visible.
- The *frenulum* is a fold of mucosa that extends along the midline anteriorly between the openings of the submandibular ducts.
- *Sublingual and submandibular glands* drain into the FOM through the Bartholin's duct and the Wharton's duct, respectively.

The Wharton's duct is about 5 cm in length and runs between the sublingual gland and the genioglossus muscle.
- The genioglossus muscle, geniohyoid muscle, mylohyoid muscle, and the anterior belly of the digastric muscle form the *muscular diaphragm* of the FOM **(Fig. 3)**.
- The paired geniohyoid muscles in the midline, genioglossus muscle, sublingual salivary glands, submandibular ducts, oral component of submandibular salivary glands, and the lingual and hypoglossal nerves are the structures that are located between the mucosa and the mylohyoid muscle.
- The tongue has eight muscles. Four extrinsic muscles (genioglossus, hyoglossus, styloglossus, and palatoglossus) are attached to bone and control the position of the tongue. Four intrinsic muscles are not attached to bone and can modulate the shape of the tongue. All the intrinsic and extrinsic muscles are innervated by hypoglossal nerve, except the palatoglossus muscle, which is innervated by vagus nerve.
- The *lingual nerve* provides sensation to the FOM. It crosses deep to the submandibular duct in the FOM laterally.
- The *glossopharyngeal nerve* supplies the somatic afferent and taste sensation to the posterior one-third of the tongue. The lingual nerve provides general somatic sensation to the anterior two-thirds of the mouth and FOM.
- *Arterial supply* to the tongue and FOM is from the lingual artery and its branches (ranine artery, dorsalis linguae, and

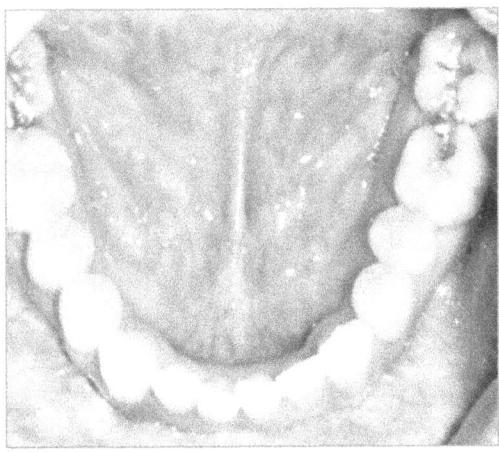

Fig. 2: Floor of mouth.

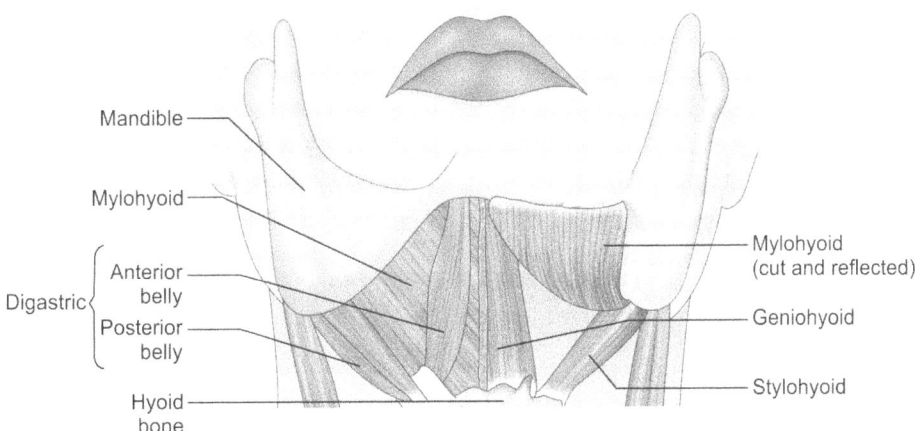

Fig. 3: Muscles forming the floor of mouth (FOM).

sublingual arteries) and the mylohyoid and submental branches of the facial artery.
- The mandible forms the outer border of the FOM and may be involved by tumors of the FOM. It may need to be divided (mandibulotomy) or resected (mandibulectomy). But, in edentulous patients, the vertical height of the mandible may not be adequate for marginal mandibulectomy: the mental foramen and inferior alveolar nerve may lie too close to the upper surface of resorbed mandible. Hence, a segmental mandibulectomy is preferred in such situations.

PRETREATMENT EVALUATION

Tumor size, the extent or depth of invasion (DOI), and the presence or absence of regional lymph node metastases are crucial for planning treatment. The DOI of early-stage squamous cell carcinoma of the oral tongue is particularly difficult to assess preoperatively.

Oral cavity cancers tend to invade soft tissue early in their natural history. Involvement of bone is usually limited to larger tumors, except for those that originate in gingival mucosa. Therefore, pretreatment imaging is required in addition to thorough inspection and palpation of the oral cavity.
- Computed tomography (CT) with intravenous contrast is commonly used to detect bone invasion.
  Limitations are being metallic dental restorations.
- Magnetic resonance imaging (MRI) provides better visualization of soft-tissue involvement, extracapsular spread and nodal involvement, gross perineural spread, and bone marrow involvement. It is limited by motion artifacts and inflammation.
- Combined positron emission tomography (PET)/CT scans increase accuracy in evaluating the extent of the primary tumor and aid in defining the target, if definitive radiation therapy (RT) is being considered. PET scanning may help to identify involved lymph nodes and to resolve any discrepancy that might arise on CT/MRI. It is also useful in post-RT ± CT evaluation and detection of distant metastasis.
- An excisional biopsy needs to be performed for smaller lesions. For deeper and more extensive lesions, an incisional biopsy is advised.
- Sentinel lymph node biopsy is an emerging technique that may provide an additional option for the assessment of regional lymph nodes.

If these initial pretreatment evaluation studies identify lymph node involvement or invasion of deeper structures, this constitutes stage III or IV disease.

HISTOLOGIC FINDINGS

- Squamous cell carcinomas constitute >90% of oral cancers.
- Adenocarcinomas are second in frequency.
- Other tumors include malignancies of the minor salivary glands such as mucoepidermoid and adenoid cystic carcinoma, melanoma, lymphoma, sarcoma, basaloid squamous cell carcinoma, and very rarely malignant hemangiopericytoma.

STAGING

The tumor, node, and metastasis (TNM) staging system of the American Joint Committee on Cancer (AJCC), 8th edition and the Union for International Cancer Control (UICC) is used to classify lip and oral cavity carcinoma.

TREATMENT OF STAGES I AND II

For stages I or II disease, surgery is generally preferred over RT because of the decreased morbidity associated with surgery. There are no randomized controlled clinical trials comparing the two and this recommendation, therefore, has largely been based upon clinical experience.

Floor of Mouth

These tumors are locally invasive. There is a high risk of neck lymph node metastases even with stages I and II.

- Surgery has been the preferred approach due to the concern of risk of radiation-induced bone necrosis and other long-term complications in patients treated with definitive RT.
- Early-stage FOM cancer can generally be managed via transoral excision. If oncologically feasible, the lingual nerve, which lies relatively superficially in the FOM, should be spared.
- Small-to-medium defects can be closed primarily, left to close by secondary intention, or reconstructed with a skin graft.
- Large defects are best repaired with a vascularized graft such as a radial forearm free tissue transfer or submental island skin flap to avoid contracture difficulty with speech and swallowing.
  Consider reconstruction for all patients who undergo resections of the FOM, unless there is a major contraindication for general anesthesia.
- *Definitive RT*—small (<1 cm) or superficial lesions (<4 mm thick) can be treated with either an intraoral cone or interstitial brachytherapy alone. An intraoral cone is more suitable for lesions located centrally or in the anterior part of the mouth.

When a boost is given with an intraoral cone, it is delivered before external beam RT, so that mucositis does not impede visualization of the lesion. When a boost is given with interstitial brachytherapy, it is delivered after external beam RT to allow for tumor shrinkage.

The use of RT as a primary option may be contraindicated in tumors that have been irradiated previously or in tumors with involvement of the mandible and with a history of poor wound healing.

Five-year overall survival rates for stages I and II cancers of 95% and 85% have been reported.

Oral Tongue

- Surgery is generally recommended for oral tongue cancer, if good functional rehabilitation can be achieved with reconstruction.
- Partial glossectomy with negative margins can preserve speech and swallowing for most cases of stages I and II lesions of the oral tongue. The choice of reconstruction and intensity of rehabilitation determine the ultimate functional outcome.
- Assessing surgical resection margins can be difficult. Deep tongue muscle margins are not found in a single plane in contrast to the radial mucosal margins.
- *Definitive RT*—small (≤1 cm) and superficial lesions can be treated with either an intraoral cone or interstitial brachytherapy alone.

Management of Neck

Management of neck is a vital component of management of oral cavity cancer. Cervical lymph node metastases are associated with inferior survival rates. Elective treatment of neck improves both disease-specific and overall survival.

- *Elective treatment* of the neck in patients with clinically N0 stages I and II oral cavity cancer was historically controversial. However, its importance for appropriately selected patient has now been established in a large randomized controlled trial (RCT) conducted at Tata Memorial Hospital, Mumbai.
- *Tumor thickness* is a useful parameter for predicting occult metastases in squamous cell carcinoma of the oral cavity, particularly for tumors arising in the oral tongue. It is now recommended for most patients with tumors ≥ 3 mm in thickness. Improved imaging techniques, including functional or molecular-based studies prior to surgery, may eventually prove useful in selecting patients for neck dissection.

  Noninvasive techniques to assess tumor thickness (digital palpation, CT, PET, MRI, and intraoral ultrasonography) and representative biopsy or frozen section analysis each have limitations. Thus, the thickness of the primary tumor is often unknown prior to surgery. Decision for neck dissection may be made empirically before surgery based upon clinical features or deferred pending final histopathologic examination.

  Sentinel lymph node biopsy is an emerging technique that may eventually be an important "middle-of-the-road" option between observation and neck dissection in patients with intermediate-thickness tumors.
- Patients may have *skip metastases* involving level III or IV without involvement of levels I and II. Thus, a selective neck dissection of levels I to IV may be more appropriate than a supraomohyoid dissection of levels I to III. Levels IIB and IV are dissected at the discretion of the surgeon. Level V dissection is generally unnecessary.
- Elective lymph node dissection for clinically N0 tumors should include at least *18 lymph nodes* as per the National Comprehensive Cancer Network (NCCN) guidelines.
- Patients with primary tumors reaching or involving the midline should be managed with bilateral neck dissection or sentinel lymph node biopsy.

Adjuvant Therapy

- Adjuvant postoperative radiation therapy (PORT) to the primary site and unilateral or bilateral neck is given to patients with high-risk features such as pathologically positive lymph nodes, perineural invasion, lymphovascular invasion, DOI >10 mm, and bony invasion.
- Concurrent chemoradiotherapy is indicated for patients who have positive or close final resection margins and with extranodal extension based on the RTOG 9501 and EORTC 22931 trials.
- Contemporary conformal RT techniques should be used to minimize treatment-related morbidity, particularly late xerostomia.

LOCOREGIONALLY ADVANCED TUMORS

- Locoregionally advanced oral cavity cancers are aggressive malignancies with high rates of recurrence following definitive treatment with either surgery or RT alone. Thus, a *combined modality approach* is generally indicated as permitted by the patient's performance status.
- Decisions about the optimal integration of surgery, RT, and chemotherapy for each patient should be made with multidisciplinary input. The management plan should be based on the likely

functional outcome of treatment as well as the expertise of the treatment team.
- *Surgery* is generally recommended as the initial therapy for locally advanced oral cavity cancers. Usually, simultaneous resection and reconstruction are feasible with acceptable functional outcomes.
- *Radiation therapy and/or chemoradiotherapy* are alternatives for:
  - Patients who refuse surgery
  - Technically unresectable tumor
  - Would have an unacceptable functional outcome with surgery
  - Medically inoperable
- The best available data for the use of *induction chemotherapy* for locally advanced oral cavity cancer does not show a survival advantage. As such, its use should be restricted to highly selected cases and/or clinical trials.

Pretreatment Evaluation

Delineation of the tumor size and extent of invasion as well as potential involvement of regional lymph nodes is essential prior to treatment in patients with oral cavity cancer.

In addition to previously mentioned investigations for early-stage tumors, patients with locoregionally advanced disease should be evaluated for the presence of distant metastases.
- CT of the chest is to screen for lung metastases.
- PET/CT can be considered to rule out distant metastatic disease or second primaries and potentially better characterize neck nodes.
- All patients should be seen preoperatively by the surgeon, radiation oncologist, and medical oncologist for preoperative treatment planning.
- Assessment of comorbidity, speech and swallowing function, nutritional status, and dental and psychosocial evaluations are also important steps in treatment planning.

Floor of Mouth

- Locally advanced cancer of the FOM is typically treated with surgical resection to achieve negative margins followed by postoperative RT with or without concurrent chemotherapy based on the final histopathology report.
- The combination of surgery and postoperative RT has been associated with better local control than either modality alone, as surgical resection alone for stages III and IV disease results in 5-year overall survival of only 46% and 26%, respectively.
- Cancer of the FOM has a high rate of mandibular invasion and cervical lymph node metastases.
- Anterior FOM cancers often involve the geniohyoid tubercle and genioglossus muscle anteriorly. Thus, surgery will frequently require segmental mandibulectomy, as marginal resection of bone is generally not possible in the coronal plane.

Oral Tongue

- Typically, 5-year disease-specific survival rates of 39% and 27% have been achieved for stages III and IV disease, respectively.
- Partial glossectomy is commonly required for locoregionally advanced disease.
- Total glossectomy is sometimes needed in cases where bilateral lingual arteries are involved by tumor.
- As with advanced FOM cancers, addition of postoperative RT or chemoradiotherapy appears to improve disease control compared with surgery alone.

- Primary treatment with concurrent chemoradiotherapy or sequential therapy may be preferred when total glossectomy is indicated, given the overall poor prognosis and poor functional outcomes associated with extensive resections. The idea is to balance the oncological and functional outcomes.

Management of Neck

- While patients with clinically involved regional lymph nodes can benefit from a complete modified neck dissection, selective neck dissection has been proved to be oncologically sound in those patients with advanced oral cavity cancer, i.e., single ipsilateral < 3 cm lymph node involvement without extranodal extension.
- Tumors that reach or cross the midline have increased chances of contralateral nodal metastases and benefit from bilateral neck treatment. Ventral oral tongue and FOM cancers are at very high risk for bilateral nodal involvement.
- If postoperative RT is planned for the ipsilateral neck, some groups advocate RT to the contralateral N0 neck rather than neck dissection. The rationale being that bilateral neck dissection followed by bilateral neck RT has a high risk of significant lymphedema.
- For patients receiving definitive RT, irradiation of the neck should follow the same indications as for neck dissection.

COMPLICATIONS
Surgical Complications

- Infection
- Bleeding
- Aspiration
- Wound breakdown
- Flap loss
- Orocutaneous fistula

Reconstructive Surgery

- Reconstructive techniques do not restore motor or sensory function.
  This is acceptable for smaller defects (e.g., hemiglossectomy reconstructed with radial forearm free flap) where the remaining normal tissue can compensate well.
- Larger defects (e.g., total glossectomy reconstructed with rectus free flap) may result in permanent debilitating functional loss.

Radiation Therapy-associated Complications

- Mucositis
- Skin reaction
- Xerostomia
- Loss of taste
- Dysphagia
- Late toxicities may include skin and soft-tissue atrophy and fibrosis, osteoradionecrosis, xerostomia, trismus, difficulty in swallowing, impaired speech, and dental caries.
  Osteoradionecrosis of the mandible is a particularly feared consequence of high-dose radiation to the oral cavity.

PROGNOSIS

The Surveillance, Epidemiology, and End Results (SEER) Cancer Statistics Review for the year 1975–2007 reported a 5-year relative survival for locally advanced oral cavity and oropharyngeal cancer of 54.7% in comparison to 82.5% for early-stage disease.

Prognostic Factors
- Presence/absence of lymph node metastasis
- Number and size of positive lymph nodes
- Presence of extranodal extension
- Ratio of positive lymph nodes to total number of excised lymph nodes
- Higher histologic grade of primary tumor
- Perineural invasion
- Large size of primary tumor

POSTOPERATIVE SURVEILLANCE
- Regular posttreatment follow-up is an essential component of patient care following potentially curative treatment of head and neck cancer.
- The intensity of follow-up is maximum during the first 2-4 years since 80-90% of all recurrences after curative treatment would occur within this time frame.
- Continued follow-up beyond 5 years is usually advised due to the risk of late recurrence and second primary malignancies.

SURGICAL TECHNIQUES
Surgical Objectives
- R0 resection
- Avoid postoperative orocervical fistulae
- Optimal cosmesis and function
- Maintain length and mobility of the tongue
- Avoid pooling of secretions and food in the reconstructed FOM
- Avoid neurovascular injury (lingual and hypoglossal nerves)
- Maintain mandibular continuity and strength
- Restore dentition

Need for tracheostomy—patients with small size tumors in the anterior FOM may not need temporary tracheostomy. However, whenever the laryngeal support of the mylohyoid, geniohyoid, and genioglossus muscles is lost and whenever a flap is used to reconstruct a FOM or tongue defect, the patient falls at risk of obstruction of airway and should have a temporary tracheostomy inserted.

SURGICAL ACCESS
- *Transoral*: Smaller tumors (T1-T2) are usually easily excised though the open mouth. In edentulous patient, the mouth is kept open wide either with a dental bite block or with a self-retaining retractor taking care to protect the teeth. However, in dentate patients, the teeth may obstruct access to the anterior FOM. In such cases, lower teeth may have to be extracted and a marginal mandibulectomy or a mandibulotomy may be required for access. This is especially required when the tumor abuts the anterior mandible.
- *Midline lip-split*: The soft tissues are stripped off the front of the mandible.
- *Visor flap*: This is performed by cutting along the gingivolabial and gingivobuccal sulci about 1 cm from the bone to permit suture placement while closing the wound and then stripping the soft tissues from the outer aspect of the mandible. Care must be taken not to transect the mental nerves, if they can be saved. The skin flap is next retracted superiorly to expose the mandible.
- *Pull through*: This may be practiced when the tumor stops some distance from the inner aspect of the mandible. Following bilateral neck dissections of levels Ia and Ib, the mandibular attachments of the anterior bellies of digastric, mylohyoid, geniohyoid, and genioglossus muscles are divided with electrocautery working from inferiorly. The mucosa of the anterior

FOM is then divided 1 cm from the inner aspect of the mandible (to facilitate later repair). This permits the surgeon to deliver the anterior FOM and anterior tongue into the neck and then to proceed with the resection.

TYPES OF GLOSSECTOMY

Type I Glossectomy (Mucosectomy)

It includes the excision of a superficial lesion with appropriate margins including mucosa, submucosa and a thin layer of the intrinsic muscles.

Closure: Primary or left raw for healing by secondary intention.

Indication: Precancerous, superficial suspicious lesions.

Type II Glossectomy (Partial Glossectomy)

It includes the excision of a lesion with appropriate margins including mucosa, submucosa, and the intrinsic muscles till the surface of the extrinsic muscles. The terminal branches of the lingual artery must be ligated and the lingual nerve is mostly preserved.

Closure: Generally primarily.

Indication: Lesions infiltrating submucosa and superficially involving the intrinsic muscles, but not the extrinsic muscles, or infiltration less than 10 mm depth.

Type III Glossectomy

Type IIIA Glossectomy (Hemiglossectomy)

It includes the excision of a lesion with appropriate margins including mucosa, submucosa, and ipsilateral intrinsic and extrinsic muscles.

The lingual artery should be ligated and removed en bloc with the lingual and hypoglossal nerves, in the specimen of the primary tumor. The base of the ipsilateral tongue is usually preserved. The tip of the tongue may or may not be preserved.

Indication: Lesions involving the intrinsic and minimally the extrinsic muscles or infiltration > 10 mm but not crossing midline.

Type IIIB Glossectomy (Compartmental Hemiglossectomy)

It includes the excision of a lesion with appropriate margins including mucosa, submucosa, ipsilateral intrinsic and extrinsic muscles, genioglossus, hyoglossus and styloglossus muscles, and the inferior portion of the palatoglossus muscle. Medially, the midline raphe is a part of the resected specimen. The lingual nerve is resected to the maximum cranial extent. The hypoglossal nerve is also removed once the ansa, the lingual artery and vein are ligated near the greater cornu of the hyoid bone, and removed en bloc.

Indication: Lesions infiltrating the intrinsic and extrinsic muscles but not crossing midline.

Type IV Glossectomy

Type IVA Glossectomy (Subtotal Glossectomy)

It implies an anterior subtotal glossectomy with preservation of bilateral base of the tongue, posterior hyoglossus muscle, along with hypoglossal and lingual nerves, from the less affected side.

Indication: Lesions that arise in the anterior 2/3rd portion of the tongue and cross midline to involve the contralateral genioglossus muscle but limited to mobile tongue.

Type IVB (Near-total Glossectomy)

Means Type IVa glossectomy along with infiltration of the ipsilateral base of the tongue.

Contralateral hyoglossus and styloglossus muscles, hypoglossal nerve, lingual nerve, and lingual artery are preserved.

Indication: Massive lesions that cross the midline to infiltrate the ipsilateral base of the tongue and the contralateral genioglossus muscle.

Reconstruction is done using a free flap

Type V Glossectomy (Total Glossectomy)

It includes the excision of a lesion with appropriate margins including anterior 2/3rd of tongue and base of the tongue. Posterior cut is at the level of vallecula; medially it includes all intrinsic and extrinsic muscles, both lingual arteries, hypoglossal, lingual nerves, and the floor of mouth.

Indication: lesions of the anterior ventral surface of the tongue, dorsum of the tongue, or the tongue base, which involve the bilateral extrinsic genioglossus, hyoglossus, and styloglossus.

Reconstruction is done using a free flap.

Depending upon the extent of the lesion, type III-V glossectomies can be written as extended to include adjacent structures such as the geniohyoid muscle, digastric muscle, the epiglottis, larynx, the lateral wall of the pharynx, or the mandible.

If some type of glossectomy is done where a structure could be preserved, then it may be written as "Glossectomy type with preservation of the structure."

TUMOR RESECTION

Neck Dissection

If a level I neck dissection(s) is done prior to resection of the primary tumor, it allows the surgeon to cut through the muscles in the FOM and tongue knowing the location of the hypoglossal and lingual nerve and lingual artery.

Mandibulectomy

- If a marginal or segmental mandibulectomy is planned, then it should be performed before resection of the FOM/tongue tumor, as it improves surgical exposure.
- If a segmental mandibulectomy is planned, then preplate the mandible with a reconstruction plate to ensure teeth alignment and a good bony contour.
- Make small sharp osteotomies to avoid inadvertent fracture of the mandible or with a powered oscillating saw.
- With marginal mandibulectomy, the cut is made obliquely to preserve the height of the outer cortex for mandibular strength, but to remove the inner cortex that abuts the tumor.
- With segmental mandibulectomy, the bone is cut at least 2 cm from visible tumor.

Tumor

- Once the mandibulectomy has been completed, bone is kept attached to the tumor specimen and delivery of the tumor into the surgical field is facilitated.
- Identify and preserve the submandibular duct(s) and the lingual and hypoglossal nerve(s), if possible. The sublingual gland may be encountered in anterior FOM cancer resections and may be sacrificed, if needed.
- Resect the tumor with at least 1 cm margins.
- Obtain frozen section confirmation of clear tumor margins, if available.

Partial glossectomy—for small tumors limited to the tongue, a partial glossectomy with a 1–2 cm margin around is sufficient with primary closure taking care not to suture the tongue to the gingival mucosa in case of extension of lesion to FOM.

Unlike the mucosal margins, taking adequate deep margins might be tricky and constant palpation for adequacy of margins usually helps.

Stay sutures are taken for adequate traction and special care to identify and preserve the lingual artery, unless it is involved with tumor.

Repair

Following resection, the surgeon carefully assesses the defect to plan how best to maintain mandibular integrity and contour, oral competence, mastication, oral transport, swallowing, and speech.

Primary closure: Avoid tethering or distorting the tongue.

Split skin graft: This may be used to cover a defect that could otherwise be left open, but for concern about a through-and-through communication to the neck or over a marginal mandibulectomy defect. The skin is sutured to the margins of the defect with absorbable sutures.

Flap Reconstruction

- Buccinator myomucosal flap
- Nasolabial flap
- Submental artery island flap
- Supraclavicular flap
- Pectoralis major flap
- Radial-free forearm flap
- Anterolateral free thigh flap
- Free fibula flap
- Titanium reconstruction plate

In case of local flaps, the pedicles are divided at 10–14 days, if teeth are present; bite blocks are inserted to prevent premature pedicle division.

Reconstruction Pointers

- Mobility of the tongue is vital for oral function.
- Length of tongue is more important than its width.
- Never suture the edge of the tongue to the gingiva; in such cases, always maintain mobility of the tongue with a flap.
- Avoid tethering the tip of the tongue.
- Some defects are best left open to heal by secondary intention to retain mobility.
- Simply shaping a flap to match the resected tissue may restore form, but may have poor functional outcome.
- Reduce the risk of orocervical fistula by approximating the mylohyoid to the digastric muscle in the neck and ensuring that the suction drain is not placed in the upper neck.

No repair: Small and/or superficial resections above the mylohyoid muscle that do not communicate with the neck dissection may be left open to heal. Resist the temptation to suture such defects, as it may alter the shape of the tongue or fix the tongue to the anterior FOM.

Resection of cancers of the FOM without taking cognizance of oral function may severely cripple the patient in terms of speech, mastication, oral transport, and swallowing.

Resecting the anterior arch of the mandible beyond the midline without reconstructing the bone with loss of the anterior attachments of the suprahyoid muscles leads to an *Andy Gump deformity* with loss of oral competence, drooling, and a very poor cosmetic outcome **(Fig. 4)**.

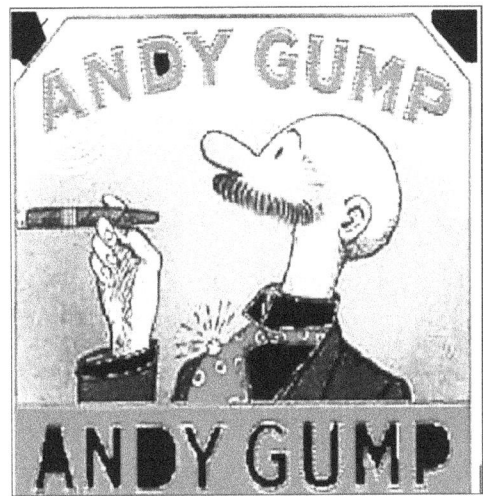

Fig. 4: Andy Gump deformity.

KEY POINTS

- The lateral border is the most common subsite of origin of tongue carcinoma.
- Bimanual examination allows assessment of extent of the primary tumor and the involvement of the structures of the submandibular triangle in case of FOM tumors and assessment of DOI in tongue tumors.
- 5-year overall survival rates for stages I and II cancers are 95% and 85%, respectively.
- Consider doing a temporary tracheostomy whenever the laryngeal support of the mylohyoid, geniohyoid, and genioglossus muscles is lost, especially when a flap is used to reconstruct a FOM defect.
- 5-year disease-specific survival rates of 39% and 27% have been achieved for stages III and IV disease, respectively, with combined modality treatment.
- Resecting the anterior arch of the mandible beyond the midline without reconstructing the bone with loss of the anterior attachments of the suprahyoid muscles leads to an *Andy Gump deformity*.

CHAPTER 19

Management of Neck in Oral Cancer

Rajeev Kumar

INTRODUCTION

The first sites of metastasis in oral cancer are the neck nodes and they are the most critical prognostic factor. Once the nodes get involved, the survival drops by 50%. Even when the nodes are clinically not detectable, 30% of oral cancers have occult metastasis in neck nodes. Neck is a small space containing major structures including trachea, esophagus, carotids, vagus, etc., which cannot be sacrificed; therefore, it is important to manage the neck with utmost care and skill. Recurrences in the neck are not easy to manage; hence, the first address to neck should be sufficient, skilful, and complete. One must also be aware of not overtreating the neck to give functional problems to the patients.

LEVELS OF NECK NODES

The levels of neck nodes are described in **Figures 1A and B**.

Seven Levels of Neck Nodes

1. *Level I—Submental and submandibular*: It contains the submental and submandibular triangles, which are bordered by the posterior belly of the digastric muscle, the midline, the body of the mandible superiorly, and the hyoid bone inferiorly. Level I is subdivided into Ia (submental triangle) and Ib (submandibular triangle).
2. *Level II—Upper jugular*: It contains the upper jugular lymph nodes and extends from the skull base superiorly to the hyoid bone inferiorly. Anterior boundaries are

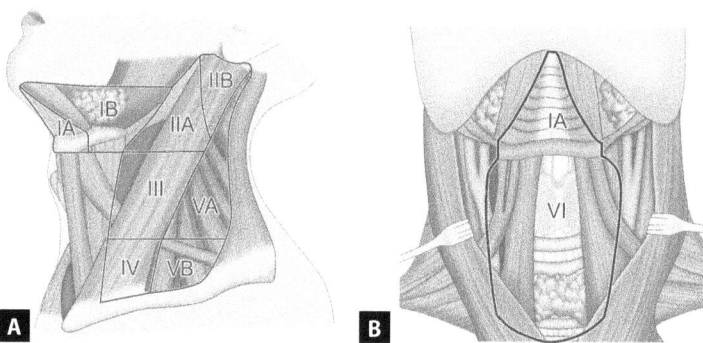

Figs. 1A and B: Levels of cervical lymph nodes. Division of nodal groups by subzones: (A) Lateral view; (B) Anterior view. (IA: submental nodes; IB: submandibular nodes; IIA: upper jugular nodes anterior to the 11th nerve; IIB: upper jugular nodes posterior to the 11th nerve; VA: lymph nodes in the posterior triangle located above the level of the inferior border of the cricoid cartilage; VB: lymph nodes in the posterior triangle located below the level of the inferior border of the cricoid cartilage)

the midline strap muscles; posteriorly, this level is bounded by the anterior border of the trapezius muscle. The spinal accessory nerve (CN XI) travels obliquely across this area and can be used to subdivide this area into IIa (anteriorly) and IIb (posteriorly).
3. *Level III—Midjugular*: It contains the middle jugular lymph nodes from the hyoid bone superiorly to the level of the lower border of the cricoid cartilage inferiorly.
4. *Level IV—Lower jugular*: It contains the lower jugular lymph nodes from the level of the cricoid cartilage superiorly to the clavicle inferiorly. Nodes that are deep to the sternal head of the sternocleidomastoid muscle (SCM) are categorized as IVa and those deep to the clavicular head of the SCM are categorized as IVb.
5. *Level V—Posterior triangle*: It contains the lymph nodes in the posterior triangle bounded by the anterior border of the trapezius muscle posteriorly, the posterior border of the SCM anteriorly, and the clavicle inferiorly. This area may be further classified into the upper, middle, and lower levels corresponding to the superior and inferior planes that define levels II, III, and IV.
6. *Level VI—Prelaryngeal (delphian), pretracheal, and paratracheal*: It contains the lymph nodes of the anterior central compartment from the hyoid bone superiorly to the suprasternal notch inferiorly. On each side, the lateral boundary is formed by the medial border of the carotid sheath.
7. *Level VII—Upper mediastinal*: It contains the lymph nodes inferior to the suprasternal notch in the superior mediastinum.

The lymph nodes in the neck are divided into five levels depending on their position. Different subsites of oral cancer drain into different levels and accordingly one can select the type of selective neck dissection (SND). They are all important for uniformity in reporting and depiction of nodal involvement. However, there are no strict boundaries for these lymph nodes and there may be some overlap.

- *Level IA nodes*:
  - Lip
  - Anterior mandibular alveolar ridge
  - Floor of mouth (FOM)
- *Level IB nodes*:
  - Oral cavity
  - Anterior nasal cavity
  - Soft tissues and structure of the mid-face
- *Level II nodes*:
  - Oral cavity
  - Nasal cavity
  - Nasopharynx
  - Oropharynx
  - Hypopharynx
  - Larynx
  - Parotid gland
- *Level III nodes*:
  - Oral cavity
  - Nasopharynx
  - Oropharynx
  - Hypopharynx
  - Larynx
- *Level IV nodes*:
  - Hypopharynx
  - Larynx
  - Cervical esophagus
- *Level V nodes*:
  - Nasopharynx
  - Oropharynx
- *Level VI nodes*:
  - Thyroid gland
  - Larynx (glottic and subglottic)
  - Apex of the pyriform sinus
  - Cervical esophagus

CLINICAL STAGING OF NECK NODES

- Regional lymph nodes (N)
- Clinical N (cN)
- *NX*: Regional lymph nodes cannot be assessed.
- *N0*: No regional lymph node metastasis
- *N1*: Metastasis in a single ipsilateral lymph node 3 cm or smaller in greatest dimension and extranodal extension (ENE)(-)
- *N2*: Metastasis in a single ipsilateral node larger than 3 cm, but not larger than 6 cm in greatest dimension and ENE(-) or metastases in multiple ipsilateral lymph nodes, none larger than 6 cm in greatest dimension and ENE(-) or in bilateral or contralateral lymph nodes, none larger than 6 cm in greatest dimension and ENE(-).
    - *N2a*: Metastasis in a single ipsilateral lymph node larger than 3 cm, but not larger than 6 cm in greatest dimension and ENE(-)
    - *N2b*: Metastasis in multiple ipsilateral lymph nodes, none larger than 6 cm in greatest dimension and ENE(-)
    - *N2c*: Metastasis in bilateral or contralateral lymph nodes, none larger than 6 cm in greatest dimension and ENE(-)
- *N3*: Metastasis in a lymph node larger than 6 cm in greatest dimension and ENE(-) or metastasis in any node(s) and clinically overt ENE(+)
    - *N3a*: Metastasis in a lymph node larger than 6 cm in greatest dimension and ENE(-)
    - *N3b*: Metastasis in any node(s) and clinically overt ENE(+)

Note: A designation of "U" or "L" may be used for any N category to indicate metastasis above the lower border of cricoids (U) or below the lower border of the cricoids (L). Similarly, clinical and pathological ENE should be recorded as ENE(-) or ENE(+).

DEFINITIONS OF NECK DISSECTION

- *Radical neck dissection*: Radical neck dissection is the removal of lymph node levels I to V along with the submandibular gland, tail of the parotid gland, SCM, internal jugular vein (IJV), and CN XI.
- *Modified radical neck dissection (MRND)*: MRND is removal of lymph nodes from levels I to V such as in the radical neck dissection, but with preservation of at least one of the nonlymphatic structures namely SCM, CN XI, and/or IJV.
    - *Type I*: The CN XI is preserved.
    - *Type II*: The CN XI and the IJV both are preserved.
    - *Type III*: It is also called functional neck dissection. The CN XI, the IJV, and the SCM are preserved.
- *Extended radical neck dissection*: Extended radical neck dissection involves removal of additional lymph node levels or groups and/or nonlymphatic structures such as muscle, blood vessels, and nerves that are not normally removed with a radical neck dissection.
- *Selective neck dissection*: SND refers to preservation of one or more lymph node levels depending on site of primary tumor and sparing the SCM, IJV, and CN XI. They can be:
    - *Supraomohyoid neck dissection*: This is the removal of lymph node groups I, II, and III.
    - *Lateral neck dissection*: This is the removal of lymph node groups II, III, and IV.
    - *Posterolateral neck dissection*: This is the removal of lymph node groups II, III, IV, and V.

If a major neck structure is removed as part of a SND, it should be indicated. For example, a lateral neck dissection with sacrifice of IJV is still a SND.

- *Salvage neck dissection*: This is a type of neck dissection in a previously treated neck, previously treated by radiation, chemotherapy, or surgery. This is performed for a persistent tumor in the neck lymph nodes in spite of treatment. This is a difficult situation particularly after radiation therapy where neck is almost woody and there are high chances of injury to major vessels with delayed healing.
- *Superselective neck dissection*: It involves complete removal of all fibrofatty tissue contents including lymph nodes of one or two contiguous levels. It is usually done for residual nodes after treatment with chemoradiation where only involved level is dissected.

IMAGING OF NECK NODES (TABLE 1)

Imaging of the cervical nodes may alter the estimated clinical stage in 20–30% of patients.

MANAGEMENT OF N0 NECK

The basic principle is to treat the nodal area when there is no clinically apparent node, but there is >15–20% chances of metastasis. It has been seen that one-third of patients with squamous cell carcinoma (SCC) of oral cavity have occult metastasis in their lymph nodes and the incidence varies according to the site of involvement.

- Floor of mouth—25%
- Oral tongue—60%
- Buccal mucosa—20%
- Retromolar trigone—20%
- Hard palate—15%
- Alveolus—15%

A study by Tytor et al. of 176 patients diagnosed with carcinoma of the oral cavity showed that the rate of metastasis in the cervical lymph node was 14% in T1 tumors, 37% in T2 tumors, and 57% in patients with large tumors >4 cm in diameter.

Brown et al. showed in their study that 71% of N0 patients who had perineural invasion developed regional metastatic disease compared to 36% of N0 patients who did not have perineural invasion. This study also demonstrated that with the presence of perineural invasion, 2-year survival reduced from 82 to 52%.

Observation versus Elective Neck Treatment for N0 Neck

There is immense controversy existing about the optimal treatment for clinically negative neck nodes. The believers of observation cite the morbidity of elective neck dissection (END). Other reason for close observation is that any appearance of cervical metastasis can be picked up earlier and then, hence, can be treated adequately. The rates of occult metastasis in the neck from oral cavity cancers are approximately 34%. Hence, it can be argued that about two-thirds of such patients would be exposed unnecessarily to the morbidity of the neck dissection.

TABLE 1: Sensitivity and specificity of different investigations.

Modality	Sensitivity	Specificity
Ultrasound	50–58%	75–82%
CT	40–68%	78–92%
MRI	55–93%	82–95%
PET	87–90%	80–93%
CT-PET	96%	98.5%

(PET: positron emission tomography)

Weiss et al. created a decision tree analysis and reached at a conclusion that observation is preferred when the chances of occult metastasis are <20%; elective treatment of neck with radiation or surgery may be preferred, if the occult metastasis chances are >20%. T1/T2 lip carcinomas, T1/T2 oral tongue carcinomas that are <4 mm thick, and T1/T2 cancers of FOM ≤1.5 mm thick have <20% occult metastasis rate to the neck.

The followers of surgery believe that dissection of lymph nodes may be used as a staging method. In the presence of extracapsular spread (ECS), a patient may be upstaged and, hence be treated with more aggressive treatment early rather than later in the disease when survival may be as good.

Another research, which compared glossectomy and neck observation versus glossectomy and neck dissection for T1 and T2 SCC of the oral tongue, reported survival of 33% in the observation group and survival of 55% in the neck dissection group. The locoregional control improved from 50 to 91% when neck dissection was done. ECS rate seen in this study was 58% in the observation group. A study, which compared 5-year survival in T1/T2 N0 SCC of the oral tongue, reported a decreased survival rate from 80.5 to 44.8%.

SENTINEL NODE BIOPSY IN HEAD AND NECK SQUAMOUS CELL CARCINOMA

Sentinel lymph node biopsy (SLNB) is indicated in early lesions T1 and T2 where there are no suspicious nodes in the neck clinically.

A European trial proved that a negative SLNB in oral cavity SCC, stages T1-2N0, was adequate to exclude metastasis in the nodes in 86% of cases, thus resulting in a negative predictive value of 95%. More research is required to ensure if SLNB alone is adequate to provide accurate staging and information to prognosticate. SLNB is still not the standard of care in head and neck squamous cell carcinoma (HNSCC).

ELECTIVE NODAL IRRADIATION

Fletcher showed that elective doses of 50 Gy to clinically N0 neck produced 95% disease control of the neck. He explained the dosimetric fact behind elective nodal irradiation (ENI) and the need for comprehensive treatment.

With 50 Gy in 5 weeks, the incidence of neck failure is 0% whereas doses of 30–40 Gy produce a regional failure in 9–10.5%.

Mendenhall reported a retrospective review of 125 patients with SCC of the head and neck with negative neck and control at the primary site. The neck failure rate was 1.9% with ENI and 18% without ENI.

The usefulness of ENI versus END showed no obvious differences according to a report by Barkley in a large retrospective study of neck treatment in 596 patients.

Elective neck dissection is the preferred management for patients of oral cavity cancer who have clinically negative neck. Elective radiotherapy to a nondissected neck to a dose of 50–56 Gy in 25–30 fractions may be effective and should be administered, if surgery is not feasible.

RECOMMENDATIONS REGARDING ELECTIVE TREATMENT OF HEAD AND NECK CANCERS (TABLE 2)

Coverage of nodal levels I to III for oral cavity cancers and levels II to IV for oropharyngeal, hypopharyngeal, and laryngeal tumors are mandatory as elective radiotherapy.

TABLE 2: Guidelines for neck treatment in patients of oral squamous cell carcinoma.

Stage N0-N1	Stage N2-N3
Levels I, II, III, and IV (for anterior tongue tumors only)	Levels I, II, III, IV, and V

Involvement of ipsilateral structures such as the parotid, the buccal mucosa, and selected tonsil cancers should be considered for ipsilateral ENI.

Elective nodal irradiation of level IV lymph nodes too must be considered in tumors involving the tip of the oral tongue because of direct drainage to this area that bypass the contiguous progression in the anterior jugular nodes.

Involvement of the ipsilateral level V lymph nodes in node-negative oral cavity tumors occur in <1% and does not need ENI.

But, with progressive involvement of levels I to III or the involvement of level IV, the risk for level V involvement increases and ENI is indicated.

MANAGEMENT OF THE CLINICALLY NODE-POSITIVE NECK (N+)

The treatment of the primary site guides treatment of the neck.

When unresectable nodal disease persists, chemoradiation is preferred.

Ipsilateral therapeutic SND for a clinically node-positive (cN+) neck should include nodal levels IA, IB, IIA, IIB, III, IV, and V. An adequate dissection should include at least 18 lymph nodes.

In patients with a cN+ in contralateral neck, a contralateral neck dissection needs to be performed. In patients with a cN0 contralateral neck, an elective contralateral neck dissection may be performed in patients of cancer of the oral tongue and/or FOM that is T3-T4 or approaches midline.

Adjuvant radiotherapy of the neck should be performed in patients with pN1, but did not undergo a good quality neck dissection.

Adjuvant radiotherapy to neck should be delivered to patients with pathologic N2 or N3 disease.

Adjuvant chemoradiotherapy using intravenous bolus cisplatin (100 mg/m^2 every 3 weeks) should be given to patients of oral cavity cancer with ENE in a positive node, irrespective of the extent of the ENE and number or size of the nodes.

Two landmark studies were conducted independently in Europe (EORTC 22931) and in the United States (RTOG 9501) studying the efficacy of addition of three cycles of cisplatin concurrent with postoperative conventional fractionation radiation for patients at high risk for recurrence. High risk included extracapsular extension and positive margins in both studies.

Concurrent weekly cisplatin may be administered with postoperative radiotherapy to patients who are considered inappropriate for standard high-dose intermittent cisplatin.

For patients who have undergone ipsilateral neck dissection only and are at considerable risk of contralateral nodal involvement as in T3-T4 cancers of the oral tongue or of FOM that approaches midline, contralateral neck radiotherapy should be administered to treat potential microscopic disease.

COMPLICATIONS OF NECK DISSECTION

Immediate/Intraoperative

- Hemorrhage—re-exploration at the earliest
- Lymphatic duct injury—occurs more on left side and identifying and repairing with nonabsorbable suture
- Airway obstruction

Delayed

- Seroma formation
- Flap necrosis
- Vascular blowout—particularly in post-radiation cases. It covers the wound with vascularized muscle flap.
- Chyle leak
- Wound sepsis, facial edema, and increased intracranial pressure—after ligation of IJV
- Shoulder pain and dysfunction
- Injury to marginal mandibular nerve, hypoglossal nerve, phrenic nerve, or vagus nerve.

KEY POINTS

- *Radical neck dissection*:
  - All node levels I-V
  - Internal jugular vein
  - Spinal accessory nerve
  - Sternocleidomastoid muscle
- *Modified radical neck dissection*:
  - All node levels I-V:
    - *Type I*: Preserve CN XI
    - *Type II*: Preserve CN XI and IJV
    - *Type III*: Preserve CN XI, IJV, and SCM
- *Selective neck dissection*: Remove only selective lymph node levels
- *Superselective neck dissection*: Remove one or two lymph node levels

CHAPTER 20

Neck Dissections in Oral Cancer

Kiran Joshi, Mudit Agarwal

INTRODUCTION

The history of neck dissection is glorious and started in 19th century. Christian Albert Theodor Billroth (1873) operated one case of tongue cancer with excision of bilateral cervical lymph node metastases. The patient was alive after 18 months of surgery without recurrence. Theodor Kocher (1880) recommended that involved lymph nodes should be removed with wider resection margins.

The concept of elective neck dissection (initially called prophylactic) was originated by *Sir Henry Trentham Butlin (1885)*. George Washington Crile (1905) described en bloc removal of all cervical lymph nodes (today called levels I-V) along the sternocleidomastoid muscle (SCM), submandibular salivary gland, tail of parotid gland, omohyoid muscle, cutaneous branches of the cervical plexus, and the internal jugular vein (IJV).

The greatest impetus to the development of radical neck dissection (RND) came from Hayes Martin (1951), who published a monumental paper entitled Neck Dissection in 1951.

The first description of modified RND was published in Spanish by Suárez (1963). Ettore Bocca (1964) from Italy reported detailed description of functional neck dissection. Medina (1989) categorized lymphadenectomies as comprehensive, selective, and extended.

Neck dissection is a well-established, oncologically sound surgical procedure which has stood the test of time for over 100 years. Weiss et al. suggested that observation is the preferred option when the probability of occult metastasis is <20%. Occult metastases rate in oral cancer remain high (20–30%). The trial by D'Cruz and colleagues showed a significant improvement in overall survival and demonstrated that elective neck dissection improved overall survival in these groups of patients by 12.5% (80% vs. 67.5%; p = 0.01). It has been estimated that the presence of lymphatic metastases decreases survival by 50% and extranodal extension further reduces survival by 50%. This has also formed the basis of change in nodal staging in the 8th edition of the American Joint Committee on Cancer (AJCC) staging manual. A single, small node (N1) converts any early primary cancer (T1-T2) to stage 3 and more than one node or a node > 3 cm (N2 or N3) to stage 4 reflecting the grim prognosis of palpable neck disease **(Tables 1 to 3)**.

TABLE 1: Level of nodes in different head and neck cancers.

Oral cavity	Levels I, II, III, and possibly IV
Oropharynx	Levels II, III, and IV
Hypopharynx	Levels II, III, and IV
Larynx	Levels II, III, IV, and possibly VI

TABLE 2: American Head and Neck Society Classification of neck dissection.

Terminology	Definition
Radical	Removal of lymph node levels I-V, sternocleidomastoid muscle, spinal accessory nerve, and internal jugular vein
Modified	Removal of lymph node levels I-V, as in radical neck dissection (RND), but with preservation of at least one of the nonlymphatic structures (sternocleidomastoid muscle, spinal accessory nerve, and internal jugular vein)
Selective	Preservation of one or more lymph node levels relative to an RND
Extended	Removal of an additional lymph node level or group or a nonlymphatic structure relative to an RND (muscle, blood vessel, and nerve); examples of other lymph node groups are superior mediastinal, parapharyngeal, retropharyngeal, periparotid, postauricular, suboccipital, or buccinators; an example of other nonlymphatic structures can be external carotid artery or hypoglossal or vagus nerves

TABLE 3: Types of neck dissections.

Radical neck dissection	N+ neck for squamous cell carcinoma where spinal accessory nerve (SAN) involved and/or extensive soft-tissue disease with the invasion of sternocleidomastoid muscle (SCM) and internal jugular vein (IJV)
Modified radical neck dissection	N+ neck for squamous cell carcinoma where SAN is free of disease
Selective neck dissection	Clinically or radiologically N0 neck and the depth of tumor invasion is >3 mm

NECK DISSECTION TERMINOLOGY

The latest classification of neck dissections was proposed by the American Academy of Otolaryngology–Head and Neck Surgery (AAO-HNS) committee (2002). It suggested the following changes in the previous classification:

- Any lymph node group outside the neck would be referred to by the name of that specific group, even though many authors suggest defining the tracheoesophageal and superior mediastinal nodes as level VII.
- Sublevels a and b were introduced in levels I, II, and IV.
- The structure(s) preserved in modified radical neck dissection (MND) should be specifically mentioned in surgical reports such as MND [preserving spinal accessory nerve (SAN)] rather than MND type I, type II, or type III.
- The levels removed in selective neck dissections should be quoted within brackets. Each dissection should be defined by the levels removed instead of the traditional classification (supraomohyoid, lateral, posterolateral, and anterior neck dissection).

NECK INCISIONS (BOX 1)

The type of skin incision depends on type of neck dissection, side of neck dissection, and primary tumor site. The standard incisions employed for classical RND range from a double trifurcate incision popularized by

Box 1: Types of neck incisions.

- *Crile*: The incision begins from the mastoid process in a curvilinear fashion up to the tip of hyoid extending superiorly to the submental area. The vertical limb starts behind the carotid artery and goes down the middle portion of the clavicle in a lazy S fashion
- *Conley*: The incision starts in the midline, 1 cm below the mandibular arch, and slopes inferiorly to a position 3 cm from the angle of the mandible. It is then curved inferiorly to the anterior border of the trapezius muscle and up to the level of clavicle at the junction of its middle and lateral third
- *Hayes Martin*: The Y-shape incision in submandibular region is met by a vertical limb, which below becomes continuous with an inverted Y in the suprascapular region
- *Apron flap incision of Latyshevsky*: Only a horizontal incision from mastoid to mastoid gently curving inferiorly over the upper border of the thyroid cartilage
- *MacFee*: Two horizontal incisions are used, one in submandibular region and other in the supraclavicular region. Most suitable incision in irradiated patient
- *Schobinger*: A curved line, starting anteriorly from the submental region, posteriorly up to the tip of the mastoid process where it is continued at right angles with respect to the vertical limb. This limb runs downward along the edge of the trapezius muscle in a curved manner down to the midline of the clavicle

Martin followed by single trifurcate incisions reported by Kocher, Crile, Schobinger, and others. All of these incisions with a vertical component in the neck give a significant esthetic deformity.

The current practice for neck dissection is to employ only a transverse incision along a suitable skin crease. If one needs to reach the submental level across the midline to the opposite side of the neck, dissecting along the same skin crease permits elevation of the upper flap up to the mental region. Similarly, to gain access to level IIb, the transverse incision is not curved toward the mastoid process but carried on laterally along the same skin crease, allowing easy access to the region of the mastoid process. This incision is adequate for a supraomohyoid neck dissection as well as a comprehensive neck dissection. Various types of incisions have been described in **Figure 1**.

Positioning

The patient is placed in a supine position with head ring and shoulder roll to extend neck and turned to the opposite side. The skin is prepped and draped to allow for full exposure of both sides of the neck with clear visualization of surrounding landmarks (e.g., the lower face including the mentum, both mastoid processes, earlobes) and the clavicles and suprasternal notch inferiorly.

Flap Elevation

The initial incision is carried through skin and platysma muscle, although the platysma is deficient in the midline and the lateral most parts of the incision. The flap is raised in the subplatysmal plane superiorly up to the lower border of mandible and inferiorly up to the level of clavicle not including the external jugular vein and the greater auricular nerves in the flap.

MODIFIED NECK DISSECTION

Incision Planning (Fig. 2)

Commonly employed neck incisions are triradiate, Macfee, and modified apron flap. The incision is marked two fingerbreadth below the lower border of the mandible and extending up to the mastoid process posteriorly and anteriorly up to the midpoint of chin. The vertical limb is given at midpoint of the horizontal incision and extends down to the clavicle.

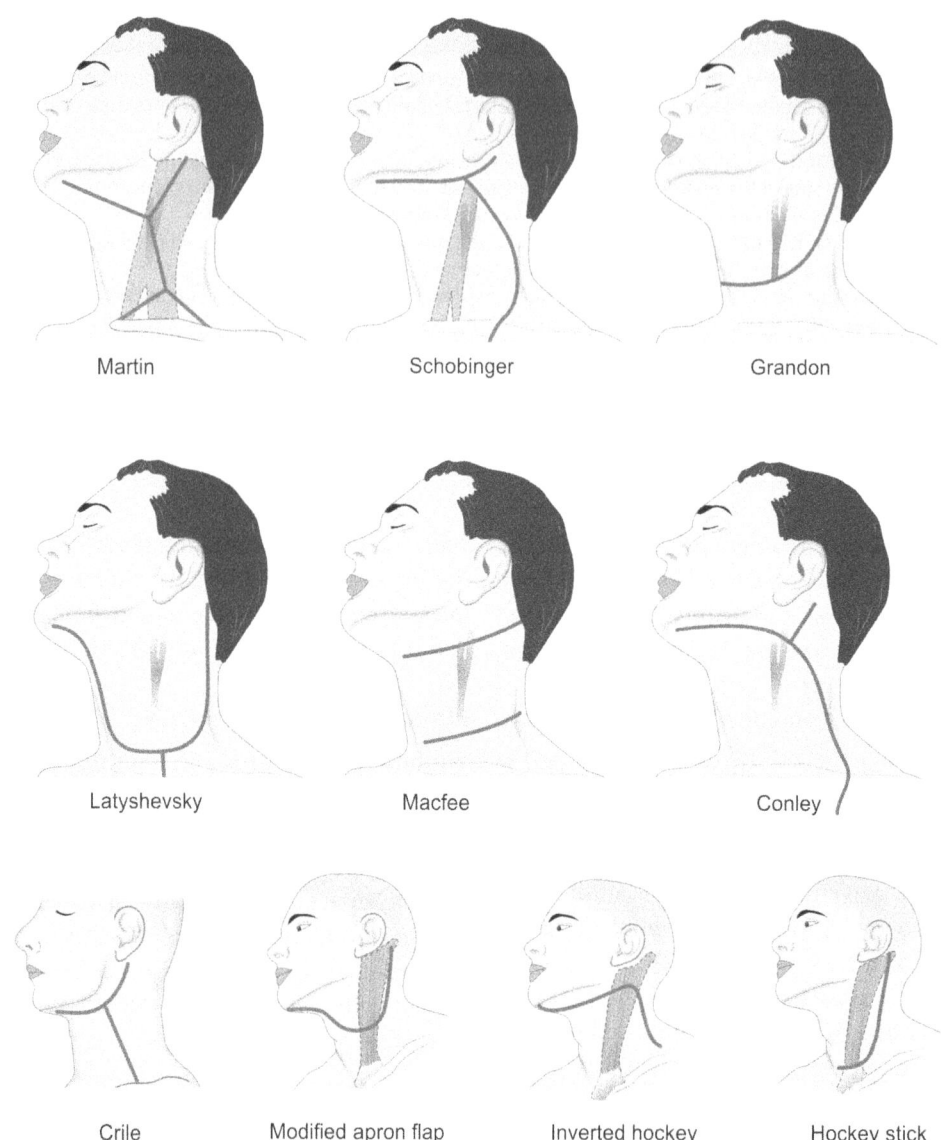

Fig. 1: Various types of neck incisions.

Surgical Steps

Step 1: Submental Triangle Clearance

Start the dissection with clearance of fibrofatty tissue and lymph nodes in the submental triangle until both anterior bellies of the digastric (the lateral borders of the triangle) and the mylohyoid muscle (the floor of the triangle) are exposed and inferiorly to the position of the upper border of the hyoid bone (the inferior border of the triangle).

Step 2: Submandibular Triangle Clearance (Figs. 3A and B)

Identification of marginal mandibular nerve—the mandibular nerve crosses the facial vein and facial artery 1 cm anteroinferior to angle of mandible. After identification of the nerve, the facial vein and artery are divided inferior to the nerve and retracted upward to protect the marginal mandibular nerve during the dissection. The perifacial lymph node clearance is done at this step.

Next, the fibrofatty tissue anterior to the gland between the anterior belly of digastric and mylohyoid muscle is removed by carefully ligating the mylohyoid vessels and nerves.

The posterior free edge of mylohyoid muscle is retracted anteriorly with right angle retractor to expose lingual nerve, submandibular duct, and hypoglossal nerve from superior to inferior direction. The duct is divided and fiber emerging from submandibular ganglion is cut, taking care of lingual and hypoglossal nerve. Facial artery that emerges at posterior border of submandibular gland from beneath the posterior belly of digastric is identified and cut.

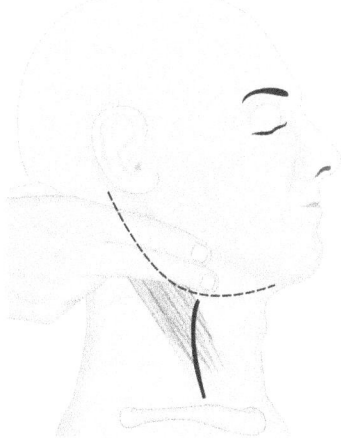

Fig. 2: Landmarks on neck.

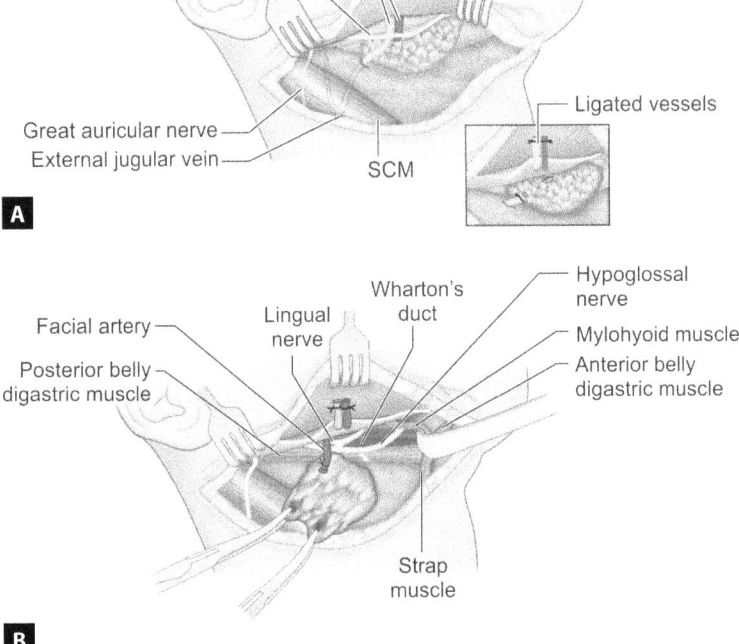

Figs. 3A and B: Submandibular dissection.
(SCM: sternocleidomastoid muscle)

Step 3: Anterior Triangle Dissection (Fig. 4)

Dissect fibrofatty tissue along with lymphatics, anteriorly from superior belly of omohyoid muscle toward carotid sheath posteriorly. Incise the fascia at anterior border of SCM and follow the medial surface of SCM until the posterior border of SCM gets exposed. Few segmental vessels entering the SCM are cauterized. Expose the posterior belly of digastric muscle along the whole length. Start dissecting the posterosuperior corner by retracting the SCM outward and posterior belly of digastric muscle upward after identifying the spinal accessory nerve, which runs along with the IJV from the jugular foramen and crosses the IJV from medially to laterally as the nerve enters the SCM at approximately the junction of the upper and middle third of the muscle. The transverse process of the atlas serves as a useful anatomical landmark for identification of nerve.

Omohyoid tendon is cut inferiorly. Carotid sheath is opened along the whole length of vessel. Fibrofatty tissue with lymphatics is dissected in the boundary made by superiorly below the posterior belly of digastric, lateral limit posterior border of SCM, and inferior limit transverse cervical vessels. Cervical plexus is divided. The level IV lymphatics adjacent to the IJV should be carefully divided between clamps and ligated with silk ligatures to avoid a troublesome chyle leak, especially on the left side, taking care of phrenic and vagus nerve.

Removal of SCM and IJV depends upon the nodal status. Divide the SCM cranially at the level of mastoid and caudally approximately 1 cm above the clavicle. The IJV is doubly ligated superiorly and inferiorly divided after ligation and transfixion with silk suture.

Step 4: Posterior Triangle Clearance (Fig. 5)

The first step is to identify the spinal accessory nerve at posterior border of SCM 1 cm above the Erb's point (exit point of great auricular nerve). The nerve is traced distally until it goes under the anterior border of trapezius muscle. Ligate the external jugular vein inferiorly. Expose the posterior border of

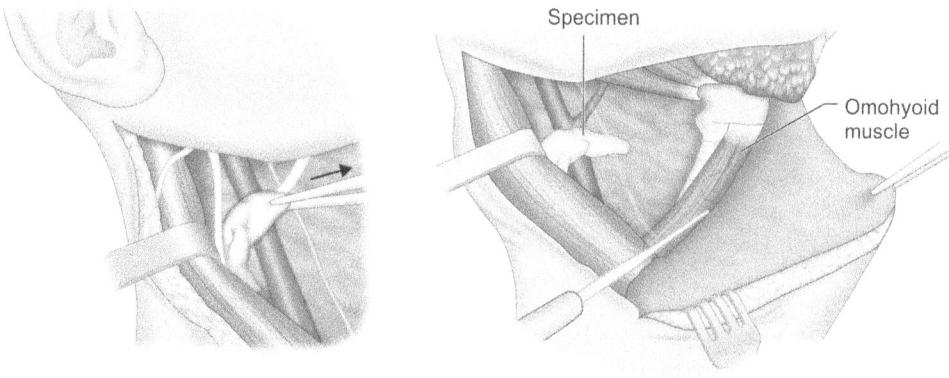

Fig. 4: Dissection of anterior triangle.

SCM and anterior border of trapezius muscle along the whole length. Dissect the fibrofatty tissue along with lymphatics between these two muscles, above the plane of prevertebral fascia, avoiding the injury to phrenic nerve, brachial plexus, and spinal accessory nerve.

The neck is washed with lukewarm saline, the anesthetist is asked to do a Valsalva maneuver to elicit unsecured bleeding vessels and chyle leakage, and a 14 no. suction drain is inserted. The neck is closed in layers with Vicryl to platysma and sutures/staples to skin.

Key Points
- Identify and protect the marginal mandibular, lingual, and hypoglossal nerves in level I.
- Identify IJV and accessory nerve at level II and make level IIb clearance safe and efficient.
- Accessory nerve can be identified 1 cm above the great auricular nerve (GAN) at posterior triangle.
- Keeping the prevertebral fascia intact is the key to avoid phrenic nerve and brachial plexus injury.
- Level IV lymphatics should be dissected with caution to avoid a chyle leak.
- Cervical plexus should be divided away from the roots to avoid injury to phrenic nerve.
- Tributaries of IJV should be divided carefully and ligated to avoid troublesome bleeding.

SELECTIVE NECK DISSECTION (FIG. 6)

Incision Planning

The neck incision is typically a transcervical horizontal skin crease (two fingerbreadth below mandible) or modified apron flap incision. The incision is extended from midline to mid-half of SCM. The transverse skin incision can be extended across to the opposite side with bilateral selective neck dissection (SND) or can be extended superiorly to split the lower lip in the midline to gain access to the oral cavity or preauricularly for a parotidectomy.

Selective neck dissection from level I-III, level I-IV, or level II-V is performed depending upon the primary tumor site in the same manner as described for modified neck dissection.

Steps

- A horizontal incision from the anterior border of the SCM to the midline of the neck just below the level of the hyoid bone is made.

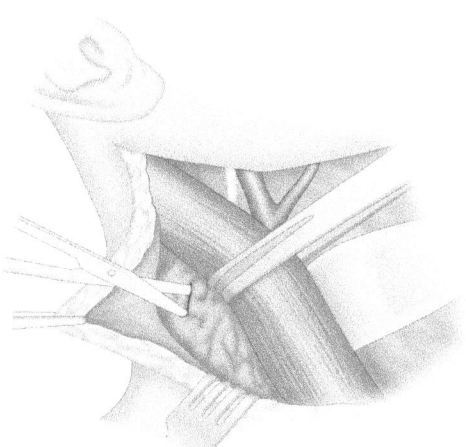

Fig. 5: Posterior triangle clearance.

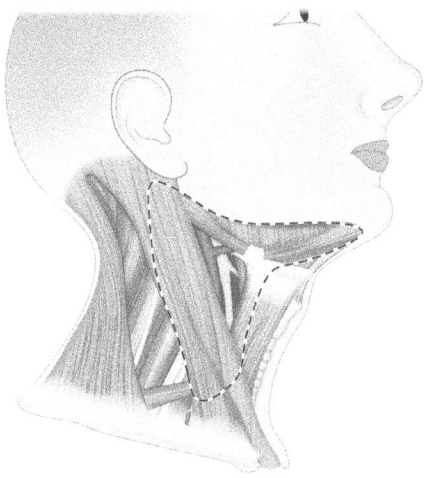

Fig. 6: Supraomohyoid neck dissection.

- Level Ia dissection clears tissue between the anterior bellies of both digastric and of the mylohyoid muscle.
- Identify marginal mandibular nerve at inferior border of mandible. Incise the fascia below marginal nerve after identifying the facial vessel.
- Facial vein and artery are ligated and retracted superiorly with marginal nerve to avoid injury.
- Fibers that travel from the lingual nerve to the submandibular ganglion are divided under direct vision, so that the lingual nerve is not injured.
- The submandibular duct is divided after identifying both the lingual (superficial to its plane) and hypoglossal (deep to its plane) nerves. Level Ib clearance performed.
- Identify the accessory nerve from its position adjacent to the IJV superiorly till its entry into the SCM.
- Incise fascia at anterior border of SCM and follow its medial surface till the posterior border.
- Dissect all fibrofatty tissue between infrahyoid strap muscle and posterior border of SCM preserving IJV and carotid artery and the posterior border of the SCM in an anterior direction preserving the branches of the cervical plexus, vagus nerve, carotid artery, and IJV.
- Establish a dissection plane between the fat of level IV, the brachial plexus, and phrenic nerve and be vigilant for the thoracic duct.

RADICAL NECK DISSECTION (FIG. 7)

Radical neck dissection is performed in same way as MND, except sacrifice of SAN, IJV, and SCM.

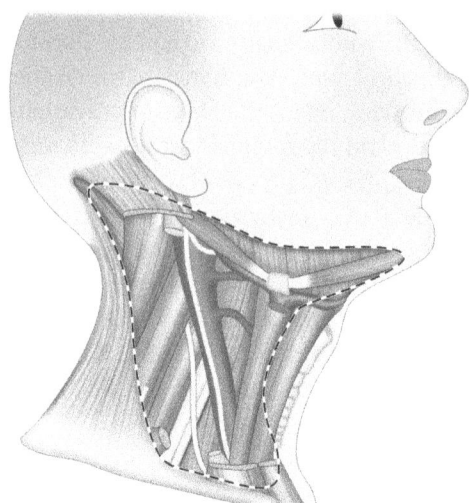

Fig. 7: Limits of radical neck dissection.

NECK DISSECTION AFTER TREATMENT WITH CHEMORADIATION

The neck evaluation, clinically and radiologically, is difficult and is to be done 6-8 weeks after completing chemoradiation. A salvage neck dissection is performed when there is an evidence of nodal disease after completion of chemoradiation. Nodal disease may be persistent or recurrent following complete treatment. The following points should be considered in such scenario:
- Avoid trifurcate junctions in the post irradiated patient
- Use scalpel for sharp elevation of flap
- Use scissor or scalpel for neck dissection.

Key Points
- Divide the lower end of the SCM without injuring the IJV.
- Isolate and ligate the IJV, taking care of vagus nerve.
- Avoid damage to the thoracic duct at level IV.
- Keep the prevertebral fascia intact to preserve the brachial plexus and phrenic nerve.
- Divide the upper end of the SCM.
- Identify and ligate the upper end of IJV.

SUBMITTING NECK DISSECTION SPECIMEN FOR PATHOLOGIC ANALYSIS

The neck specimen should be either divided into levels and sublevels or tagged by the surgeon in the operating room before submitting to pathologist to know the total number of lymph nodes in each level and sublevel, the number of lymph nodes with evidence of metastases, and whether there is any evidence of extracapsular extension. To minimize the error, each neck level can be submitted to the laboratory in separate containers.

THEN AND NOW

Lymphoscintigraphy—Directed Neck Dissection

The sentinel node is the first node reached by the lymphatic stream, assuming an orderly and sequential drainage from the tumor site, and should be predictive of the nodal stage. According to the literature, sentinel node biopsy is a reliable technique in selected cN0 cases, but the procedure is still experimental and should not be performed outside validation trials. Lymphoscintigraphy can supply complete mapping of the lymphatic drainage before surgery in order to plan reliable SND tailored to each patient. Dynamic lymphoscintigraphy seems to be able to show the lymphatic stream from the primary tumor and could allow a SND to be tailored thus, reducing the related morbidity.

Robotic Neck Dissection

Minimally invasive neck dissection (MIND) uses endoscopic equipment or advanced robotic technology to access the neck without large incision to provide less morbidity, better cosmesis, and maintaining the oncology safety. The advent of minimally invasive surgical techniques began as early as in the 1980s soon followed by the introduction of surgical robotics in 1985. The initially introduced transaxillary approach was successful in lateral neck dissection, but yielded difficulties in exposure and dissection of the upper neck levels that are especially important in treatment of oral cancer. So, retroauricular approach is being used more commonly for robotic neck dissection for oral cancer. This approach was initially described by Terris et al. and popularized in South Korea. The retroauricular incision is placed just 5 mm inside the hairline (**Figs. 8 and 9**). Then, skin flap is raised with cautery up to the midline and inferiorly to the clavicle. Self-retaining retractor (Chung's retractor) is used to hold the skin flap. Robot is docked, dissection started with levels Ia and Ib, and then followed by levels IIa, IIb, III, and IV. Free-flap vascular anastomosis is feasible by retroauricular approach for intraoral defects. Robotic neck dissection is usually performed for N0 or N1 neck nodes. Nikolaus et al. compared robotic versus conventional neck dissection and found intraoperative and postoperative complications were similar, but nodal yield was more in robotic arm.

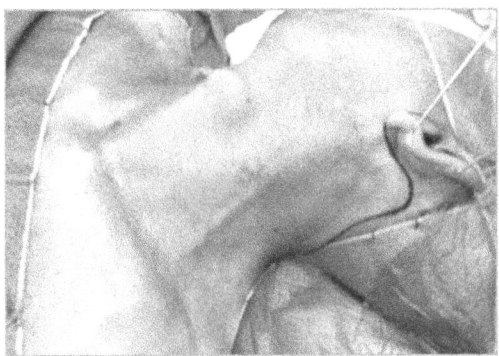

Fig. 8: Retroauricular approach.

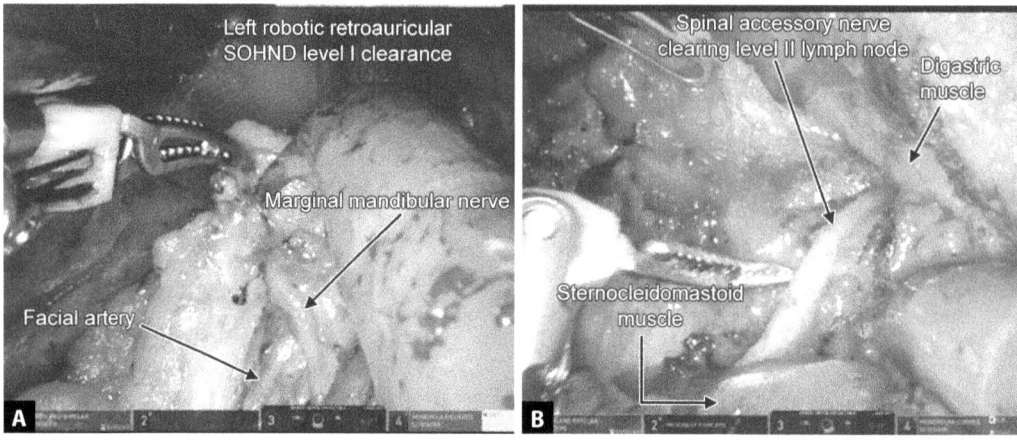

Figs. 9A and B: Robotic neck dissection.
(SOHND: supraomohyoid neck dissection)

The duration of surgery was more in robotic group. Recurrence rate was similar in both groups. The cosmetic satisfaction was significantly better in robotic group.

Although the feasibility of the procedure has been shown, its oncological safety and useful in practice are other issues that need to be addressed.

KEY POINTS

- Decisions are more important than incisions. When not to operate, it is most important.
- Know the anatomy of neck before surgery.
- Dream about surgery (rehearse surgical steps a day before).
- Use of clips, diathermy, or suture is a matter of preference (know where not to use diathermy).
- Always put pectoralis major myocutaneous flap (PMMF) over irradiated neck to safeguard great vessels.
- Incisions are a matter of preference. Good exposure is the key.
- Prefer putting clips/fine ligature in thoracic duct area.
- Check for venous bleeding before closure (head low and Valsalva).
- Never keep drains over vessels.
- Caution anesthesiologist while dissecting at carotid bulb.

CHAPTER 21

Complications of Surgery and Reconstructive Procedures

Kripa Shankar Mishra, Rajan Arora, AK Dewan

INTRODUCTION

According to *Murphy's law*, "things will go wrong in any given situation, if you give them a chance." This is a reminder that unless attempts are made to avoid it, complications are likely to occur. The more experience we gain in the practice of our art, the less likely these complications become. Complications are an essential component of preoperative counseling and obtaining an informed consent. While doing consultation of a patient, always explain the procedure, risk associated, success and failure rates, and possible complications to safeguard all. *"When you explain the possibility of a complication before the surgery, it is called informed consent. When you explain a complication after it has happened, it is called an excuse."*

CLASSIFICATION

We can divide complications into two groups as intraoperative complications and postoperative complications. Further, postoperative complications can be divided into three parts in a chronological order—immediate, intermediate, and late. Intraoperative complications can be discussed under two subheads—local and systemic.

Intraoperative Complications

Local Complications

- *Ligature slip*: Use strong ties to ligate major arteries and veins and apply at least two clips to their major branches to avoid risk of bleeding due to slippage of ligature and clips during tissue retraction and lavage of the surgical field.
- *Bleeding*: The major sources of bleeding in oral surgery and neck dissection may be the following vessels and their branches:
  - Facial artery
  - Lingual artery
  - Maxillary artery
  - Pterygoid plexus of veins
  - Internal jugular vein (IJV)

  To avoid bleeding from these vessels, use tie and clips of a proper size and avoid using a high-energy cautery near any major vessel that may lead to wall necrosis and secondary hemorrhage.
- *Nerve injury*:
  - In neck dissection, the most common encountered nerve is the marginal mandibular division of the facial nerve that runs 1 cm below the lower border of the mandible (**Fig. 1**).

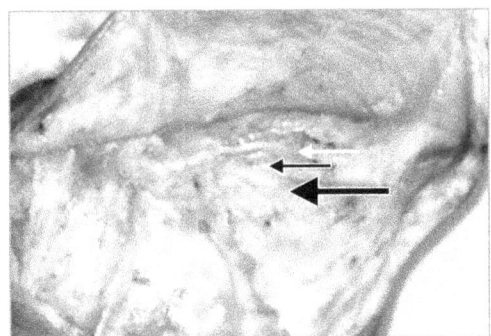

Fig. 1: White arrow—mandibular nerve; thin black arrow—facial artery; thick black arrow—digastric tendon.

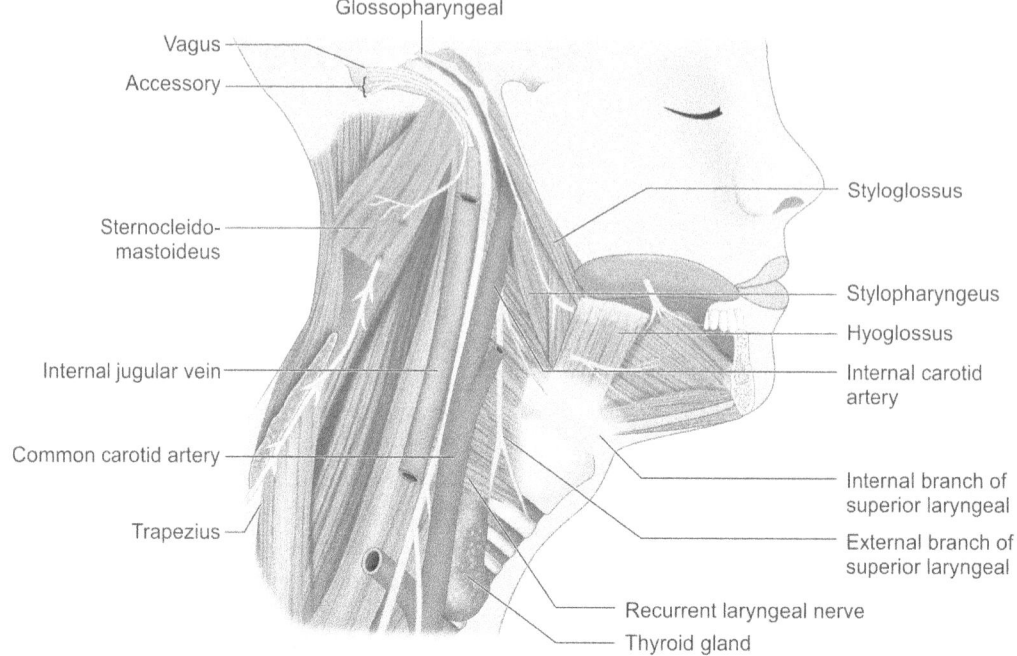

Fig. 2: Spinal accessory nerve.

It supplies muscles of the lower lip. Injury to this nerve causes a distorted smile and deviation of the angle of mouth. To avoid injury to this nerve, a neck incision should be given, two finger-breadths below the lower border of the mandible.
- *Spinal accessory nerve (SAN)*: The safest identification of SAN is in the posterior neck triangle where it may be recognized exiting from the posterior border of the sternocleidomastoid muscle (SCM) at Erb's point. At the level of clavicle posteriorly it pierces the trapezius muscle **(Fig. 2)**.

An injury to this nerve causes difficulty in abduction of arm called shoulder dysfunction syndrome. If the nerve is not involved in disease, it should be preserved carefully.
- *Greater auricular nerve that* causes postoperative paresthesia/anesthesia of the external ear. Careful lymph node dissection can prevent injury to this nerve **(Fig. 3)**.

Other nerves that rarely get injured are the vagus nerve and sympathetic trunk that lie in the carotid sheath.
- *Carotid sinus syndrome*: Excessive manipulation of carotid bulb during surgery can lead to bradycardia and hypotension.
  - ↑ Carotid arterial pressure = ↓ Pulse and BP
  - It is advised to handle carotid bulb with care.
  - Use lignocaine spray or inject lignocaine in the adventitia to regain the pulse and blood pressure toward normal.
- *Thoracic duct injury*: Careful dissection of level IV lymph nodes on the left side of neck can prevent this problem. On table, forced Valsalva and Trendelenburg

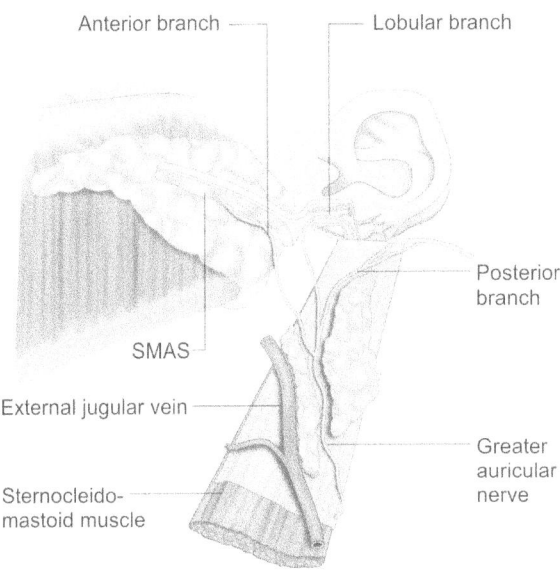

Fig. 3: Greater auricular nerve: Landmark and innervation.

positions of the patient will help in detecting this problem. Taking deep bites with suture may prevent this problem.
- *Air embolism*: Due to injury to IJV, air may get sucked in suddenly.
  Prevention: Apply pressure over the injured site, place clamps on both the sides of the injury site, and keep the patient in Trendelenburg or left lateral position.

Systemic Complications

- *Hypothermia*: Use of a rectal temperature probe for intraoperative monitoring, warmer to keep the patient's body warm, and infusion of warm fluid can check this problem easily.
- *Deep vein thrombosis (DVT)*: Prolonged surgery may need DVT prophylaxis in the form of DVT pump or injection of low-molecular-weight heparin subcutaneously.

Postoperative Complications

Postoperative complications can be classified into three types: (1) Immediate, (2) Intermediate, and (3) Late.

Immediate Local Complications

Immediate local complications are complications that occur within 24 hours.
- *Bleeding*: It may present as oozing from the suture line or excessive drain output or swelling in neck and cheek **(Fig. 4)**. A restless patient with falling BP and increasing heart rate may be an indication of bleeding from the surgical field; hence, postoperative monitoring of vitals is very crucial. The staff should inform the concerned surgeon immediately.
  Prevention: Meticulous dissection and use of clips and sutures to ligate major vessels instead of using cautery at high voltage can prevent bleeding. The anastomotic site of vessels and vascular pedicle should be checked before neck closure.
- *Airway obstruction*:
  – Edema due to extensive resection of tissues
  – Blood or mucus secretions plugging endotracheal tube
  – Compression of airway due to hematoma

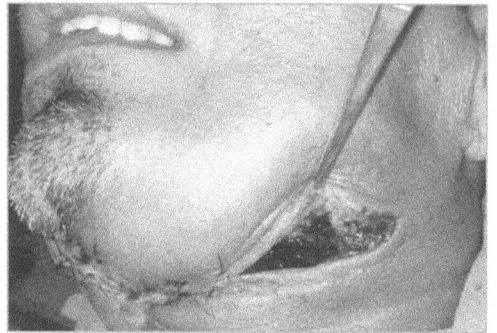

Fig. 4: Neck hematoma.

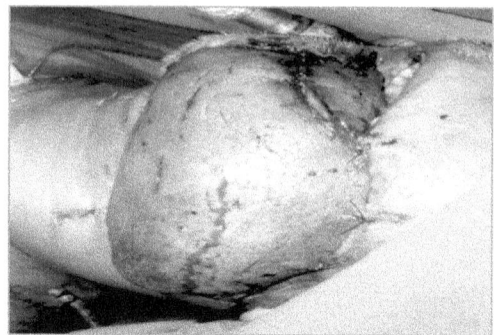

Fig. 5: Flap after venous thrombosis.

Prevention: Meticulous dissection, hemostasis, and postoperative steroids may reduce edema. Judicious use of elective tracheostomy may avoid this situation. Aphorism, "if a tracheostomy comes in one's mind then that is the time to do it."

In the postoperative period, if the patient is in respiratory distress, prefer tracheostomy over difficult intubation; otherwise there may be compressive injury to vessels of the free flap.

- *Vascular compromise of the flap*: Vascular pedicle kink/torsion/compression may occur due to change of neck position in the postoperative period; to prevent this, check the ideal position of head in which lie of vascular pedicle is uncompromised during closure of the neck. The tunnel size for vascular pedicle should be two finger-breadths wide to accommodate the postoperative edema.

Venous congestion is the most common cause of flap-related re-explorations. The flap will appear as dark and edematous in case of venous congestion **(Fig. 5)**. On pinprick, there will be dark and brisk bleed; blood spontaneously will be coming out from the prick site.

Arterial thrombosis is less common than venous thrombosis, but chances of flap salvage remain lower because its clinical presentations are late. The flap will appear

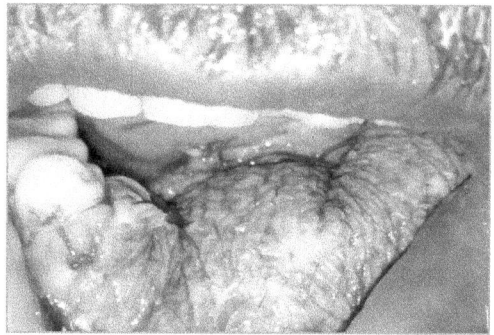

Fig. 6: Pale flap after arterial thrombosis.

pale with reduced turgor **(Fig. 6)**. On pinprick, there will be very delayed bleed in partial thrombosis and no bleed in complete thrombosis. In very late cases, the flap will show shedding of the epithelium with exposed dermis underlying.

In all complications, the level of suspicion should be high and re-explorations should be done early to successfully salvage the flap.

Immediate General Complications

- *Shock*: A *restless patient* should always be assessed for impending shock. It may be due to massive blood loss and insufficient volume replacement. Treatment is immediate replacement of blood with packed red blood cell transfusion and IV fluids.
- *Cardiac arrhythmias*: These occur due to physiological changes in the body.

Maintaining fluid and electrolyte balance in coherence with controlled blood pressure is must to prevent cardiac arrhythmias.

Intermediate Complications

Intermediate complications are those complications that occur from 24 hours to 1 week.
- *Seroma*: It may need repeated aspiration or placement of a suction drain. Chin strap application will reduce repeated collection.
- *Chyle leak*:
  - It usually occurs while dissecting level-IV lymph nodes on the left side of neck.
  - This should be recognized at the time of surgery. Head down and Valsalva will exaggerate the leak and will help on table identification of the problem.
  - In the postoperative period, it will present as high drain output or collection in the neck.
  - *Small leaks (<400 mL/day)*: These can be managed conservatively, NPO low-fat diet and pressure on supraclavicular fossa.
  - *Major leaks (>600 mL/day)*: These may need ligation of the thoracic duct with the help of video-assisted thoracoscopic surgery (VATS).
- *Failure of suture line healing*: Minor wound breakdown is not uncommon.
  - This can be prevented by use of a meticulous surgical technique, appropriate incisions, prophylactic antibiotics, and placing drains to avoid collections in the surgical field.
  - General factors are poor nutrition, uncontrolled diabetes, anemia, renal failure, and hepatic dysfunction.
- *Necrosis of cheek/neck skin flap* (**Fig. 7**): Predisposing factors are as follows:
  - Less than 90° angle between incision lines
  - Preoperative radiotherapy
  - Use of a monopolar cautery near skin
  - Constant traction by sutures anchoring skin to drapes
  - Drying of tissue in the absence of regular saline irrigation
- *Partial flap necrosis*: It occurs due to a large flap on a small perforator or compression of flap margins due to tight suturing. Taking sutures at a long distance for outer defects can prevent this problem.
- *Orocutaneous fistula*: The following factors may be responsible:
  - Poor suturing technique
  - Previous radiotherapy
  - Postoperative anemia, hypoalbuminemia
  - Inadequate control of diabetes
  - Untreated hematoma, seroma, or abscess
- *Flap failure*: Small defects can be managed with secondary suturing/grafting or secondary healing. Large defects may need a second free flap or pedicled flap according to the general condition of the patient.

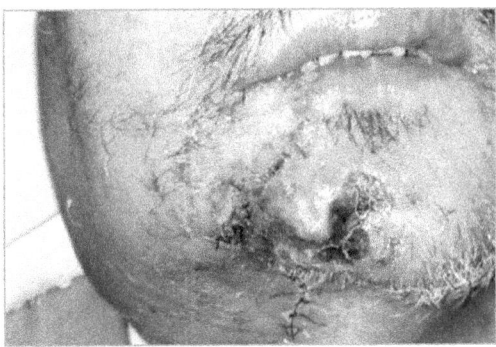

Fig. 7: Necrosis of chin skin.

Intermediate General Complications

- *Lung collapse/bronchopneumonia*: Early ambulation and chest physiotherapy can prevent this problem.
- *DVT*: If the patient is not allowed for early ambulation, then mechanical or chemoprophylaxis should be given to prevent DVT and thromboembolism.

Late Complications

Late complications are complications that happen after 1 week, usually after discharge.

- *Sialocele*: It can be prevented by intraoperative parotid duct stenting and suturing of the injured parotid tail.
  Treatment is glycopyrrolate, chin strap application, repeated aspiration, or drainage with minivac drain.
- *Oral incompetence/drooling of saliva/deviation of angle of mouth*: It may occur due to injury of the marginal mandibular nerve or due to resection of the lip.
  It can be prevented by intraoperative placement of a sling between the lower lip and the periosteum of maxilla to keep neocommissure high up against the gravity.
  In the postoperative period, use of a chin strap with lip support and physiotherapy will reduce this problem.
- *Deviation of jaw/malocclusion*: It occurs due to segmental mandibulectomy.
  Prevention: If possible, bony reconstruction should be done like a free fibula flap to replace the resected mandible.
  If bony reconstruction is not possible, then use a recon plate with a soft-tissue flap.
  If both options are not possible, then bite guide application is useful to prevent this problem.
- *Vascular blow-out*: It is an uncommon but lethal problem and specially occurs in the radiated neck where the vessel wall becomes fragile and inadequate soft-tissue coverage of vessels invites this problem. Intraoperative coverage with *pectoralis major* muscle can prevent this problem.
- *Trismus*: It occurs due to contracture of split-thickness skin graft (SSG) or short flap.
  Whenever possible, the flap should be used to cover the deep defects and flap size should be adequate.
  If there is submucosal fibrosis, the opposite side should also be managed with contracture release with or without coronoidectomy and coverage with FTG or nasolabial flap.
- *Poor speech*: It occurs due to resection of the anterior part of the tongue; the flap used for reconstruction should be pliable, so that tongue mobility can be achieved.
- *Difficulty in swallowing*: Resection of the base of tongue affects swallowing; the reconstructed tongue should be of adequate volume to help in swallowing.
- *Unwanted hairs in the flap*: As the skin maintains the same property as of the donor site, the problem of hairs in the oral cavity is a very common complaint.
  Prevention: Plucking or trimming of the hairs as well as LASER hair removal is the solution.
- *Plate exposure*: Postradiation exposure of miniplate and recon plate is not a very uncommon problem (**Fig. 8**). It can be prevented by covering the plate under muscle or de-epithelialized part of the flap.
- *Osteoradionecrosis*: Sometimes, after radiation, part of native mandible or reconstructed mandible gets necrosed. A thin cheek flap may be the region behind this; hence, extra cover is to be given

Complications of Surgery and Reconstructive Procedures

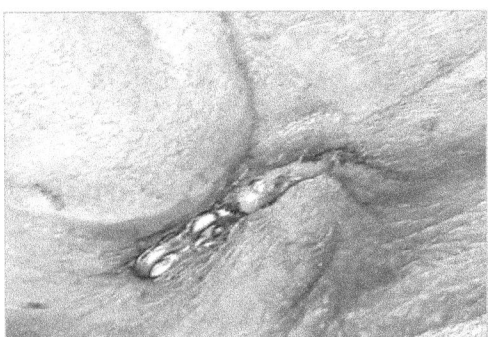

Fig. 8: Plate exposure.

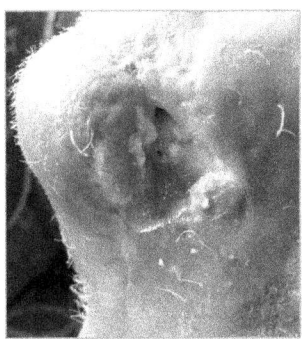

Fig. 9: Plate exposure, osteoradionecrosis, OCF.

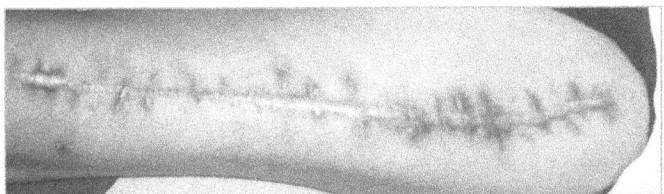

Fig. 10: Hypertrophic scar.

over the mandible to avoid this problem. Hyperbaric oxygen may help in wound healing after debridement **(Fig. 9)**.

- *Fracture of the mandible*: In case of marginal mandibulectomy, when the patient starts taking solid, sometimes the mandible gets fractured.
  Prevention: Keep the mandible height at least 1 cm and keep the cut margins of the mandible sloppy during marginal mandibulectomy.
- *Bulky flap*: The flap choice should be matching to the defect.
- *Hypertrophic scars*: In the postoperative period, massage of the scar line should be advised **(Fig. 10)**.
- *Primary recurrence*: Within 2 years of initial treatment, regular follow-up is must for early detection of the problem.

This chapter will not be complete without mentioning this line *"prevention is better than cure."*

KEY POINTS

- Detailed preoperative counseling.
- Stick to the basic rules and principles of surgery.
- Optimize patient before surgery.
- Plan good and easy incision.
- Judicious use of cautery in the vicinity of vessels and skin.
- Give sufficient time for preoperative planning.
- Low threshold for re-exploration.
- Treat every unfortunate event with high suspicion.
- Manage complications with more passion and care.

CHAPTER 22

Principles of Surgical Reconstruction in Oral Cancers

Rajan Arora, Ravi K Singh

INTRODUCTION

- Reconstruction of oral defects may require anything from simple direct suturing to complex composite free tissue transfers (free flaps) in single stage to multiple stages.
- The selection of the most appropriate reconstructive technique requires a careful assessment of the risks and benefits of each procedure in the light of the patient's clinical status.

RECONSTRUCTIVE PARADIGM

- Surgical decision-making in general surgery has been simplified to some extent by outcomes-based algorithms that lead to clear-cut approaches and procedures for a wide range of problems; in plastic surgery, it is complicated by the wide range of procedures suitable for a given problem.
- In the past, the reconstructive ladder became a much-publicized tool to aid surgeons in decision-making **(Fig. 1A)**.
- The ladder simply attempted to provide surgeons with a progressive approach to wound management, beginning with simple solutions to more complex options.
- Due to advances in plastic surgery and emerging tools of reconstruction in some instances, this reconstructive ladder can be reversed, also known as a reconstructive elevator **(Fig. 1B)**.
- In an attempt to clarify some of these issues, the reconstructive pie was proposed **(Fig. 1C)**.
- The pie concept allowed for a free flow between skin grafts, local flaps, pedicled

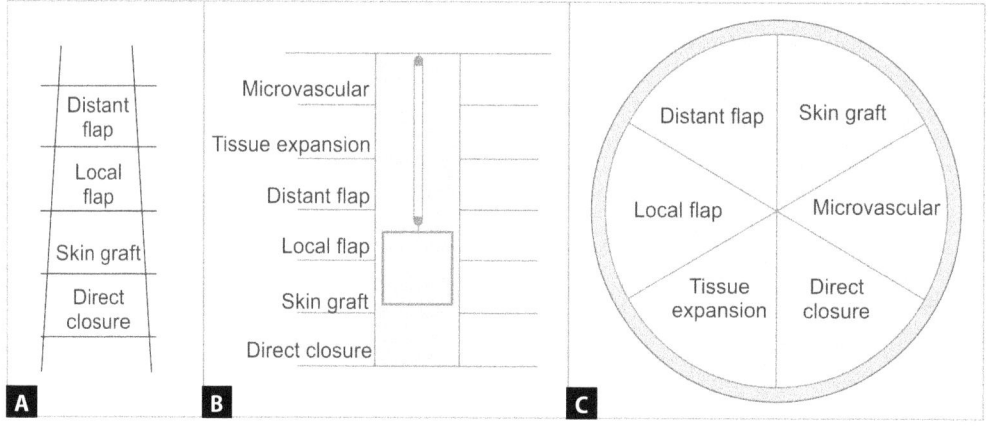

Figs. 1A to C: (A) Reconstructive ladder; (B) Reconstructive elevator; (C) Reconstructive pie.

flaps, tissue expansion, and free tissue transfer.
- This model does not give the surgeon any guidance other than to suggest that any of the above options may be useful.

"When considering reconstructive options, it is imperative to keep in mind that safe wound closure should be based on the selection of the most appropriate technique, whether simple or complex, to achieve effective wound healing, while taking into account local wound requirements and complexity."

ORAL CAVITY RECONSTRUCTION

Anatomy of the Oral Cavity

The oral cavity consists of the lips, buccal mucosa, maxillary and mandibular alveolar ridges, retromolar trigone (RMT), floor of mouth, hard palate, and oral tongue **(Fig. 2)**.

Common Defects

Typical oral cavity defects include:
- Buccal mucosa
- RMT
- Floor of mouth
- Varying extents of the tongue including partial, subtotal, and total glossectomy

Composite defects are common with inclusion of multiple oral cavity components and may also involve the palate, oropharynx, mandible, and lips.

Reconstruction of these more complex defects requires additional functional and aesthetic considerations, but the basic reconstructive principles of the oral cavity will remain the same.

Defect Analysis

It includes an evaluation of:
- Size
- Location
- Wound characteristics
- Adjacent tissue
- Potential donor sites

Wound bed assessment should include all tissue components, including:
- Tissue quality
- Skin

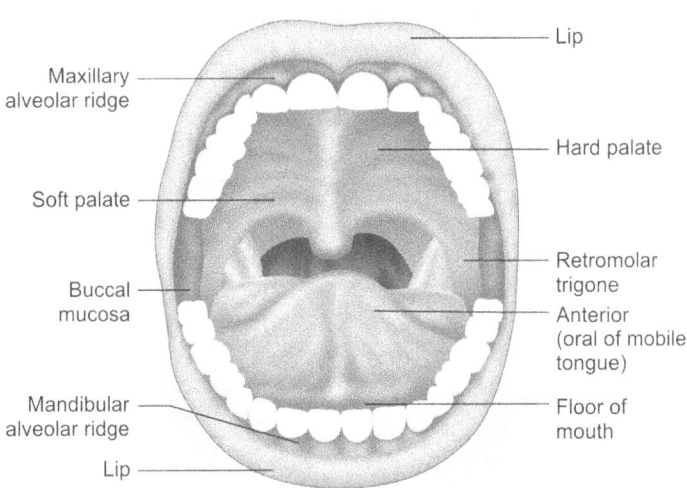

Fig. 2: Graphical depiction of structures of the oral cavity.

- Subcutaneous tissue
- Mucosa
- Vasculature
- Nerve supply
- Cartilage
- Bone

Wound characteristics include assessment of:
- Vascularity to the region
- Infection
- Desiccation
- Tissue viability and presence of slough or eschar
- Quality of granulation (if any)
- Presence or absence of radiation injury
- Degree of fibrosis and scarring
- Presence or absence of malignancy

Systemic Factors

- *Patient's pathology*: Congenital or acquired. Acquired problems may arise from:
  - Trauma
  - Infection
  - Radiation therapy
  - Neoplasia
  - Vascular or autoimmune causes
- Defects may be stable or unstable and may range from physically deforming to life threatening.
- A seriously ill patient may not tolerate such a complex intervention. It should be remembered that organ failure or a major medical morbidity takes precedence over defect reconstruction.
- Patients with severe neurologic impairment or a limited lifespan as a result of organ failure are not good candidates for complex reconstructions.
- Systemic factors that impact wound healing and flap survival include smoking, obesity, immunocompromised states, steroid usage, and cardiopulmonary impairment; these are listed as high-risk patients.

Local Factors

Patients may be in good general health but have local wound conditions that place them at high risk for failure. These are:
- Wound contamination
- Infection
- Radiation therapy
- Poor vascularity
- Extensive scarring
- Exposure of underlying tissues such as bone, joint, tendons, viscera, or body cavities.

Timing of Closure

- The timing of wound closure is critical to a successful outcome. Operating on an unstable patient with hypoperfusion may result in potential flap loss.
- Tumor excision followed by immediate reconstruction in cancer treatment has allowed primary closure with functional reconstruction in complex situations, with improvement in patient outcomes and reduced morbidity.
- Negative pressure wound therapy (NPWT) attempted in unstable patients or in a patient not suitable for immediate reconstruction is followed by definitive procedure on a later date

SYSTEMATIC APPROACH TO WOUND CLOSURE: SURGICAL OPTIONS

Split-thickness Skin Grafts (Fig. 3)

Advantages

- Split-thickness skin grafts (STSG/SSG) are used for superficial, granulating clean wounds overlying stable surfaces.
- They are simple and easily performed.
- They tend to shrink, contracting the original wound size in both area and depth, and can produce quite good aesthetic outcomes.

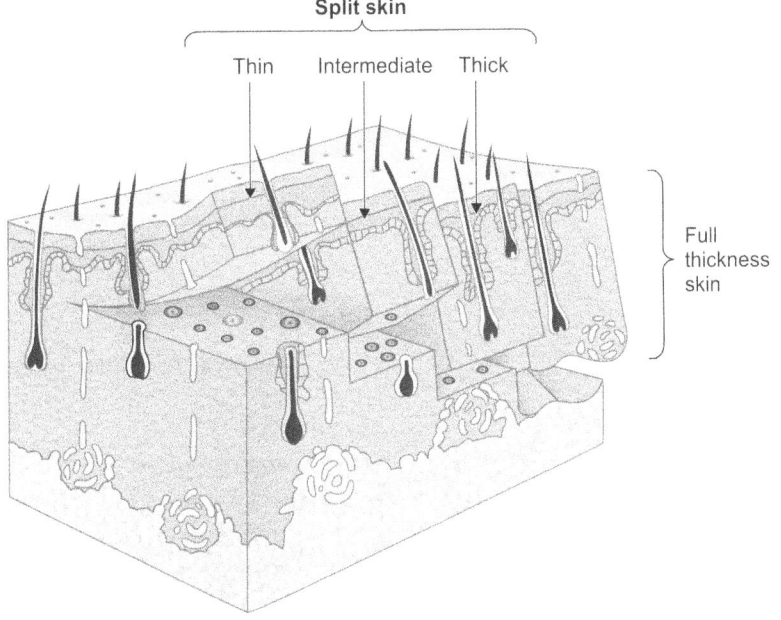

Fig. 3: Split-thickness and full-thickness grafts.

Disadvantages

- Their inherent tendency to contract makes them a poor choice for use across joints and for correcting contractures. They may cause trismus after grafting of RMT or buccal mucosa.
- Poor color match
- Painful donor sites
- Not applicable for exposed vital structures (organs, nerve, tendon, and bone)

Skin graft can be harvested by:
- Humby skin grafting knife **(Fig. 4)**
- Power-driven dermatome **(Fig. 5)**

Full-thickness Skin Grafts (Fig. 3)

Advantages

- More aesthetically pleasing
- Good color and contour match
- Less amount of contracture
- Provide better texture on the face

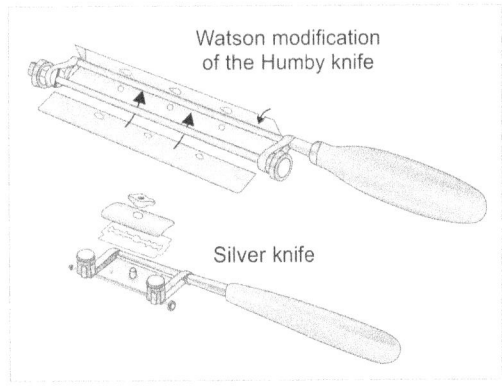

Fig. 4: Humby knife.

Disadvantages

- Limited-size graft and large full-thickness graft (FTG) may require other second procedures for donor closure.
- Slower to develop a blood supply, and take is correspondingly slower
- Highly vascular bed is needed.

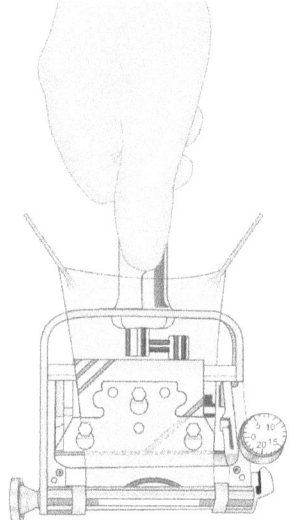

Fig. 5: Power-driven dermatome.

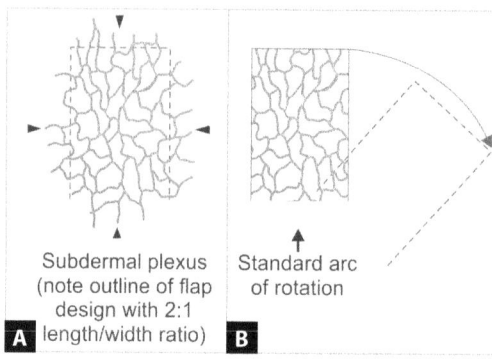

Figs. 6A and B: Random pattern flap.

CLASSIFICATION OF FLAPS

Flaps can be classified by the five "C"s:
1. Circulation
2. Composition
3. Contiguity
4. Contour
5. Conditioning

Circulation Flaps

Circulation flaps can be further subcategorized into:
- Random flaps
- Axial flaps (direct, fasciocutaneous, musculocutaneous)

Random Flaps
- No directional blood supply; not based on a named vessel **(Figs. 6A and B)**
- These include most local flaps on the face.
- These should have a maximum length: breadth ratio of 1:1 in the lower extremity, as it has a relatively poor blood supply.
- These can be up to 6:1 in the face, as it has a good blood supply.

Axial Flaps

Direct cutaneous flaps:
- These contain a named artery running in subcutaneous tissue along the axis of the flap. Examples: Deltopectoral (DP) flap, based on perforating vessels of the internal mammary artery
- These flaps can include a random segment in their distal portions after the artery tapers out.

Fasciocutaneous flaps:
- These are based on vessels running either within or near the fascia.
- The fasciocutaneous system predominates on the limbs.
- Fasciocutaneous flaps are classified by Cormack and Lamberty as given in the following text.
  - *Type A*: Dependent on multiple nonnamed fasciocutaneous vessels that enter the base of the flap, e.g., local flaps of legs
  - *Type B*: Based on a single fasciocutaneous vessel, which runs along the axis of the flap, e.g., scapular/parascapular flap and perforator-based flaps
  - *Type C*: Supplied by multiple small perforating vessels, which reach the flap from a deep artery running along a fascial septum between muscles,

e.g., radial forearm flap (RFF) and lateral arm flap
- *Type C flaps with bone*: Osteofasciocutaneous flaps, originally classified as type D, e.g., RFF raised with a segment of radius, lateral arm flap raised with a segment of humerus

Musculocutaneous:
- These flaps are based on perforators that reach the skin through the muscle.
- The musculocutaneous system predominates on the torso.
- Muscle and musculocutaneous flaps were classified by *Mathes and Nahai* in 1981 (**Fig. 7**) as given in the following text.
  - *Type I*:
    - Single vascular pedicle
    - *Examples*: Gastrocnemius, tensor fasciae latae (TFL), abductor digiti minimi
    - Good flaps for transfer—the whole muscle is supplied by a single pedicle.
  - *Type II*:
    - One dominant pedicle(s) and other minor pedicle(s)
    - *Examples*: Trapezius, soleus, gracilis
    - Good flaps for transfer—can be based on the dominant pedicle after the minor pedicle(s) are ligated.
    - Circulation via minor pedicles alone is not reliable.
  - *Type III*:
    - Two dominant pedicles, each arising from a separate regional artery or the opposite sides of the muscle
    - *Examples*: Rectus abdominis, pectoralis minor, gluteus maximus
    - Useful muscles for transfer—can be based on either pedicle
  - *Type IV*:
    - Multiple segmental pedicles
    - *Examples*: Sartorius, tibialis anterior, long flexors, and extensors of the toes

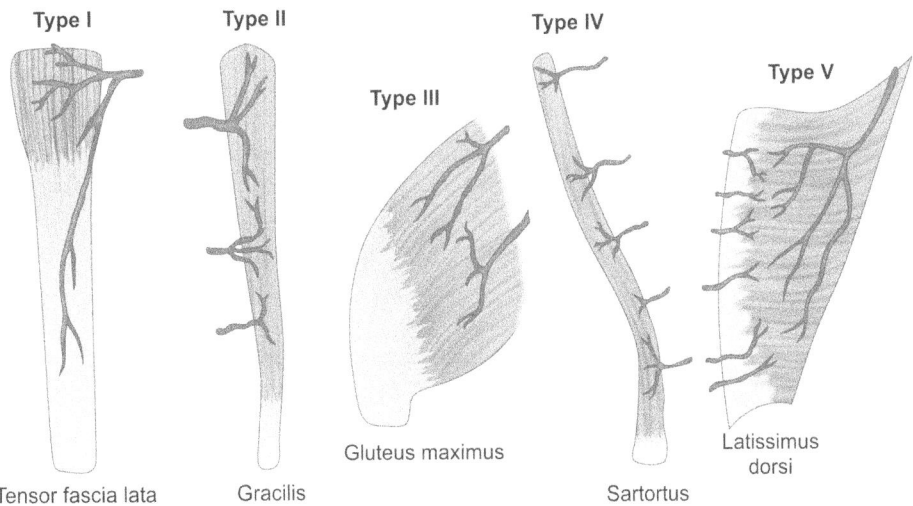

Fig. 7: Mathes and Nahai classification of muscle flaps.

- Seldom used for transfer—each pedicle supplies only a small portion of muscle
- Type V:
  - One dominant pedicle and secondary segmental pedicles
  - *Examples*: Latissimus dorsi, pectoralis major
  - Useful flaps—can be based on either the dominant pedicle or the secondary segmental pedicles

Composition

Flaps can be classified by their composition as:

- *Cutaneous*: Contains skin and subcutaneous tissue only (e.g., DP flap)
- *Fasciocutaneous*: Skin + subcutaneous tissue + fascia (local flaps of arms and legs)
- *Fascial*: Fascia only (TFL flap)
- *Musculocutaneous*: Skin + subcutaneous tissue + fascia + muscle [pectoralis major myocutaneous (PMMC) flap]
- Muscle only (PMMC flap)
- *Osseocutaneous*: Skin + subcutaneous tissue + bone (e.g., fibula flap)
- *Osseous*: Bone only (fibula bone)

Contiguity

Flaps can be classified as **(Figs. 8A to C)**:
- *Local flaps*: Composed of tissue adjacent to the defect
- *Regional flaps*: Composed of tissue from the same region of the body as the defect, e.g., forehead flap, PMMC flap, DP flap
- *Distant flaps*:
  - Pedicled distant flaps come from a distant part of the body to which they remain attached.
  - Free flaps are completely detached from the body and anastomosed to recipient vessels close to the defect.

Local Flaps

- *Advancement flaps* (simple, modified, V-Y, keystone, bipedicled)
- *Pivot flaps* (transposition, interpolation, rotation, bilobed)

Contour

Flaps can be classified by the way they are transferred into the defect.

Advancement

- Stretching the flap
- Excision of Burow triangles at the flap's base
- V-Y advancement
- Z-plasty at its base
- Careful scoring of the undersurface
- Combinations of the above

Transposition

The flap is moved into an adjacent defect, leaving a secondary defect that must be closed by another method.

Rotation

- The flap is rotated into the defect.
- Classically, rotation flaps are designed to allow closure of the donor defect.
- In reality, many flaps have elements of transposition and rotation and may be best described as pivot flaps.

Arc of Rotation

- The extent that a muscle may be elevated from its anatomic location and its subsequent ability to reach adjacent defects without devascularization determines its arc of rotation.

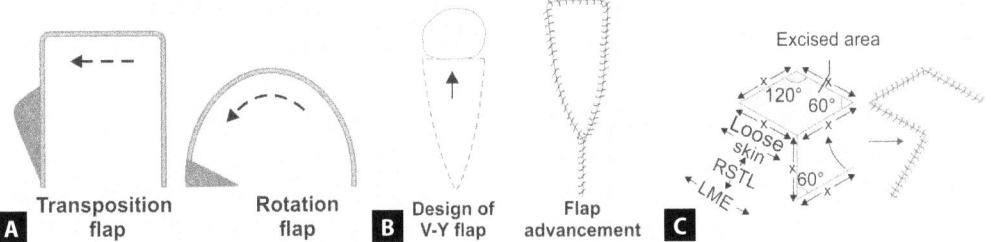

Figs. 8A to C: (A) Transposition and rotation flap; (B) V-Y advancement flap; (C) Rhomboid/Limberg flap.

- The dominant vascular pedicle's entrance site into the muscle determines the point of rotation.
- Only muscle distal to the point of rotation is used as a transposition flap.
- These local flaps can be either transposition or rotation advancement flaps. Examples of such procedures are Limberg flaps for various oral defects.

Interpolation

The flap is moved into a defect either under or above an intervening bridge of tissue, e.g., PMMC flap.

Propeller Flaps

- When the design is an ellipse and the flap is transposed based on that perforator, it is known as a *propeller flap* (**Figs. 9A and B**).
- Propeller flaps are a type of perforator flap. They are called propeller flaps because the flaps rotate around the pedicle in the same way a propeller rotates around its hub.

Axial Perforator-based Cutaneous Flaps

- Cutaneous flaps with a known axial or perforator inflow have a longer arc of rotation, and some have the option of being converted to free flaps.
- Examples include the groin, radial forearm, and supraclavicular flaps.

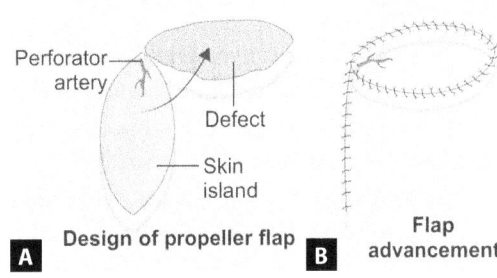

Figs. 9A and B: Propeller flap.

Composite Flaps

- Complex defects require three-dimensional planning of multicomponent of flaps to achieve optimum results; called composite flaps, these may be local or free flaps.
- A full-thickness mandibular defect may require skin, bone, and intraoral lining, all of which can be supplied with a fibular or iliac crest composite free flap.

Free Flaps

- Microsurgical reconstruction has become a mainstay of modern plastic surgery.
- It completely transformed our ability to reconstruct defects by bringing the most appropriate tissue components into the field rather than being limited by what local tissues had to offer.
- The potential for complex three-dimensional reconstruction advanced exponentially as a consequence of the microsurgical revolution.

Perforator Flaps

- The analysis of cutaneous perforator blood supply before raising the flaps should be done with the help of Doppler and CT angiography.
- These flaps contain a reliable blood supply and they also spare the underlying musculature from being violated.

Tissue Expansion

- The original concept devised by Radovan incorporates the insertion of an inflatable silicone balloon into the subcutaneous tissues adjacent to a given defect.
- The healthy skin is sequentially expanded and stretched until the desired surface area is attained; then the expander is removed and the stretched skin is advanced into the defect.
- Tissue expansion has limited utilization in oral cancers.

PRINCIPLES OF CLOSURE

Simple Linear Wounds

- Clean linear wounds, such as excisions for small skin cancers or benign lesions, are often best closed with direct linear suturing.
- Wound approximation devices used to reduce wound diameter by progressive, continuous wound-edge traction over days or weeks, obviating the need for more extensive procedures.
- NPWT devices are also immensely helpful in reducing wound surface area before closure.

Fresh Lacerations

Clean, freshly lacerated tissues are best treated with primary closure, without tension.

Clean Granulating Wounds

- Larger surface granulating wounds are usually closed with split-thickness skin grafts, depending on surface area involvement.
- Grafting should be deferred in pus discharging and unhealthy wounds to avoid graft loss.

Contaminated Traumatic Wounds

- All contaminated wounds must be thoroughly debrided and lavaged to remove impacted dirt and debris.
- All contaminated or devitalized tissue must be removed before definitive closure is contemplated.

Infected Wounds

- Infected wounds should be drained of all pus, and all necrotic material should be debrided back to healthy bleeding.
- Antibiotic therapy is *never* a substitute for adequate surgical drainage and debridement; e.g., the treatment of osteomyelitis includes resection of any necrotic bone back to healthy punctate bleeding.
- Wound closure should be delayed until a stable, clean wound bed has been achieved and surrounding inflammation has resolved.

Necrotic Wounds

- Wound necrosis creates an ideal milieu for bacterial proliferation as necrotic tissue is avascular and antibiotics cannot penetrate the mass of dead tissue.
- Adequate debridement is essential to achieving a clean, stable wound before closure.
- When assessing wounds containing necrotic tissue, the regional blood

flow should be assessed carefully; a revascularization procedure before reconstruction may make the difference between success and failure.

Chimeric Flaps

- The term *chimera* refers to a beast in Greek mythology that was a composite of a lion, a goat, and a serpent.
- In a similar fashion, the chimeric approach can provide a multiplicity of tissues on one vascular pedicle.
- A classic example of this is the anterolateral thigh (ALT) flap, whose vascular axis, the lateral circumflex femoral artery, can supply multiple muscles, fascial tissue, multiple cutaneous skin paddles, and vascularized bone all on one vascular pedicle for reconstruction of complex maxillary and mandibular defects.

PRINCIPLES OF RECONSTRUCTION

Flap Design

- Flap design should take into account the size of the defect in relation to the tissue available from a given flap as well as the arc of rotation of the flap when pedicled flaps are used.
- Flaps should be designed slightly larger than the defects they are designed to close.
- Skin flaps designed to fit a particular anatomic defect should be designed around a template of the defect.

TECHNICAL CONSIDERATIONS

Precise anatomic knowledge is essential if many of these complex reconstructive procedures are to be accomplished successfully.

Pedicle Identification and Elevation

- Based on external landmarks, flap elevation is commenced and dominant pedicle identification should be performed and confirmed before any minor pedicles are divided.
- Doppler studies or preoperative multi-detector CT (MDCT) scans or magnetic resonance angiography (MRA) can be very helpful in confirming the presence or absence of pedicles.
- Intraoperatively, indocyanine green fluorescence imaging is very helpful in locating perforators as well as delineating zones of perfusion.
- Once a pedicle has been identified, every effort should be made to preserve its integrity during flap elevation and to prevent twisting or kinking during flap transfer.

POSTOPERATIVE MANAGEMENT

Positioning

- Although every effort may have been made to prevent intraoperative compression within tunnels or around pedicles, incorrect postoperative positioning can induce similarly disastrous results.
- Free flaps in oral cancers may be compressed because of neck flexion; the problem could be avoided by using neck rolls, head rings instead of a large pillow to provide cervical support.
- A Trach-Tie supporting a tracheostomy can occlude the pedicle of any flap traversing the neck.

Dressings

- Tightly applied dressings over the flap can compress the pedicle and strangulate the flaps.

- Patients with flaps of oral cavity should be placed in an upright position to promote venous return and minimize swelling, as inadequate venous return and edema may compromise flap circulation.

Suction Drains

- Closed suction drains are always used after flap surgery.
- Although they will not necessarily prevent hematomas, they reduce fluid accumulation and prevent seromas.
- Drain management should be individualized to each patient situation.
- In general, drainage should be <10–20 mL per 24-hour period before drains are removed.

Perioperative Antibiotics

- Administration of perioperative antibiotics is considered the standard of care for most major procedures.
- According to many recent studies, postoperative antibiotics have not been shown to be beneficial beyond the first 24 hours and may in fact increase complication rates.
- Antibiotics should only be given postoperatively if a wound is contaminated or frankly infected. In such circumstances, it is not usual to perform a flap; reconstruction should be delayed until sepsis has been controlled.
- There are no substantive data to show that the presence of drains warrants administration of long-term antibiotic cover.

Mobilization

After extubation and weaning from anesthesia, the patient should be encouraged for early mobilization to prevent DVT, but it should be guarded, supervised, and with support.

Rehabilitation

- Early oral liquid followed by a semisolid diet is advised for early recovery in the postoperative period.
- Speech therapy, tongue movement, jaw exercises, and neck movement are usually to be avoided till 3 weeks postoperatively.
- Customized chin and lip support is advised after 3–4 weeks depending upon healing and postoperative recovery.
- Massage with lubricants, physiotherapy, and pressure garments for donor site is advised.

PRINCIPLES OF MICROVASCULAR ANASTOMOSIS

Alexis Carrel described the triangulation technique of blood vessel repair in 1902. He was awarded a Nobel Prize in 1912.

SURGICAL TOOLS

- Magnifying loupes (magnification usually between ×2.5 and ×4.5)
- Microscopes (small vessels are best repaired under an operating microscope; able to magnify between ×6 and ×40)
- Microinstruments
- Microsutures
- Surgical stool/chair with elbow support
- Anastomotic devices

Instruments

- Forceps—four pairs of jeweler's forceps
- Vessel dilators
- Microdissecting scissors

- Needle holders
- Single and double microvascular clamps of varying sizes

Irrigating Solutions
- Heparin dissolved in Hartmann's procedure or saline to a concentration of 100 units/mL
- Topical papaverine or lignocaine (4%) to relieve vessel spasm

Sutures
- Monofilament, micropoint, rounds body 8, 9, 10 and 11-0 nylon
- Half-circle or compound-curve atraumatic needles of 50–130-μm diameter

Coupling Devices
- Commercially available devices that may save time over hand-sewn anastomosis.
- Mostly used for end-to-end or end-to-side venous anastomosis.

TECHNIQUE

Acland described five factors that influence microvascular patency:
1. Surgical precision
2. Vessel diameter
3. Blood flow into the anastomosis
4. Tension at the anastomosis site
5. Use of anticoagulants or thrombolytic agents

PRE-REQUISITES FOR SUCCESSFUL MICROVASCULAR ANASTOMOSIS

- Obtain adequate access. Do not operate down a hole.
- Operate in a dry field.
- Position and secure the flap before starting the anastomosis.
  - The flap should be tacked into position before starting the anastomosis.
  - Position the pedicle with care, ensuring that it is:
    - Correct length to lie at the anastomosis site without tension
    - Not twisted or kinked
    - Not compressed
- Prepare the vessels for anastomosis by stripping the loose periadventitial tissue.
- Flush the vessel with heparin solution. Excessively powerful irrigation can cause intimal trauma.
- Limit vessel distension with the dilating forceps: Excessive dilatation causes intimal tears or vessel spasm.
- Perform a forward-flow test prior to anastomosis: Proximal arterial flow is tested by releasing the clamps on the artery.
- Never start the anastomosis until you are happy with the setup.

POINTS OF TECHNIQUE

- The needle should be held halfway along its length.
- The most difficult sutures are generally inserted first.
- The needle should be accessible within the visual field when tying knots.
- Triangulation, bisecting, and posterior wall first techniques can be used.
- Interrupted or continuous sutures can be used.
- Do minimum vessel handling after anastomosis to avoid spasm.

TABLE 1: Postoperative monitoring.

Clinical monitoring of free flap or vascular anastomosis; still the most reliable method	Equipment for monitoring microcirculation
• Color • Temperature • Tissue turgor • Capillary return • Bleeding on pinprick	• Doppler monitoring of perforator site • Implantable Doppler probe • SPY Elite System (indocyanine green-based fluorescent angiography)

KEY POINTS

- Oral cancer defects are complex with complicated function and anatomy, and the reconstruction of these oral defects focuses not only on aesthetic results but also on functional restoration. Surgical decision-making is complex and must be individualized for each patient.
- Equal weight should be given to patient assessment, surgical planning, intraoperative execution, and postoperative care, because a deficiency in any one area may ultimately lead to failure of the reconstruction.
- There is always a learning curve to improve outcomes, and everyone should follow the basics principles and essential steps.

CHAPTER 23

Reconstructions of Oral Mucosal Defects

Rajan Arora

INTRODUCTION

Oral cancers form bulk of the head and neck cancers. Given the complex anatomy of the region, a variety of functional and aesthetic deficits are put into motion after resection. Thus, the need for an immediate reconstruction forms an essential part of the current treatment protocol. Recent advances such as microvascular free tissue transfers and compatible osteointegrated implants have enabled reconstructive surgeons to give a better final outcome, thus improving the quality of life.

SURGICAL ANATOMY

Gingivobuccal complex includes:
- *Buccal mucosa*: Cheek, vestibule, and retromolar trigone
- *Gums*: Superior and inferior alveoli

Buccal mucosa includes:
- *Cheek*: Superiorly and inferiorly attached to alveoli and posteriorly to retromolar trigone.
- *Retromolar trigone*: Triangular area over ramus ascending from behind the third molar to maxillary tuberosity.
- *Vestibule*: Superior and inferior mucosal folds between gums and buccal mucosa.

Blood supply:
- *Artery*: Facial and buccal artery (from the pterygoid branch of the maxillary artery).
- *Vein*: Pterygoid plexus to facial vein to internal jugular vein.

Innervation:
- *Sensory*: Maxillary and mandibular divisions of trigeminal nerves.
- *Motor*: Masticators by mandibular nerve, buccinator by the buccal branch of the facial nerve.

GOALS OF RECONSTRUCTION (BOXES 1 AND 2)

As per the current trends in reconstruction, use of "the reconstructive ladder" is severely limiting. To provide a customized treatment to every single patient based on his/her needs, body habitus, comorbidities and wishes, it is essential to have a more open-ended approach.

RECONSTRUCTION OPTIONS

Local Flaps
- *Buccal fat pad flap* **(Fig. 1)**:
  - *Vascular supply*: Branches from superficial temporal artery, facial artery, maxillary artery.

Box 1: Goals of reconstruction.
- *Functional*:
  - Adequate mouth opening
  - Isolated oral and nasal cavity
  - Continuous alimentary tract
  - Swallowing
  - Stable occlusion
- *Aesthetic*:
  - Restoration of facial contour
  - Restoration of volume
  - Restoration of dimensions
- Minimize complications and morbidity
- Faster recovery
- Maximize quality of life

Box 2: Factors affecting reconstruction.

- Size:
  - *Small*: <3 cm
  - *Medium*: 3–6 cm
  - *Large*: >6 cm
- Depth:
  - Superficial (lining only)
  - Moderate depth (lining + soft tissue)
  - Composite/3D (lining + soft tissue/bone/skin)
- Site (alone or in combination):
  - Buccal mucosa
  - Retromolar trigone
  - Gingival mucosa
  - Oral commissure
  - Gingivobuccal sulcus
- Position of defect:
  - Anterior
  - Lateral
  - With or without vestibulum
  - With or without lip/hard palate/soft palate
- Patient factors:
  - Age
  - Past radiation
  - Comorbidities
  - Blood dyscrasias
  - Body performance status

- *Dimensions*: Buccal fat pad consists of main body and four extensions, namely buccal, pterygoid, superficial, and deep temporal. The body and the buccal extension can be harvested.
- *Harvesting essentials*:
  - Access via either vertical incision lateral to the anterior ascending mandibular ramus or horizontal incision along the superior vestibular sulcus.
  - Fat pad is expressed gently after fascia incision.
  - Avoid use of suction device.
- *Advantages*: Easily available, quick and easy dissection, low morbidity, very low failure rate.
- *Disadvantages*: For small-to-medium defects, cannot provide bulk. Low arc of rotation, can alter face contour, cause minimal trismus, needs bite block for 12 days, not reliable in extensive neck dissection and post radiation.

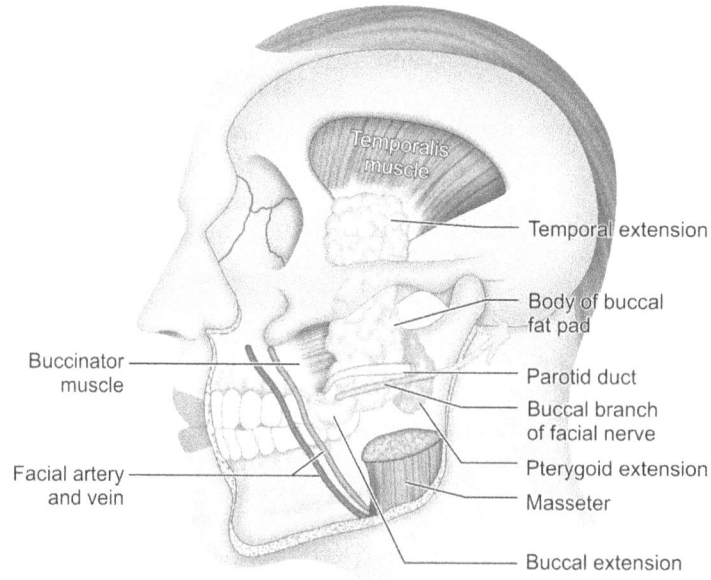

Fig. 1: Buccal fat pad flap.

- *Tongue flap*:
    - *Vascular supply*: Lingual artery
    - *Harvesting essentials*:
        - Flap is usually posteriorly based, dorsal or lateral in orientation.
        - Attempt should be made to preserve tip.
        - Posterior limit is circumvallate papillae.
        - Donor area should preferably be closed primarily.
    - *Advantages*: Locally available, robust blood supply, single-stage procedure, quick harvest.
    - *Disadvantages*: Decreased bulk of residual tongue, restriction of mobility of tongue, altered speech and swallowing.
- *Masseteric flap*:
    - *Vascular supply*: Artery—masseteric branch of facial artery, vein—facial vein
    - *Harvesting essentials*:
        - Can be harvested as cross-over or islanded flap.
        - Parotid gland and facial nerves should be protected.
        - Dissection is done below upward.
        - Spontaneous epithelization or skin grafting can be done.
    - *Advantages*: Ease of harvest, quick dissection, minimal technical support needed, reliable blood supply, acceptable donor site morbidity.
    - *Disadvantages*: Limited availability due to inclusion in the resected field.
- *Facial artery myomucosal flap (Fig. 2)*:
    - *Vascular supply*: Artery—facial artery, vein—buccinator venous plexus
    - *Dimensions*: Maximum 3 cm × 7 cm, boomerang shaped
    - *Harvesting essentials*:
        - Flap can be either antegrade or retrograde.

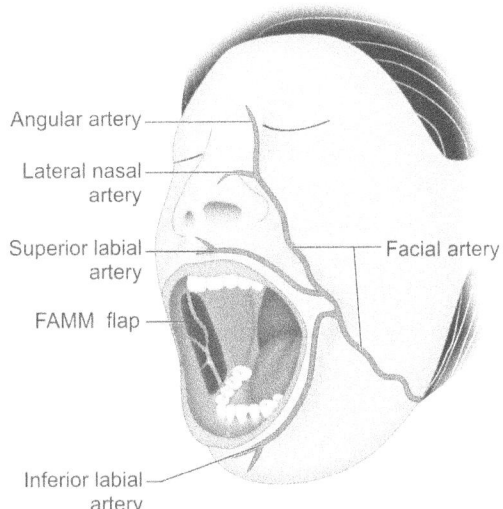

Fig. 2: Facial artery myomucosal (FAMM) flap.

- Flap consists of buccal mucosa and buccinator muscle segment.
- Flap is harvested centered on artery, distal to proximal.
- Pivot point is lower retromolar trigone in antegrade flap and upper gingival sulcus at the level of alar rim in retrograde flap. Donor defects are closed primarily.
- Care is taken to protect Stenson's duct.
    - *Advantages*: Axial flap with excellent venous drainage and adequate mobility of almost 180°.
    - *Disadvantages*: Cheek tethering, injury to Stenson's duct, bite block for 10 days, tortuous facial artery prone to injury.

Regional Flaps

- *Nasolabial flap*:
    - *Vascular supply*: Artery—angular branch of the facial artery, infraorbital artery, transverse facial artery, vein—associated venae comitantes.
    - *Dimensions*: Single—2 cm across 3 cm, bilateral—5 cm across 5 cm.

- *Harvesting essentials*:
    - It can be inferiorly or superiorly based.
    - It can be axial or random, islanded or pedicled.
    - Upper edge should be at least 15 mm away from medial canthus.
    - Flap inset should be tension free.
- *Advantages*: Versatile, robust supply, ease of harvest, acceptable donor scar.
- *Disadvantages*: Limited tissue, pin cushioning effect of cheek, asymmetry of cheek, prone to venous congestion, discharging sinus at the entry of flap.

- Submental flap:
    - *Vascular supply*: Artery—submental artery (dominant), suprasternal artery (minor).
    - *Dimensions*: Upper limit—mandibular arch, lateral limit—mandibular angle, width—redundant skin allowing primary closure.
    - *Harvesting essentials*:
        - Angle of mandible is kept as a pivot for flap designing across midline.
        - Dissection proceeds from the inferior to the superior direction for pedicle identification.
        - Flap is raised medial to lateral.
        - Branches to submandibular glands should be carefully ligated.
    - *Advantages*: Axial blood supply, donor site hidden in the crease.
    - *Disadvantages*: Marginal mandibular nerve and facial veins prone to injury, not preferable in post radiation, extensive neck dissection and where facial artery is damaged or injured, intraoral hair (in males), preferably done in females.

- Island platysma:
    - Similar to submental flap
    - *Harvesting essentials*:
        - Inferior border of mandible is the pivot point.
        - Flap is planned on distal insertion of sternocleidomastoid.
        - Flap is harvested before tumor resection and neck dissection.
        - Dissection proceeds from the clavicle upward in the subplatysmal plane.
        - External jugular vein is included in the flap.
    - *Advantages*: Wide muscle available, axial blood supply, donor site hidden in the crease.
    - *Disadvantages*: Flap elevation before tumor resection may lead to discrepancy between the defect and flap.

- Forehead flap (**Fig. 3**):
    - *Vascular supply*: Artery—inferior branch of the superficial temporal artery.
    - *Dimensions*: Entire forehead skin between the hair line superiorly and the brow line inferiorly.
    - *Harvesting essentials*:
        - Flap is raised above periosteum.
        - Can be unilateral, islanded, bilobed based on both branches of the artery.
        - Donor site is covered with split-thickness skin graft.
    - *Advantages*: Wide hairless skin, constant blood supply, rapid harvest.
    - *Disadvantages*: Poor donor scar, loss of brow function.

- Temporalis muscle flap:
    - *Vascular supply*: Deep temporal artery

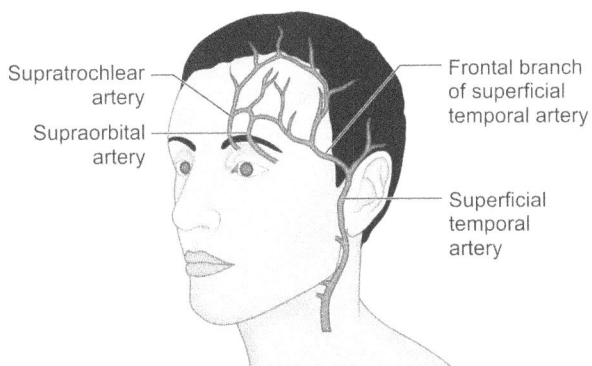

Fig. 3: Forehead flap.

- *Harvesting essentials*:
  - Hemicoronal or coronal incision for access.
  - Superficial temporal fascia with its blood supply and can be used separately.
  - Muscle is exposed after incision of deep temporal fascia.
  - Subperiosteal dissection done to free the muscle.
  - Muscle is passed under the arch with the help of sutures.
  - Greatest arc of rotation is at the coronoid process.
  - Donor is closed with or without implant for contour effect.
- *Advantages*: Robust supply, easily available, long reach, adequate bulk.
- *Disadvantages*: Frontal branch of facial nerve prone to injury, maxillary artery prone to injury during dissection near the coronoid process, contour deformity of skull, local site alopecia.
• *Pectoral major myocutaneous flap*:
  - *Vascular supply*: Artery—pectoral branch of the thoracoacromial artery (dominant), lateral thoracic and internal mammary artery (minor). The vascular course is cephalocaudal, deep to the muscle.
  - *Harvesting essentials*:
    - Skin paddle is marked over the caudal medial aspect of the muscle.
    - Medial and lateral minor perforators are cautiously ligated.
    - Pivot point is at the clavicle.
    - Laterally, the horizontal fibers of the muscle are cut to increase the mobility.
    - Donor site closure is either primarily or with a skin graft.
  - *Advantages*: Bulk tissue available, less donor site morbidity, useful in vessel-depleted neck.
  - *Disadvantages*: Reach of this flap is poor above the upper alveolus, precarious blood supply in extended distal skin paddle, can be too bulky in obese individuals, pedicle compromise in case of inset under strain or external compression.

Free Flaps

These can be single or double paddle and may or may not include bone or muscle depending on defect.
• *Free radial artery forearm flap (RAFF) (Fig. 4)*:
  - *Type*: Fasciocutaneous, osteofasciocutaneous, with/without tendon (palmaris longus), can be sensate.

- *Vascular supply*: Artery—radial artery, vein—paired vena comitantes, cephalic vein.
- *Dimensions*: 12 cm (4-30 cm) across 5 cm (4-15 cm) in the adult.
- *Harvesting essentials*:
  - Allen's test is essential to establish patency of arch before harvest.
  - Distal third forearm consists of maximum perforators.
  - Flap harvest is optimum under tourniquet.
  - Cephalic vein, if included, should be harvested beyond its communication to venae comitantes in the proximal forearm.
  - For bone harvest, a 10-12-cm maximum unicortical bone can be harvested.
  - For sensate flaps, the lateral antebrachial cutaneous nerve can be harvested.
- *Advantages*: Reliable blood supply, long pedicle, pliable flap, can be used as a flow through flap, multiple skin paddles, good caliber for anastamoses.
- *Disadvantages*: Poor donor scar, hair in mouth, secondary fractures of donor bone in elderly, single vessel donor arm.

- Free anterolateral thigh (ALT) flap **(Fig. 5)**:
  - *Type*: Fasciocutaneous, adipofascial, myofasciocutaneous, chimeric.
  - *Vascular supply*: Artery—descending branch of the lateral circumflex femoral artery, vein—venae comitantes.
  - *Dimensions*: 21 cm (4-35 cm) across 8 cm (4-25 cm) in an adult.
  - *Harvesting essentials*:
    - Anatomical landmarks for septum—anterior superior iliac spine to the superolateral border of patella.
    - Longitudinal flap allows better donor closure.
    - Attempt should be made to include more than one perforator.
    - Eccentric flap design can help in increasing pedicle length and flap reach.
    - Fascial cuff should always be included around the flap.
    - Harvest is medial to lateral.

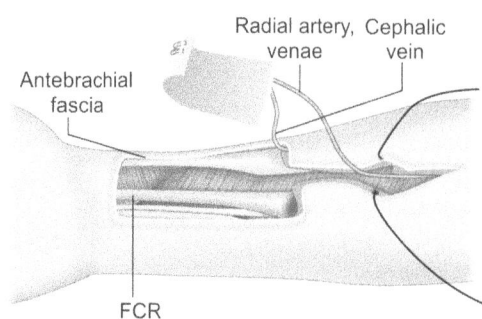

Fig. 4: Radial artery forearm flap. (FCR: flexor carpi radialis muscle)

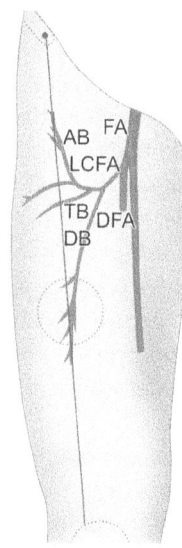

Fig. 5: Surface markings of free anterolateral thigh flap. (AB: ascending branch; DB: descending branch; DFA: deep femoral artery; FA: femoral artery; LCFA: lateral circumflex femoral artery; TB: transverse branch)

- In adipofascial flaps, a minimum 3-mm fat layer is preserved over fascia for vascular supply.
- Vastus lateralis muscle can be harvested for bulk.
- Lateral femoral cutaneous nerve can be harvested for a sensate flap.
- Multiple perforator allows flap to be divided into two or more paddles.
- *Advantages*: Constant anatomy, ease of harvest, long reliable pedicle, large caliber vessels, versatile thickness allows primary thinning of flap, allows two-team approach, less donor site morbidity.
- *Disadvantages*: Color mismatch, presence of hair, skin graft required for donor defects > 8–9 cm, bulky in obese patients and may need secondary corrective procedures.

- *Medial sural artery perforator (MASAP) flap* **(Fig. 6)**:
  - *Type*: Fasciocutaneous
  - *Vascular supply*: Artery—medial sural artery, a branch of popliteal artery, vein—venae comitantes.
  - *Dimensions*: 12 cm across 8 cm in the medial half of the upper third of posterior calf.
  - *Harvesting essentials*:
    - Vascular axis—midpopliteal crease to medial malleolus.
    - First perforator enters 8 cm along the line from crease.
    - Motor nerve to medial belly of gastrocnemius should be spared.
  - *Advantages*: Two-team approach possible, better alternative to RAFF.
  - *Disadvantages*: Poor donor scar in case of wide flaps, posterior scar unacceptable to female patients, short pedicle.

- *Thoracodorsal artery perforator flap*:
  - *Type*: Fasciocutaneous
  - *Vascular supply*: Artery—septocutaneous perforators from the descending branch of the thoracodorsal artery, vein—venae comitantes.
  - *Dimensions*: 15 cm across 8 cm on a single perforator.
  - *Harvesting essentials*:
    - First perforator is 6–8 cm below the posterior axillary fold, 2 cm inside the margin of latissimus dorsi muscle.
    - Anterior to posterior dissection helps identifying and tracing the perforator back to main vessel.
    - Thoracodorsal nerve is to be preserved.
  - *Advantages*: Reduced donor site morbidity by preserving nerve and muscles, thin pliable flap, nearby flap territories undisturbed, hidden donor scar.
  - *Disadvantages*: Inconsistent anatomy of perforators, pedicle prone to injury during intramuscular dissection, can cause breast deviation in females.

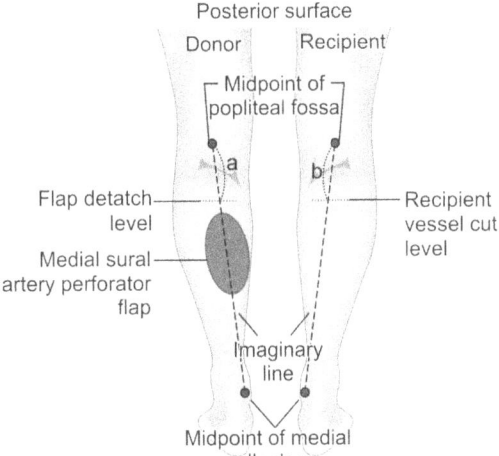

Fig. 6: Medial sural artery perforator flap.

- *Profunda artery perforator flap*:
  - Type: Fasciocutaneous
  - Vascular supply: Artery—perforator to profunda femoris artery, vein—paired vena comitantes.
  - Dimensions: 1 cm below gluteal crease, 6 cm minimum width for primary closure.
  - Harvesting essentials:
    - Dominant perforator is 2–4 cm posterior to gracilis muscle.
    - Posterior limit of incision is midgluteal crease.
    - Posterior cutaneous femoral nerve should be preserved by dissecting deeper to Scarpa's fascia.
  - Advantages: Hidden donor site, minimal lymphedema risk, two-team approach, long pedicle.
  - Disadvantages: Inconsistent anatomy, may need preoperative CT or MRI, narrow flap, bulky in obese cases.
- **Free fibula flap (Fig. 7)**:
  - Type: Osseous, osteomuscular, osteocutaneous.
  - Vascular supply: Artery—dominant nutrient artery, branch of peroneal artery, minor periosteal branches of peroneal artery, vein—venae comitantes.
  - Dimensions: Skin—12 cm (maximum 32 cm) across 6 cm (maximum 14 cm), bone—midsegment after leaving 6 cm on each side.
  - Harvesting essentials:
    - Rule out evidence of vascular disease and trauma preoperatively.
    - Flap elevation is under tourniquet control.
    - Anterior approach is preferred and flap is mobilized distal to proximal.

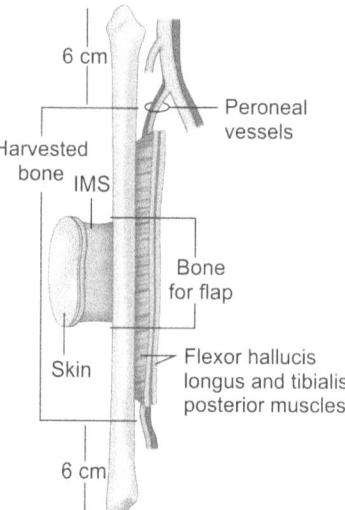

Fig. 7: Free fibula flap. (IMS: intermuscular septum)

- Flap is centered on posterior intermuscular septa, i.e., over the posterior border of fibula.
- Common peroneal nerve must be identified and preserved.
- Posterior tibial artery must be confirmed before ligation of peroneal artery.
- Flow to the distal foot should be confirmed by clamping the peroneal artery distally.
- Including flexor hallucis longus muscle reduces the chances of injury to pedicle.
- Superficial peroneal nerve should be preserved in the proximal part of the peroneus longus muscle.
- For plate fixation, unicortical screws are preferred.
- Advantages: Two-team approach feasible, vascularized bone, versatile, allows craniofacial contouring by osteotomies, large caliber vessels, limited functional disability.

- *Disadvantages*: Obvious donor scar, tedious and technically difficult harvesting technique, ankle function limitation in aggressive physical activities.

POSTOPERATIVE CARE

Monitoring: Intensive care unit (ICU) stay for 3–5 days with vitals and flap monitoring helps in reducing chances of early complications.

Airway: Elective tracheostomy is indicated in extensive resection requiring bulky flap, mandibular resection crossing midline, palatal resection, and major tongue reconstruction.

Feeding: Nasogastric tube feed is continued for 5–7 days till patients can tolerate their own saliva.

Position: A 15–30° head elevation reduces venous congestion and bleeding. Head turning is advised as per the direction of the vascular pedicle of flap.

Prophylactic antibiotics: These are given for 5 days postoperatively.

Blood thinners: Low-molecular-weight heparin is given for 5 days as a counter measure for deep venous thrombosis. Anticoagulants also prevent thrombosis of new anastomotic vessels.

Physiotherapy: Jaw-stretching exercises should be started after initial wound healing and continued.

Dental rehabilitation: It is considered in vascularized bone transfer.

Prosthesis: Bite guide avoids deviation of jaw and should be applied for 6–8 weeks.

KEY POINTS

- Small superficial defects of cheek can be left to heal by secondary intention.
- Superficial small-to-moderate-sized defects can be primarily closed by local tissue advancement.
- All superficial defects in the cheek region can be safely skin grafted with minimal scarring and contracture.
- Large defects with loss of muscle or in retromolar trigone can cause severe trismus if left to heal by secondary intention or skin grafts.
- In case of loss of oral commissure, maximum efforts must be made to restore it in the primary reconstruction.
- Defects should be measured at their maximum dimensions in the largest possible mouth opening for planning reconstruction.
- Efforts should be made to recreate the sulcus to avoid any postoperative restrictions.
- Location of salivary duct post resection and its reconstruction by stenting or sialodochoplasty in the event of segment loss reduces chances due to salivary leak.
- Cases with submucous fibrosis may need contralateral intervention (release + skin grafting/coronoidectomy/flap cover) for adequate restoration of mouth opening.
- The choice of flaps in case of postradiation reconstruction should consider the size of the irradiated territory (local flaps) and vascular status of neck (free flaps).
- For complex defects, free flaps should be preferred over local and regional flaps for better functional and aesthetic outcome.
- Preoperative planning, meticulous intraoperative execution, and postoperative monitoring with low threshold for complications form the pillars of a successful reconstruction.

24. Reconstruction of Soft Tissues and Bony Defects of Oral Cavity

Rajan Arora

INTRODUCTION

Composite resection is the standard treatment approach for cancer of the oral cavity. This results in considerable functional and cosmetic deformity. The role of the reconstructive surgeon is to provide diverse reconstructive options to enable an aesthetic and functional reconstruction while minimizing the morbidity of the patient.

Goals of the reconstruction include:
- Restoration of the anatomic structure (form)
- Providing function that enhances the patient's quality of life

For oral cavity, the functional goals of reconstruction are:
- Intelligible speech
- Isolation of oral cavity from sinuses and nasal cavity
- Unrestricted mouth opening
- Stable occlusion and mastication
- Swallowing
- Avoiding aspiration
- Coverage of the neck and restoration of the watertight seal of the oral cavity to prevent leakage of saliva and to prevent life-threatening complications such as blowout of the great vessels of the neck.

WORKUP OF PATIENTS UNDERGOING RECONSTRUCTION

- Preoperative workup by the extirpation surgery team is quite extensive.
- Other investigations that may aid in deciding the choice of reconstruction include CT angiography and magnetic resonance angiography (MRA) to assess the arterial anatomy prior to harvest of a free fibular flap. CT angiography is done for preoperative imaging of perforators in the anterolateral thigh (ALT) flap or the deep inferior epigastric artery perforator (DIEP) flap.
- Prefabricated mandible templates based on CT scan data are also used to aid in shaping the neomandible from fibula, scapula, and radius bone after extirpative surgery.

Selection of Reconstructive Options

For primary reconstruction of an ablative defect, the optimal reconstructive option needs to be decided before operation and it should be based on:
- Prognosis
- General medical condition of the patient
- History of previous surgery or head and neck radiation
- Plan of postoperative irradiation
- An accurate preoperative prediction of the size, depth, location, and extent of the ablation

Before deciding on a reconstructive solution, the surgeon should consider the facility available and his/her own experience, comfort, skill, and knowledge of the local, regional, and distant anatomy.

Reconstructive Techniques

The reconstructive technique is selected according to the complexities of the defect.
- Direct closure
- Closure by secondary intention
- Skin grafting
- Application of local flaps
- Regional flaps
- Distant flaps
- Free flaps

Direct Closure

Direct closure is where ample of soft tissue can be mobilized to achieve closure without compromising oral function, e.g., tethering of tongue, trismus due to shortening of mucosa.

Closure by Secondary Intention

This closure happens by allowing the wound to granulate/epithelialize, e.g., tongue and floor of mouth. The wound heals with contracture and scarring but must not jeopardize function by impairing the motility of the tongue.

Skin Grafting

- Good for small defects which cannot be closed directly, e.g., anterior buccal mucosal defects.
- Can be used after partial maxillectomy where maxillary prosthesis is planned.

Local Flaps

Indications:
- Small defects where the bone gets exposed after the ablation
- Where a vascularized bed is needed, such as in irradiated bed

Local flap provides thin and sensate cover of similar tissues for small defects.

It may not be a viable option where the area adjacent to the defect is included in the radiation field in previously irradiated patients.

For example, the tongue flap is a versatile flap to cover small intraoral defects, but care must be taken not to compromise tongue function or facial artery musculomucosal (FAMM) flap which is a reliable axial pedicle flap to cover moderate intraoral defects.

Regional Flaps

These flaps are from other parts of the face, e.g., nasolabial flap, forehead flap, and temporalis muscle flap.

Submental flap, particularly in females, is useful for floor reconstruction.

There may also be a concern about using a flap from the lymphatic drainage territory of the tumor site.

Distant Flaps

These flaps are from distant sites such as:
- Chest [deltopectoral flap and pectoralis major myocutaneous (PMMC) flap]
- Neck (sternocleidomastoid muscle flap, less reliable than the other flaps)
- Shoulder (supraclavicular artery island flap)
- Back (trapezius musculocutaneous flap)

Free Flaps

Free flap is an island flap detached from one part of the body with its feeding vessels and reattached at the distant recipient site by microvascular anastomosis.

Nowadays, it is the gold standard for the reconstruction of the soft tissue and bony defects of the head and neck region.

Advantages:
- Single-stage procedure
- Faster recovery
- Effective in poorly vascularized sites, e.g., postradiotherapy

- Success rate is predictable than axial flaps.
- Donor site is selected to minimize morbidity.
- Wide range of donor sites is available.
- More appropriate flap with replacement of lost tissue with similar components. Allow the option of incorporating any tissue type, e.g., skin, muscle, tendon, or bone.
- It can be tailored to the specific defect.
- Restoration of otherwise lost function

Disadvantages:
- Microvascular equipment and expertise required
- Long operations
- Failure is usually total
- Technique relies on suitable vessels at the recipient site

Radial artery forearm flap (RAFF) is a thin and pliable flap for reconstruction of oral mucosa, lip, and tongue.

Anterolateral thigh flap is now a workhorse flap for reconstruction of any kind of soft-tissue defects. It can be thinned and may be used in place of RAFF.

Free fibular osteocutaneous flap is a flap of choice for mandibular reconstruction. Provide good quality and quantity of bone stock with a reliable skin paddle.

Although various other donor sites are available, most of the oral defects can be reconstructed with these three flaps.

COMPONENT-WISE RECONSTRUCTION OF ORAL DEFECTS

Defects of oral cavity can be divided into three groups:
1. Only soft-tissue defects
2. Soft tissue with bone
3. Only bony defects

Defects Needing Soft-tissue Reconstruction Only

Buccal Mucosa Defects

Depending upon the size of the defect, small defects can be closed directly, left for healing with secondary intention or split skin grafted.

Moderate-sized defects with exposed bone can be covered with local flaps, e.g., nasolabial or tongue flap.

Larger defects including marginal mandibulectomy (also in case of excision of lesion of RMT area) are covered with either regional flap, e.g., PMMC flap, or if expertise is available can be reconstructed with RAFF or anterolateral thigh flap.

Palatal Defects

Soft palate: It is a dynamic structure and difficult to reconstruct.

A thin flap such as RAFF is best suited for this defect.

Hard palate: Reconstruction of the hard palate is frequently achieved with prosthesis.

An obturator attached with dental prosthesis is being used to plug the palatal hole after lining the defect with simple split skin graft.

An isolated hard palate defect can be covered with free RAFF or ALT flap to separate the nasal cavity from the oral cavity.

Tongue, with or without floor of mouth: The tongue is a unique muscular structure within the oral cavity. It plays an important role in articulation of speech, appreciation of taste, and initiation of swallowing.

Priorities of reconstruction of tongue include airway protection, swallowing, and articulation of speech.

Functional reconstruction of this dynamic structure is difficult to achieve.

The most appropriate reconstructive choice depends on the size of the tongue defect.

Smaller defects can be closed primarily.

For partial glossectomy, a thin pliable flap such as free RAFF is the flap of choice but reconstruction should not affect the mobility of the remaining healthy tongue.

After hemiglossectomy, free ALT is the flap of choice because of its bulk.

Near total glossectomy leads to a permanent swallowing problem. Bulky flaps such as free ALT or rectus abdominis myocutaneous flap help in swallowing of food in such situations.

Defects Needing Both Soft Tissue and Bone

Segmental Mandibulectomy with the Buccal Mucosa or Floor of Mouth

Resection of buccal mucosa or floor of mouth with segmental mandibulectomy needs composite tissue for reconstruction including both skin paddle and a piece of bone. In such situations, the flap of choice is a free fibular osteocutaneous flap. The main advantage of this flap is that it not only bridges the bony gap, but also provides the good-quality bone stock for dental rehabilitation.

Other options for reconstruction of soft tissue and mandibular defect are reconstruction plates with a PMMC or any soft-tissue free flap.

Posterior segmental mandibulectomy may not require bony reconstruction, and a soft-tissue defect reconstructed with a pectoralis major flap is sufficient.

Maxillectomy with or without an orbital floor requires a free fibular osteocutaneous flap for the reconstruction. Sometimes, it can be reconstructed with temporalis muscle with skin graft, but in such cases dental rehabilitation is not possible.

Defects Needing Bone Only

In *mandibular excision for ameloblastoma*, where the mucosa is not at all involved, simple bony reconstruction with a free fibula flap without a skin paddle is enough. Iliac crest and scapula vascularized bone flaps are other examples of free flaps for bony reconstruction.

WORKHORSE FLAPS FOR RECONSTRUCTION

These are the common flaps used for reconstruction of most of the three-dimensional soft-tissue and composite defects of oral cavity.

Pectoralis Major Muscle/ Myocutaneous Flap

Based on the thoracodorsal branch of the thoracoacromial trunk, the pectoralis major flap can be used as only muscle flap for the coverage of the large vessels of neck after neck dissection and for the coverage of primary closure of pharynx after total laryngectomy in postradiation patients.

It is also used as a myocutaneous flap (single- or double-skin paddle) for the reconstruction of oral as well as through and through orocutaneous defects. The skin paddle over the muscle is supplied by the perforators of the branches of the thoracodorsal artery. These can be raised along the superior and lateral borders of the muscle.

Inclusion of the sixth rib with the flap can also be used to bridge the bony defect of the mandible although it is not a good choice for the bony reconstruction.

The main advantage of this flap is that it is easy to harvest and can be used as a good option for reconstruction of composite defects of oral cavity in those centers where microvascular reconstructive facilities are not available.

Deltopectoral Flap

It is one of the pedicled fasciocutaneous flaps based on the anterior intercostal perforators of the internal mammary artery.

The main disadvantage of this flap is that it may need delaying procedure to enhance its length and also requires one more stage to divide its pedicle to complete the inset of flap.

Free Radial Artery Forearm Flap

In 1981, Yang first described the radial forearm flap in China. For this reason, it is also known as the "Chinese flap."

As the name suggests, it is based on the radial artery of the forearm **(Fig. 1)**.

Indications—Reconstruction of:
- Oral cavity
- Tongue reconstruction
- Pharyngeal reconstruction
- Soft palate
- Cutaneous defects
- Base of skull
- Small-volume bone
- Soft-tissue defects of face

Advantages:
- Thin, pliable skin. Reconstitution of contours, sulci, and vestibules is easy.
- Highly tolerant to radiation therapy.
- Composite flap can be raised with bone, tendon, brachioradialis muscle, and vascularized nerve.
- Sensory recovery is reported in patients even when a neural anastomosis is not performed.
- Skin from the entire forearm can be harvested.

Disadvantages:
- Unsightly appearance of donor site—due to split skin graft
- Loss of sensation over the dorsum of hand—sometimes, the sensory branch of the radial nerve is injured while raising the flap.

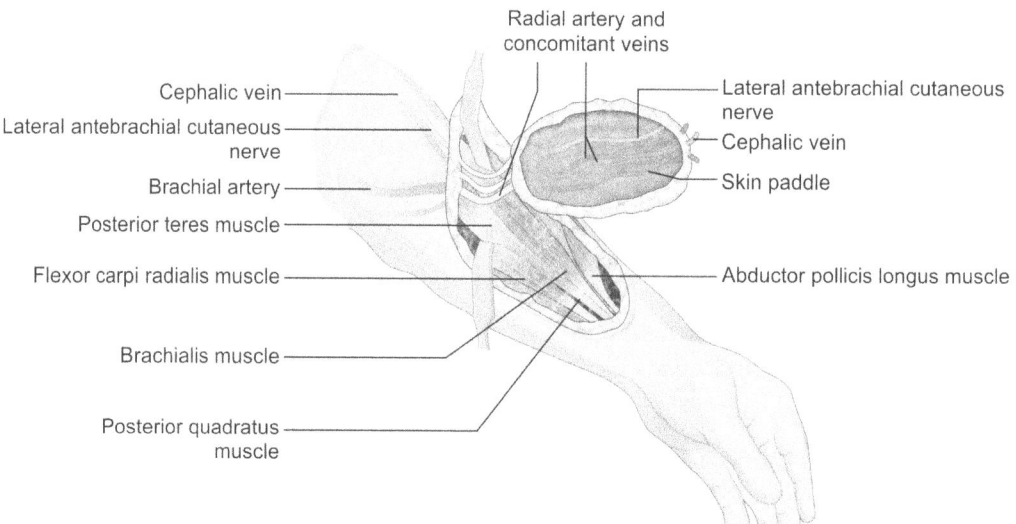

Fig. 1: Radial artery forearm flap.

Free Anterolateral Thigh Flap (Fig. 2)

This was first reported by Song et al. A vascular pedicle is formed by the descending branch of the lateral circumflex femoral artery.

Indications:
- Buccal mucosa defect
- Through and through oral defects
- Upper/lower lip reconstruction
- Reconstruction of neopharynx
- Tongue—partial or total
- Orbital defects
- Palatal reconstruction after partial maxillectomy to fill the cavity after total maxillectomy In high-risk patients for mandibular reconstruction instead of free fibula we use ALT with reconstruction plates to save time.
- External skin defects

Types of ALT: This flap can be raised as:
- Fasciocutaneous flap
- Musculocutaneous flap
- Fascial flap
- Adipofascial flap
- Chimeric flap—skin paddle + muscle, two skin paddles on two different perforators
- Muscle-only flap
- Flow-through flap

Advantages:
- Almost all the defects of head and neck can be reconstructed with this flap.
- We can harvest a large skin paddle.
- Long skin paddle on multiple perforators.
- Small skin paddles on different perforators (chimeric).
- Pliability is good.
- No major artery is sacrificed.
- We can harvest muscle with skin to obliterate cavities and for contouring.

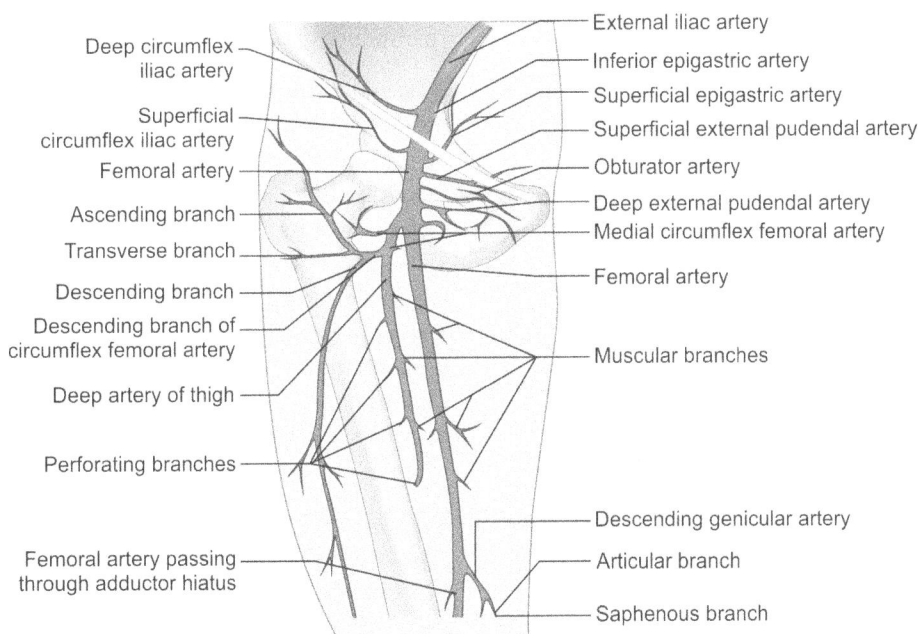

Fig. 2: Anterolateral thigh flap.

- If we can close the donor area directly, donor site morbidity is minimal.
- It can be thinned.

Disadvantages:
- Rarely perforators are not found—in that case anteromedial thigh (AMT) flap or tensor fascia-lata flap can be harvested through the same incision
- Difficult to dissect

Free Fibula Osseous and Osteocutaneous Flap

- Taylor first described a vascularized free fibula in 1975.
- Hidalgo did the first mandibular reconstruction in 1989.

The vascular pedicle consists of peroneal artery and its venae comitantes.

Indications:
- Mandibular reconstruction
- Maxillary reconstruction

Advantages:
- 25 cm of bone stock can be harvested.
- Enough for whole mandibular recon
- Ideal for osseointegrated implant placement
- It can be used as a vascularized bone.
- It can be raised as osteocutaneous flap, osteomyocutaneous flap and, can be raised with two skin paddles.

Disadvantages:
- In 5-10% of cases, blood supply to skin paddle is inadequate.
- Donor site problems
- Edema
- Weakness in dorsiflexion of the great toe
- Skin graft is required to cover the donor site.
- Poor donor site appearance

Technical considerations:
- May need angiography or MRA to rule out *peronea magna* (dominant peroneal artery with absent posterior tibial vessels).
- 6-7 cm segment preserved proximally and distally to protect common peroneal nerve and ensure ankle stability.

SECONDARY SURGERY

For the complications: Reconstruction of the head and neck defect does not end at the primary surgery. Unfortunately, every surgeon will experience several reconstruction failures, e.g., disruption of the suture line, partial or total flap failure leading to an orocutaneous fistula. Pooling of secretions and infection in the neck can lead to life-threatening complications such as carotid artery blowout. Early debridement and coverage of exposed vital structures with local, regional, or free flaps are required in such cases depending upon the extent of the defect. Some cases do heal with conservative treatment only.

Secondary surgery to enhance function or aesthetics after reconstruction: Patients may also require secondary surgery to enhance function after reconstruction. Debulking of flaps results in enhanced facial contour, symmetry, and aesthetic outcome and can be performed under local anesthesia. Secondary vestibuloplasty allows for delayed osseointegrated implants. Other procedures may include scar revision or resurfacing of an unsightly skin-grafted donor site using modalities such as tissue expanders.

Secondary surgery for recurrences: A significant number of cancer patients may present with a recurrence requiring further reconstruction.

In this subgroup of patients, the neck is often scarred due to previous surgery and radiation. Recipient vessels for free flaps are hard to find and are often encased in scar. Often, vessels from the contralateral neck or vein grafts may have to be used.

KEY POINTS

- Composite resection is the standard treatment approach for cancer of the oral cavity with considerable functional and cosmetic deformity.
- The goal of the reconstruction includes restoration of the anatomic structure (form) and function that enhances the patient's quality of life.
- Reconstruction also prevents life-threatening complications such as blowout of the great vessels of the neck.
- Optimal reconstructive method depends on the prognosis of the disease, general condition of the patient, history of previous surgery or radiation, plan of postoperative irradiation and preoperative prediction of the size, and location and extent of the ablation.
- Reconstructive technique ranges from direct closure, skin grafting to transfer of local to distant flaps.
- Nowadays, a free flap is the gold standard for the reconstruction of the composite defects of the head and neck region.
- *Advantages*: Free flap is a single-stage procedure, recovery is fast, effective for postradiotherapy sites, allows incorporation of any kind of tissue, e.g., skin, muscle, tendon, or bone, and restoration of otherwise lost function is possible.
- *Disadvantages*: Requirement of microvascular equipment and expertise, duration of surgery is long, and technique relies on suitable vessels at the recipient site.
- Common pedicled workhorse flaps for reconstruction of oral cavity are PMMC and DP and free workhorse flaps are RAFF, ALT, and free fibula flap.
- Almost all the defects of the oral cavity can be reconstructed with these flaps.

Adjuvant Treatment in Oral Cavity Cancer

Abhinav Dewan, Swarupa Mitra

INTRODUCTION

- For early stage oral cavity cancers (OCC), a single-modality treatment with surgery or radiotherapy (RT) has been demonstrated to be equally effective for local control (LC) (80–90% for T1–2 lesions).
- For T3–4 tumors, treatment with single modality leads to significantly higher failure rates. Surgery followed by postoperative treatment has become the accepted standard of care for advanced-stage OCC.
- Selected high-risk patients with head and neck squamous cell carcinoma (HNSCC) are planned for postoperative radiation therapy (PORT), with or without concurrent chemotherapy, following primary surgical resection with the aim of improving LC and overall survival (OS). The rationale for this approach is to eradicate microscopic deposits of cancer cells using RT.

FACTORS WARRANTING POSTOPERATIVE ADJUVANT THERAPY

- Patients who have undergone gross total resection of the primary disease may be at a high risk of recurrence depending upon the clinicopathological factors. Adjuvant RT generally in conjunction with chemotherapy can improve the likelihood of LC and disease-free survival (DFS).
- Adjuvant chemoradiation is generally restricted to patients thought to be at the highest risk of locoregional recurrence (LRR) and should be used with caution because of the morbidity of adding chemotherapy to PORT. RT alone remains an option for patients with an intermediate risk of recurrence or for individuals who cannot tolerate concurrent chemotherapy (CCT).
- The National Comprehensive Cancer Network (NCCN) enlists the following as poor risk indicators for adjuvant therapy:
  - Positive/close margins
  - Extranodal extension (ENE)
  - Lymphovascular invasion (LVI)
  - Perineural invasion (PNI)
  - Advanced T-stage (pT3-4)
  - High grade
  - Advanced N stage (N2-3)
  - Involved nodes in levels IV and V
- Other prognostic factors that are frequently discussed in multidisciplinary tumor boards are presence of worst pattern of invasion (WPOI), depth of invasion (DOI), recurrent disease, nodal yield, nodal ratio in neck dissection specimen, nodal diameter >3 cm, tumor spillage, and tumor multicentricity.

Primary Tumor Risk Factors

Margins

- The goal of surgery is complete resection of the tumor with negative margins.

- A positive margin is a poor prognostic factor in head and neck cancer (HNC); it increases the chances of recurrence substantially and decreases survival.
- For the oral cavity, a close margin is typically defined as <5 mm.
- As a standard, a minimum tumor margin of 5 mm is considered acceptable and presence of lesions (i.e., severe dysplasia/carcinoma in situ and invasive carcinoma) within this distance should be reported and are associated with a significant risk of local recurrence.

Worst Pattern of Invasion

- Adequacy of margins also depends upon WPOI at the tumor–host interface.
- WPOI at the deep tumor is a strong prognostic indicator of LC for oral cancers in early stages.
  - Type 1: Tumor invasion in a broad and pushing manner
  - Type 2: Pushing "fingers" or separate bigger tumor islands
  - Type 3: Invasive tumor islands of >15 cells/island
  - Type 4: Even smaller tumor islands of ≤15 cells down to even isolated single invasive cells
  - Type 5: Dispersed pattern of tumor invasion having a distance of 1 mm or more of normal tissue between the tumor satellites of any size
- During pathological reporting, the highest POI score has been deemed as the WPOI.
- WPOI-5 is a proved marker for poor locoregional control (LRC) in early stage oral cancer and predicts 42% LRR, and hence supporting an adjuvant treatment

Depth of Invasion

- DOI is the distance from the basement membrane perpendicularly down to the deepest microscopic edge of the tumor (Fig. 1).
- It is a critical predictor of disease-specific survival (DSS) for oral cavity squamous cell carcinoma (OCSCC) for all T-stages.
- Thin and superficially invasive lesions have a lower risk of lymphnodal (LN) metastasis, are highly curable, and offer an excellent prognosis.
- Thicker lesions that deeply infiltrate the underlying soft tissues have a significantly increased incidence of LN metastasis and an adverse impact on prognosis.
- Risk of LN metastasis and survival rates in relation to tumor thickness for T1-2 SCC of the tongue and floor of mouth (FOM) are shown in **Figure 2**.
- Review of literature on the thickness of primary tumor for selection of elective treatment of the neck indicates that the lesions thicker than 4 mm have a progressively increased risk of LN metastasis.
- For pT1 cancers of tongue and FOM, a DOI of ≥4 mm is statistically associated with a poorer prognosis, worser LRC [hazard ratio (HR) 1.67], and increased risk of dying from cancer (HR 2.44).
- Depth of invasion of ≥4 mm is a predictor for nodal relapse rate (24%) and confers four times more risk than seen for tumors with DOI < 4 mm.
- The American Joint Committee on Cancer (AJCC), 8th edition, has now incorporated DOI as an important determinant of T-staging for OCSCC.

Perineural Invasion

- Presence of PNI and LVI is a prognostic indicator for tumor control and survival.
- PNI is the presence of microscopic tumor cells within any of the three layers of the nerve sheath or presence of tumor cells

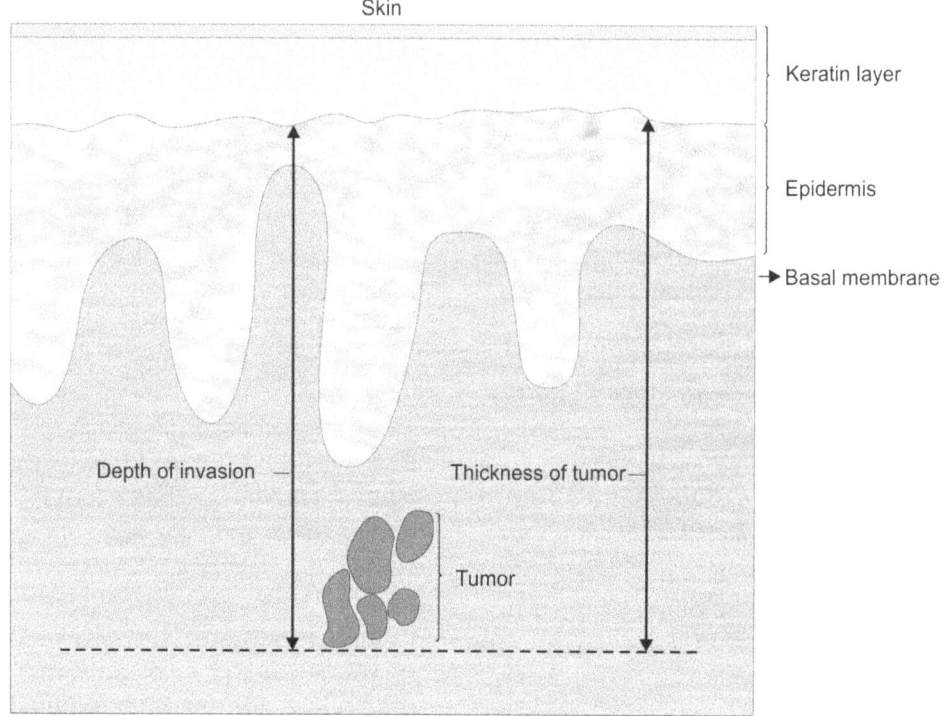

Fig. 1: Depth of invasion versus tumor thickness.

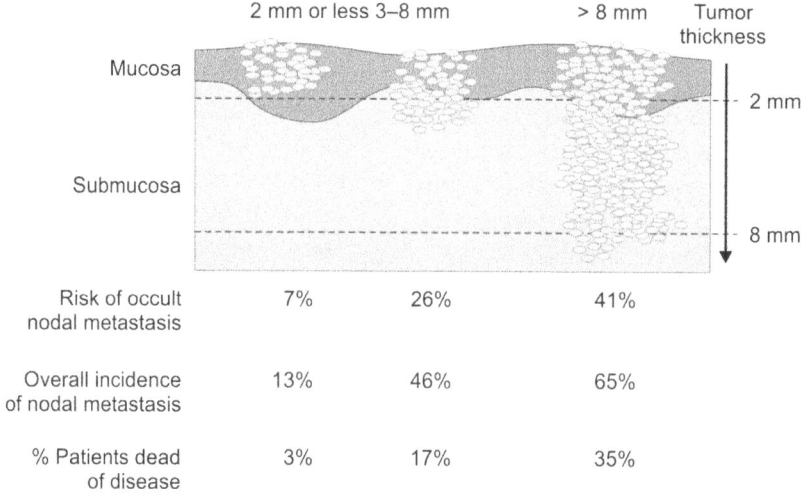

Fig. 2: Incidence of lymph nodal metastasis and survival in relation to thickness of the primary lesion for T1 and T2 squamous cell carcinoma of the tongue and floor of mouth.
Source: Shah JP, Patel SG, Singh B. Jatin Shah's Head and Neck Surgery and Oncology, 4th edition. Philadelphia: Mosby; 2012.

surrounding at least one-third of the circumference of a nerve. It is found to be associated with an increased risk of lymph node metastasis and poor DSS and OS in OCSCC.
- PNI is associated with a worse 5-year DSS when compared to patients without PNI (76% vs. 92%; $p < 0.003$). Moreover, on a multivariate analysis, PNI predicts regional LN metastasis (55% vs. 21%; $p = 0.017$).
- Elective treatment of the neck in patients of early OCSCC with PNI can reduce the rate of recurrence in the neck from 85.7 to 16.2% ($p = 0.001$). Elective neck treatment for improving DSS as well as neck control is indicated for patients with cN0 but with PNI-positive tumors.
- Due to the lack of conclusive evidence that RT improves LC in PNI +ve tumors in the absence of any other adverse pathological features, use of adjuvant RT for OCSCC remains controversial and is not universally recommended.

Lymphovascular Invasion

- LVI has been seen to cause worse LRC and OS.
- It is recommended to give adjuvant RT in patients with LVI but node-negative disease.
- *Advantages of PORT*:
  - No delay in surgery caused
  - Allows complete evaluation of tumor and lymph nodes before treatment
  - Residual microscopic disease can be effectively treated improving the local and/or regional control
  - Reduced RT dose
- *Disadvantages of PORT*:
  - There could be a delay in initiation of RT, if postoperative recovery is complicated by fistula or other wound problems.
  - Scarring and vascular modifications due to surgery may decrease tissue oxygenation and thus may adversely affect RT tumor cell kill.

FUTURE DIRECTIONS

Genetic Factors

- Even with negative margins, local recurrence rates of up to 10–30% have been reported.
- A genetic predisposition within the tumor area has been found in 20–60% of such patients that may remain undetected by conventional histopathology.
- The novel technologies could identify any precursor lesions in addition to the residual cancer cells present in the tumor field.
- Presence of TP53-mutated DNA at tumor-free surgical margins has been found predictive for LRR [relative risk (RR) 7.1; $p = 0.021$] and may be useful to decide on postoperative RT.

Nodal Risk Factors

- LN involvement was an established indication for adjuvant RT many years ago, since surgery alone historically was associated with high risks of recurrence in such patients.
- The number of metastatic nodes and the overall yield of nodes after neck dissection have prognostic significance.
- The number of nodes harvested, irrespective of whether they are malignant, impacts the survival. Many studies suggest that harvesting <18 LN in a neck dissection leads to poorer survival, while others show that survival improves with even more extensive neck dissections with up to 35 nodes.

- Patients with inadequate LN dissection and with a high risk of microscopic nodal involvement should be planned for adjuvant RT.
- According to many studies, the LN ratio (involved LN/LN removed) is a prognostic indicator for OS in patients who have been treated with upfront surgery.
- Conversely, patients who have single nodal involvement with adequately dissected neck have excellent outcomes with surgery alone, and RT may be deferred in these patients.

Extranodal Extension

- Presence of ENE is considered a significant predictor of distant metastasis and OS.
- Clinically, ENE is characterized by tissue invasion and fixity to skin, dermis, and muscle and/or infiltration of nerves by involved nodes.
- CT and MRI are useful in detecting clinical ENE but may not be reliable in predicting lesser degrees of ENE.
- The maximum information on ENE is based on pathologic findings.
- *Microscopic ENE*: ENE 2 mm or less beyond nodal capsule.
- *Major ENE*: ENE > 2 mm beyond nodal capsule. It is then said to be ENE positive.

COMPOSITE ANALYSIS OF RISK FACTORS

Three risk groups have been identified based on the historical data (RTOG 8503/MD Anderson Cancer Centre/University of Pennsylvania/EORTC 22931/RTOG 9501):

- *Low risk*: No LN involvement, no ECE present, and surgical margins are not involved histologically
- *Intermediate risk*: LN positivity, involved lymph nodes at more than one level, level IV or V nodal involvement, N2/3 disease, perineural or perivascular invasion, pT3/T4 disease, invasion of cartilage, bone, or soft tissues by the primary tumor, WPOI 4-5 (controversial), DOI ≥ 4 mm (tongue)
- *High risk*: Positive margins, ECE, and presence of more than two adverse features are the most unfavorable parameters associated with a significant increase in LRR and mortality. This group typically constitutes indication for CCT.

Postoperative Radiation Therapy Alone

- PORT alone is inferior to concurrent chemoradiotherapy following gross tumor resection for high-risk disease.
- Patients at higher risk for recurrence based on PNI or LVI, two or more involved lymph nodes, or T3 and T4 tumors are considered to be at an intermediate risk and may be treated with postoperative RT alone.

Future Directions for Intermediate-risk Postoperative Patients

- *RTOG 0920*: Randomizing patients with intermediate risk to RT alone or to RT plus cetuximab.
- Eastern Cooperative Oncology Group (ECOG)-American College of Radiology Imaging Network (ACRIN) Cancer Research Group-Phase III trial of intermediate-risk patients having disruptive p53 mutations, which predict poorer prognosis, to be treated with either RT alone or RT plus cisplatin and postsurgical resection in order to improve DFS in this cohort.
- *NRG-HN003*: Investigating the inclusion of pembrolizumab to RT and cisplatin in high-risk patients.

- *LCCC1725* phase II study of adjuvant RT with durvalumab and tremelimumab for medium-risk patients.
- *PATHWay*: Randomized, double-blinded phase II study of 1-year duration of pembrolizumab or placebo.

Adjuvant Chemotherapy: For Whom should Chemotherapy be added to Adjuvant RT?
- Adjuvant RT has been seen to improve outcomes. But with RT alone, there is a probability to failure to cure in higher risk patients with positive margins/ECE.
- *Two landmark, large, randomized trials studied if there was any benefit of addition of chemotherapy*: EORTC 22931 and RTOG 9501 (chemotherapy regimen used in both the studies was 3 weekly bolus cisplatin 100 mg/m^2 and the inclusion was the presence of criteria of positive margin and ENE)
- In summary, for those patients who are fit and the surgical pathology report shows positive margins or ENE, the addition of cisplatin to adjuvant RT gives approximately a 48% reduction in the risk of LRR and a 30% improvement in DFS and OS.
- Patients with multiple positive lymph nodes but without positive margins or ENE do not benefit.
- It is still not clear, if patients with stage III or IV cancer, involved level 4 or 5 LN, or perineural or vascular invasion would benefit from chemotherapy.

Concurrent Chemotherapy Regimen
- High-dose bolus cisplatin (100 mg/m^2 on days 1, 22, 43) is the standard drug regimen to be given concurrently with RT.
- Weekly cisplatin regimens (35–40 mg/m^2)
- Many HNSCC patients may be poor candidates for cisplatin due to their advanced age, baseline renal dysfunction, known auditory deficits including hearing loss and/or tinnitus, and poor performance status. Cisplatin may be administered with dose modification or replaced with carboplatin in such patients.
- The role of cetuximab is not established in the postoperative setting and should only be used as part of a postoperative adjuvant strategy in the context of a clinical trial.
- Various phase III clinical trials assessing the role of cetuximab and docetaxel in the adjuvant setting include RTOG 0920, RTOG 1216, and RTOG 0234.

Initiation and Treatment Delays
- The overall duration of treatment by RT is a major determinant for outcome of HNSCC. This is reflected by reduced LCR when the same dose is delivered over a longer time. Moreover, a higher dose needs to be delivered to increase the tumor control probability when the treatment of duration is prolonged.
- The explanation for this outcome is that the surviving clonogenic tumor cells undergo repopulation very rapidly in response to the cell kill by the fractionated RT.
- This is the rationale for shortening the overall duration of RT without decreasing the dose of RT to improve LCR.
- In the absence of wound healing issues or medical contraindicated, PORT should be started no later than 6 weeks after surgery and should be completed in a timely manner.
- LRC is better for patients who complete postoperative RT within 100 days or less from the date of surgery in comparison to patients treated over a longer period of time.

- Ang et al. emphasized that surgery and adjuvant RT should be considered a combined treatment package and should ideally be completed within 11 weeks.
- The time interval between surgery and initiation of RT as well as the duration of PORT appears to have an impact on outcome.

Adjuvant Radiotherapy Doses

Adjuvant RT doses for HNC depend upon the clinical and pathologic findings are described in **Table 1**.

Schedule

- Conventional postoperative RT schedules typically deliver 54–66 Gy in 1.8–2 Gy daily fractions, over 5–7 weeks.
- Altered-fractionation RT schedules including accelerated RT and hyperfractionation have been investigated to overcome accelerated repopulation and to safely escalate the dose. These strategies have demonstrated improved LRC, but the survival benefit has not been established. The added cost and logistical challenges of multiple fractions per day and additional toxicity have limited their implementation.

TABLE 1: Adjuvant RT doses.

Pathological features	RT dose
Primary disease (CTV-primary):	
High-risk features (margin positive)	66 Gy
Intermediate-risk features	60 Gy
Infratemporal fossa (in case of RMT/upper GBS/upper alveolus involvement)	54 Gy
Nodal disease (CTV-node):	
High-risk features (ENE+)	66 Gy
Involved nodes (ENE−)	60 Gy
CTV-low risk (prophylactic CTV/pathologically uninvolved nodal region)	50–54 Gy

(CTV: clinical target volume; ENE: extranodal extension; GBS: gingivobuccal sulci; RMT: retromolar trigone)

Target Volume Delineation for Intensity-modulated Radiotherapy

- Preoperative imaging, clinical examination, intraoperative findings, and histopathology results are needed for target volume delineation.
- The basic steps for identifying the postoperative bed at-risk are based on the fundamental principles of delineation of CTV for definitive RT:
  - *Head and neck cast fabrication and CT simulation* (3-mm slice thickness with IV contrast)
  - *Co-registration* of the images of the preoperative diagnostic CT/MRI scans with the simulator CT scan
  - *Re-creating the preoperative primary/nodal gross tumor volumes (GTV)*: Location of the preoperative primary tumor and involved node(s) (GTV-P/GTV-N) has to be re-created on the simulator CT scans co-registered diagnostic images.
  - *Clinical target volume (CTV)*: It includes the GTV + volume of normal tissue at risk for microscopic tumor infiltration. This is the volume that has a probability of tumor recurrence. In the postoperative setting, CTV includes the primary and nodal beds, with a recommended margin to account for microscopic spread, all pathologically involved nodal levels, as well as other nodes at risk.
  - *Delineation of the primary tumor and involved nodal CTV (CTV high-risk)*: CTV high-risk (CTV-HR) corresponds to the preoperative GTV-P plus a margin for microscopic spread. A 10–15-mm margin is generally taken for the CTV-HR in the postoperative setting, due to the uncertainties in defining the tumor bed following

surgery. CTV-HR should be edited for anatomical barriers such as bone, fascia, and air and for organs at risk (OARs).

A radiation oncologist should acknowledge the fact that most of the oral cavity structures are midline and CTV-HR should include a generous coverage of the oral cavity. For oral tongue/FOM, CTV-HR usually includes the entire oral tongue and FOM complex. Infratemporal fossa (ITF) is added to the target volume when it is pathologically involved and also when treatment is being given for primaries in the retromolar trigone, upper gingivobuccal sulcus, and upper alveolar region.

Nodal CTV (CTV-N) corresponds to the preoperative GTV-N along with a margin, of generally 10 mm, for microscopic disease spread, edited for anatomical barriers.

Nodal CTV should be extended to include the following (**Table 2**):
- All pathologically involved nodal levels. When a pathologically involved node lies between two contiguous nodal levels, or is a boundary node, both levels will be included in the CTV.
- When a pathological lymph node is found abutting or invading a muscle not removed in the neck dissection, this muscle too may be included in the CTV, at least for the entire invaded level.
- Postoperative changes, e.g., seroma
- *Low-risk clinical target volume (CTV-LR)*: Prophylactic or elective CTV must include all the uninvolved nodes which are at risk. These will vary according to the site of the tumor and its laterality and extent of neck dissection.

TABLE 2: Nodal stations to be included.

	Levels to be included in CTV-node-low risk	
Nodal category	I/L Neck	C/L Neck[a]
N0-1 (in levels I, II, III)	I, II,[b] III, Iva,[c] +IX[d]	Ib,[e] II,[b] III, +Iva[c]
N2a-b	I, II, III, Iva,[f,g] Va,b,[g,h,i] +VIIb,[i] +IX[d]	Ib, II,[b] III, +Iva[c]
N2c	According to N category on each side of the neck	
N3	I, II, III, Iva,[f,g] Va,b, +VIIb[j] +IX[d]	Ib, II,[b] III, +Iva[c]

[a]Unilateral neck treatment is recommended for N0-N2a lateralized tumors of upper and lower alveolar ridges, lateral floor of mouth, and buccal mucosa. It could be considered for N0-N1 lateral border of oral tongue carcinomas not reaching the midline by <1 cm.
[b]Level IIb can be omitted, if no cervical lymph nodes are involved on the same side.
[c]For cancers of the anterior tongue and of the oral cavity extending to the oropharynx (e.g., anterior tonsillar pillar, tonsillar fossa, base of tongue); for N1 tumor with involvement of level III.
[d]For tumor of the buccal mucosa.
[e]Contralateral level Ib is included for all cases of carcinoma of the tongue/FOM and may be included for other sites after due risk assessment.
[f]Level IVb should be included in case of involvement of level IVa.
[g]Ipsilateral SCF (level IVb and level Vc) when level IVa or V is involved.
[h]Level V could be omitted, if only levels I to II were involved.
[i]Level VIIb should be included in case of level II involvement.

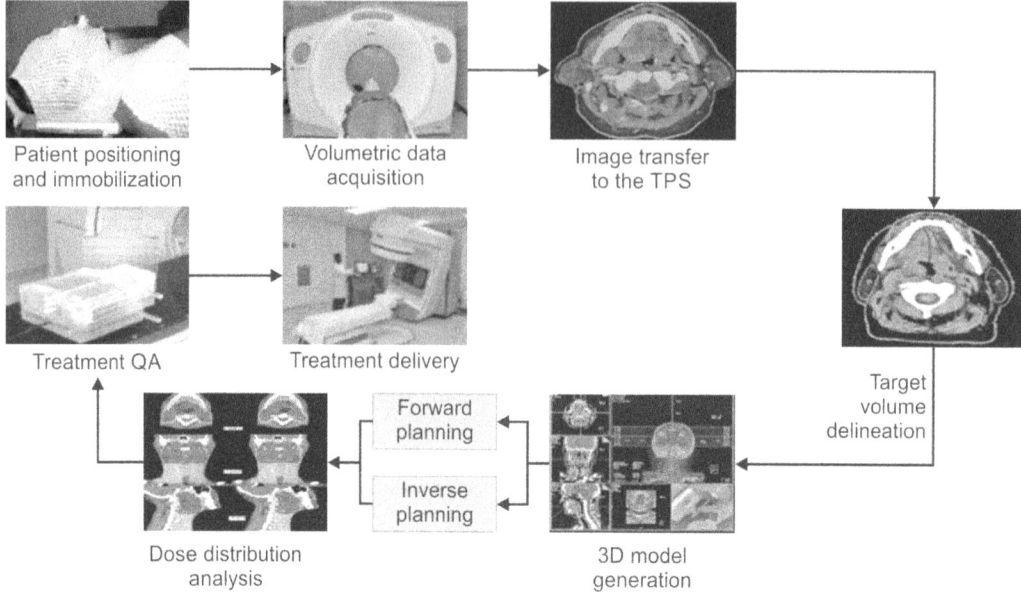

Fig. 3: Workflow of IMRT planning.
(QA: quality assurance; TPS: treatment planning system)

- *Planning target volumes (PTV):* Defined by an isotropic margin added to each CTV. The magnitude of margin varies among different institutes (usually between 3 and 5 mm).

- Optimally, all patients should be planned using intensity-modulated RT (IMRT; **Fig. 3**) or rotational arc techniques [rapid arc/volumetric modulated arc therapy (VMAT)].

KEY POINTS

- Selected patients with HNSCC treated with primary surgical resection who are at an increased risk of LRR are treated with postoperative RT with or without chemotherapy with the aim of improving LRC and survival.
- Adjuvant treatment is recommended for patients at high risk of recurrence with adverse histopathological features.
- Adjuvant chemoradiation is recommended in case of positive margin and ENE.

26 Radiotherapy in Oral Cancer

Munish Gairola, Parveen Ahlawat, Sarthak Tandon

INTRODUCTION

The treatment for oral cancers is complex and involves a multidisciplinary approach. Not only is the treatment of these cancers complex, but oral cancers also have probably the highest incidence of treatment-related morbidities among all the cancers. Various goals to be aimed for the treatment of the patients with oral cancers should be high locoregional control and survival rates in patients with limited disease, increased survival in patients with advanced disease, better organ-function preservation, increased therapeutic ratio, and minimum morbidities maintaining a good quality of life.

TREATMENT GUIDELINES FOR ORAL CANCERS

Early Stage Oral Cancer

Single-treatment modality is preferred, either primary surgery or radical radiotherapy (RT).

In practice, surgery is preferred over RT for the following reasons:

- A surgically resected specimen can be studied for complete and true extent of the disease by providing pathological staging. If pathological staging reveals it to be pT3, pT4, or pN, then positive adjuvant treatment is indicated for such patients.
- A surgically resected specimen can be studied for various risk factors for recurrence such as lymphovascular invasion, perineural invasion, and worst patterns of invasion or depth of invasion. The presence of any of these risk factors warrants adjuvant therapy. Thus, surgical resection allows us to further individualize adjuvant treatment.
- Advancements in surgical procedures have enabled us to achieve good local control, cosmesis, and functional outcomes.
- RT-associated late toxicities and probability of radiation-induced malignancies can be avoided.

On the other side, RT has an edge over primary surgical resection in terms of better organ preservation, function preservation, and cosmesis. The superiority of one modality over the other for early oral cancers has not been compared in randomized controlled trials (RCTs) but based upon retrospective evidences. Both modalities appear to provide similar outcomes. In a scenario where both surgery and RT are expected to provide equal efficacy, the modality which is expected to give lesser morbidity, better quality of life, and better organ preservation should be used.

Locally Advanced Resectable Oral Cancer

A combined modality treatment (surgery followed by adjuvant RT) is the preferred strategy.

Indications of adjuvant RT:
- Pathological T3 or T4 primary
- Pathological neck positivity
- Microscopic resection margin positivity
- Initial (frozen section) microscopic margin positive although revised margin free
- Microscopic close margin (close margins ≤4 mm)
- Perineural invasion (extratumoral)
- Lymphovascular invasion
- Depth of invasion >4 mm for tongue and floor of mouth (FOM) and >7 mm for buccal mucosa, gingivobuccal sulcus, and retromolar trigone
- Bone involvement
- Moderate-to-high-grade dysplasia or severe dysplasia at margin.

Indications of adjuvant chemoradiation:
- Microscopic margin positivity
- Extranodal extension

Locally advanced unresectable oral cancers: Radical concurrent chemoradiation (CCRT) is the standard of care.

Locally very advanced unresectable oral cancers or metastatic cancers: Cure is very unlikely in these cancers. Hence, these patients should not be subjected to radical treatment-related severe morbidities. The intent in such a scenario is palliation from pain, bleeding, odorous discharge, infection, airway obstruction, difficulty in chewing/mixing food/deglutition and swallowing, local tumor progression, and occasionally symptoms caused by distant metastasis such as painful bony metastasis. Various options to achieve palliation are palliative RT, palliative chemotherapy, targeted therapy, and immunotherapy alone or in combination. The best supportive care is adopted when there is disease progression.

RADIOTHERAPY FOR ORAL CANCERS

Two types of RT can be used for oral cancers:
1. Brachytherapy
2. External beam radiotherapy (EBRT)

Brachytherapy

Brachytherapy is a form of highly conformal RT in which a radioactive source (such as Iridium 192 or Cesium 137) is inserted into the tumor or kept in close proximity of the tumor for a certain time period during which the radioactive source emits radiation from inside out. This allows a very high dose of radiation delivery to a very small region in much lesser time than EBRT. This form of RT results in much lesser radiation-induced tissue damage and toxicity.

Brachytherapy can be used as:
- *Monotherapy*, in which the full dose of radiation is delivered through brachytherapy only, without utilizing any contribution from EBRT. It is done for intact T1 and small T2 tumors with a low risk of lymph node involvement. It is also used as salvage brachytherapy for reirradiation purpose.
- *Brachytherapy boost (combined EBRT + brachytherapy)*, in which brachytherapy is delivered to the primary tumor after 1–2 weeks of completion of EBRT. It is used for intact T1/T2 tumors which carry a substantial risk of microscopic nodal involvement. It can also be used for patients with T3/T4 tumors with or without clinical nodal involvement which would otherwise require too morbid surgical resection causing poor functional or cosmetic results.

Types of Brachytherapy

Depending upon the patterns of placement of radioactive source, brachytherapy for oral cancers can be classified into the following:
- *Interstitial implant brachytherapy*: In this, few hollow plastic tubes are inserted through the tumor in the operating room under general anesthesia. The radioactive source is then passed through the tubes. While passing through the hollow tubes, the radioactive source keeps emitting radiation, thus causing tumor cell kill. It is commonly used for buccal, lip, tongue, and FOM cancers **(Figs. 1 and 2)**.
- *Surface mold brachytherapy*: In this, a customized applicator is made with specialized polymers, acrylic resin, or wax (used in dentistry) in which the plastic catheters are embedded. This applicator is fitted over the surface of the tumor. Once fitted, the radioactive sources are then passed through the catheters emitting radiation. It is commonly used for palatal tumors and superficial buccal or lip cancers **(Figs. 3A to C)**.
- *Intraoperative brachytherapy*: In this less commonly used technique of brachytherapy, an applicator is directly placed over the postoperative bed in

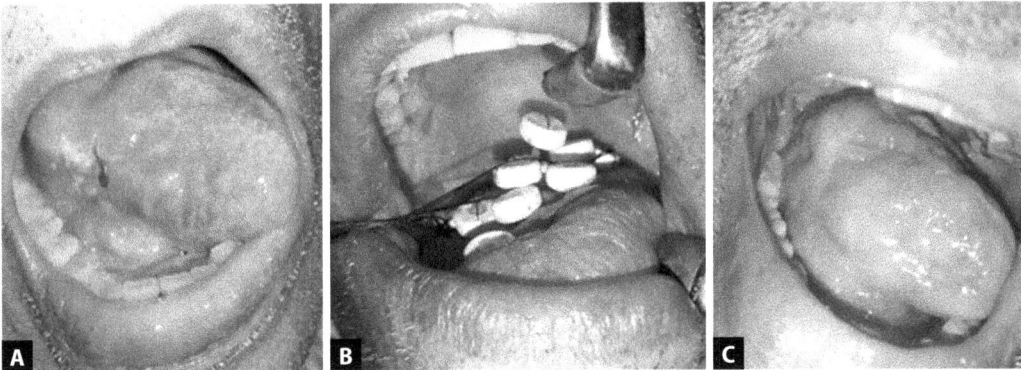

Figs. 1A to C: Interstitial implant brachytherapy for tongue carcinoma. (A) Pretreatment lesion in the right lateral border of the tongue; (B) Brachytherapy implant in place; (C) Post-treatment—complete response.

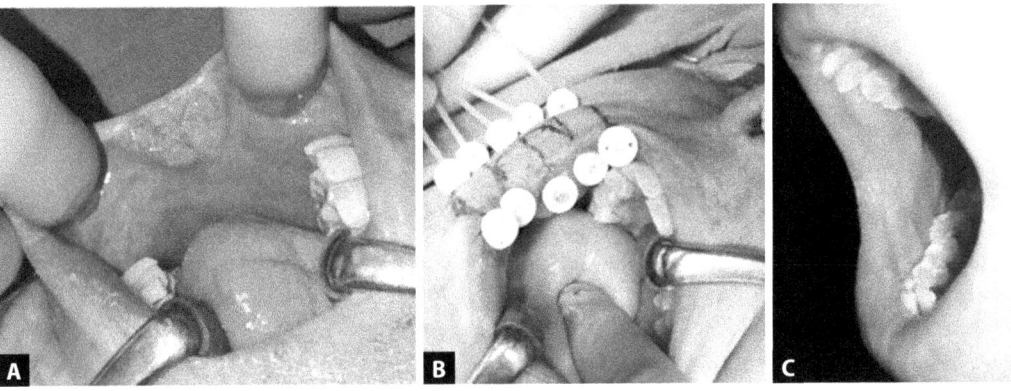

Figs. 2A to C: Interstitial implant brachytherapy for angle of mouth and buccal mucosa carcinoma. (A) Pretreatment; (B) Brachytherapy implant in place; (C) Post-treatment—complete response.

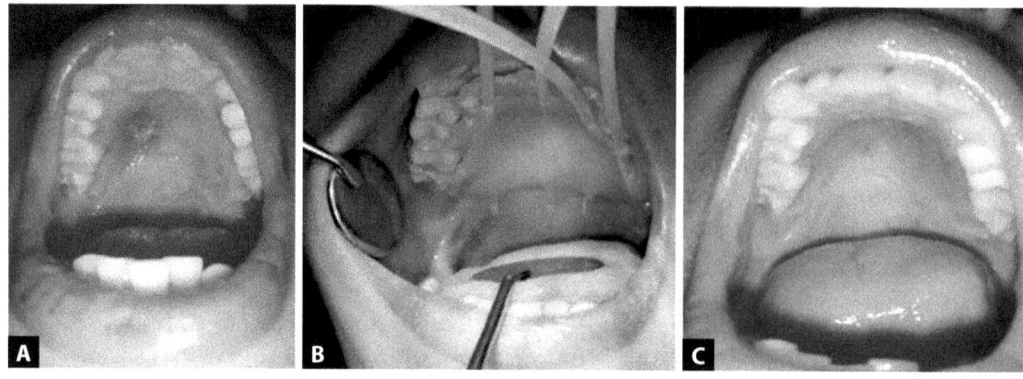

Figs. 3A to C: Surface mold brachytherapy. (A) Pretreatment lesion over the hard palate; (B) Surface mold in place; (C) Post-treatment—complete response.

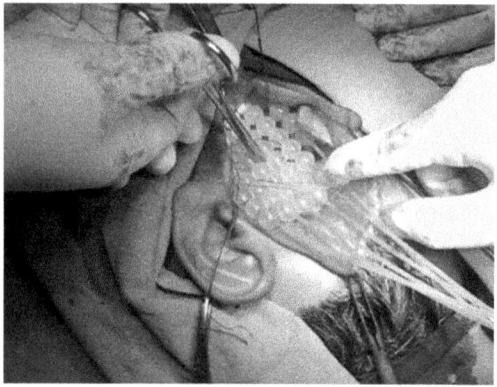

Fig. 4: Intraoperative brachytherapy for parotid bed tumor.

the operation theater itself and then the patient is transferred to the brachytherapy suite where the RT source is passed through the applicator emitting radiation. One common scenario where it is used is isolated nodal recurrence **(Fig. 4)**.

Selection Criteria for Brachytherapy

The following criteria must be fulfilled in order to perform a successful brachytherapy treatment:
- Early stage primary—T1 or T2
- Well-defined border of tumor
- Tumor should be at least 5 mm away from the mandible.
- Tumor should be accessible for insertion of the applicator or interstitial needles.
- Adequate mouth opening

Advanced tumors such as T3/T4 can also be taken up for brachytherapy, but it needs to be given as a boost after the completion of EBRT.

Brachytherapy Doses

Monotherapy:
- Dose 36 Gy: 4 Gy per fraction, two fractions per day
- Dose 45 Gy: 5 Gy per fraction, two fractions per day
- Dose 48 Gy: 6 Gy per fraction, two fractions per day.

Brachytherapy boost (combined EBRT + brachytherapy): 18 Gy–3 Gy per fraction, two fractions per day. This is given after the delivery of 50 Gy of EBRT.

Advantages of Brachytherapy

- *Reduced radiation toxicity:* Since brachytherapy gives a very sharp dose fall-off radiation beyond the edge of tumor, the surrounding normal organs such as normal mucosa, skin, bone, parotid gland, spinal cord, eye, brainstem, and lip

are spared from excessive radiation dose, thereby leading to reduced toxicity.
- Better functional preservation
- Better cosmesis
- Potential surgical disfigurement may be avoided.
- Better quality of life

Adverse Effects of Brachytherapy

- *Procedural complications*: Bleeding, infection, airway issues, venous thrombosis, etc.
- *Acute toxicity*: Mucositis, pain, dysgeusia
- *Late toxicity*: Mucositis, persistent ulcer, erosion, atrophy, dysgeusia, soft-tissue necrosis, and mandibular complications such as bone exposure and osteoradionecrosis.

External Beam Radiotherapy

External beam radiotherapy is a method of delivering a beam of high-energy rays (electromagnetic: X-rays and gamma rays, or particulate: electron, proton, and neutron) to the tumor. Unlike brachytherapy where the source emits radiation inside out, radiation in EBRT is generated outside the body, targeted onto the patient, and finally penetrates into the tumor. There are various machines which are used to produce these high-energy beams, for example linear accelerators for X-rays (most commonly used machine), telecobalt machine for gamma rays, and cyclotron for proton beam.

Techniques of EBRT

Radiotherapy techniques have changed significantly over the past few decades, largely due to our better understanding of radiophysics and radiobiology, technological advancements, and incorporation of imaging, computers, and engineering in RT techniques. It has evolved from the conventional technique using simple treatment fields to highly complex and conformal techniques. Following are the various planning techniques for oral cancers which have evolved over the last few decades:

- *Conventional RT using manual surface markings*: In this technique, various surface bony and soft-tissue landmarks (zygoma, zygomatic arch, mastoid process, external auditory canal, masseter muscle, etc.) are used to localize the area to be targeted and RT is delivered using very simple treatment fields, generally two opposed lateral **(Fig. 5)**. Very large regions of adjacent normal tissues are also irradiated unwantedly, thereby leading to very high radiation toxicity.
- *Conventional RT using two-dimensional orthogonal X-rays*: In this technique, two orthogonal X-rays of the head and neck regions are obtained and the target region is identified based on bony landmarks visible on X-ray films **(Figs. 6A and B)**. This is a slightly better technique than the previous technique, largely because it identifies the target with slightly more accuracy; however, it still irradiates a

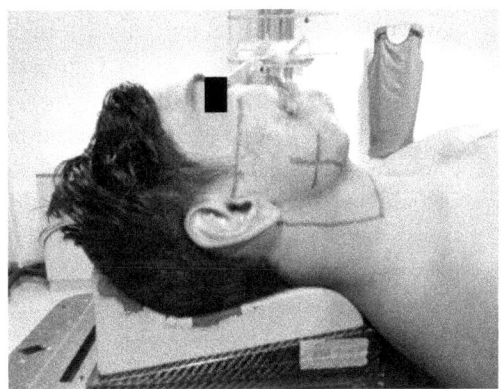

Fig. 5: Conventional radiotherapy using manual surface markings for carcinoma buccal mucosa.

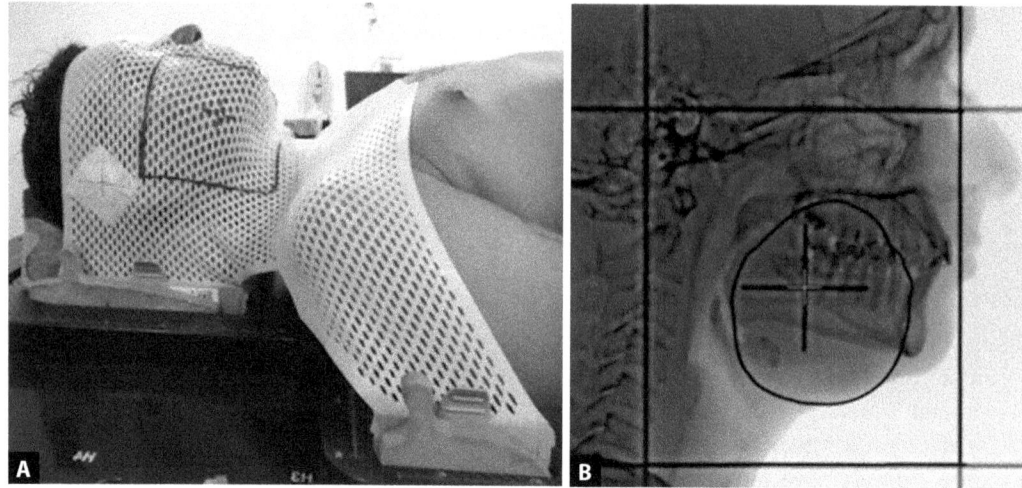

Figs. 6A and B: Conventional radiotherapy using two-dimensional orthogonal X-rays for a patient with carcinoma buccal mucosa.

large region of the adjacent normal tissues, thereby causing high toxicity. Conventional RT techniques though simple are still the most common techniques in resource-limited countries such as India.
- *Three-dimensional conformal RT (3D-CRT)*: In this technique (introduced in the 1980s), CT images are acquired and the target area (primary and nodes) and adjacent normal structures such as parotids, spinal cord, mandible, constrictor muscles, larynx, and optic pathways are outlined on each CT slice (the process called contouring). Complex RT planning is then done using computers wherein multiple fields (having the same intensity across each field) are placed so as to deliver higher doses to the target and lesser doses to the surrounding normal tissues (called forward planning). This technique allows lesser radiation toxicity than conventional techniques.
- *Intensity-modulated radiotherapy (IMRT)*: There was a paradigm shift in RT when this technique was first introduced in the early 1990s. It is a further refinement of the 3D-CRT technique wherein treatment planning is done using computer-controlled multileaf collimators (MLCs) and advanced treatment planning optimization algorithms that are able to create multiple radiation fields, each with a nonuniform intensity providing desired RT dose variation inside the radiation field. As opposed to previous RT planning techniques, where the dose distribution can only be modified by means of a trial-and-error approach (changing, for instance, the field weight, angle, and shape), with IMRT, the radiation oncologist designates the doses and dose constraints for the tumor and the surrounding normal organs. The treatment planning system utilizes various algorithms that determine the best optimum radiation beam parameters such as shape and intensity profiles, number of beams, and direction of beams, so as to achieve the prescribed normal tissue tolerance while delivering full dose to targets (inverse planning).

Head and neck cancers are ideal sites for IMRT because of the complex anatomy of the head and neck region wherein targets and the normal surrounding structures are in very close proximity to each other.
- *Image-guided radiotherapy (IGRT)*: It is a step further to IMRT using modern imaging modalities for adjusting target motion and positional uncertainties. This technique minimizes the errors such as variations in daily patient setup errors which are very common in oral cancer patients. Thus, accurate and precise delivery of RT may allow better cure rates and lesser radiation toxicity.

Work Flow for IMRT/IGRT

Following are the steps involved in IMRT/IGRT treatment:
1. *Positioning and immobilization*: In this first step of IMRT, the patient's head and neck region is fixed (immobilized) to the CT couch ensuring that immobilization is comfortable and reproducible during daily treatment sessions. For oral cancer IMRT, the immobilization is done using a thermoplastic cast made of a special material which when heated in warm water becomes soft and pliable and then can be molded into any shape. When adequately warmed, it is kept over the head and neck region and allowed to take shape of the contour of the patient's head and neck region (**Fig. 7**).
2. *Planning CT*: Following patient positioning and immobilization, CT images with IV contrast and slice thickness 3 mm are acquired with mask on, called planning CT (**Figs. 8A and B**).
3. *Contouring (target delineation)*: Planning CT is transferred to computers having

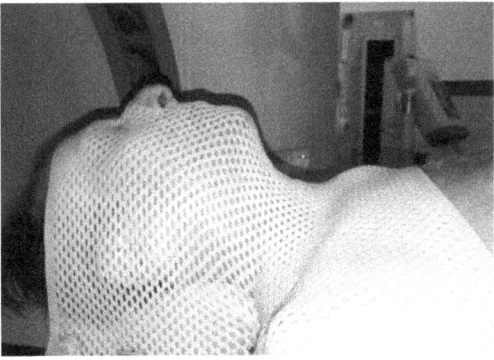

Fig. 7: Immobilization for oral cancer. Image-guided radiotherapy with a thermoplastic cast.

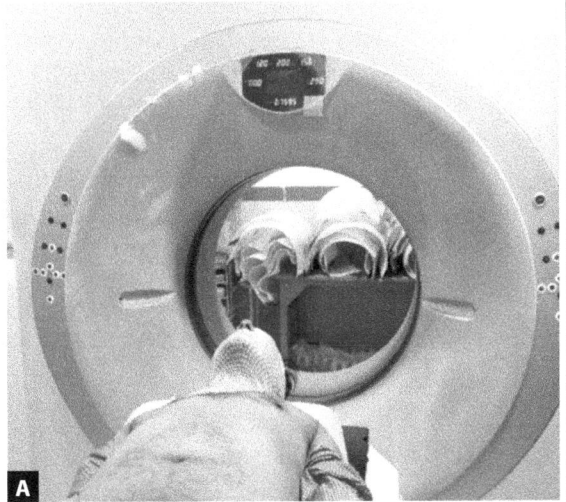
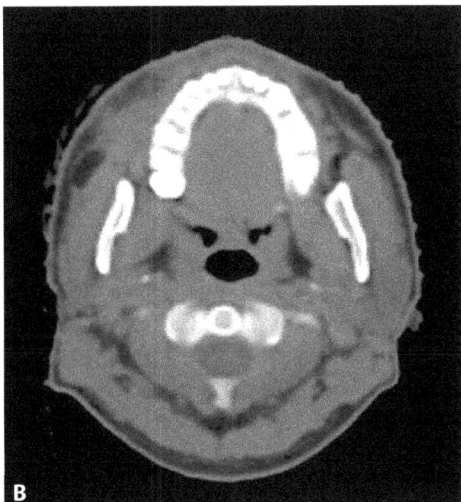

Figs. 8A and B: Planning CT.

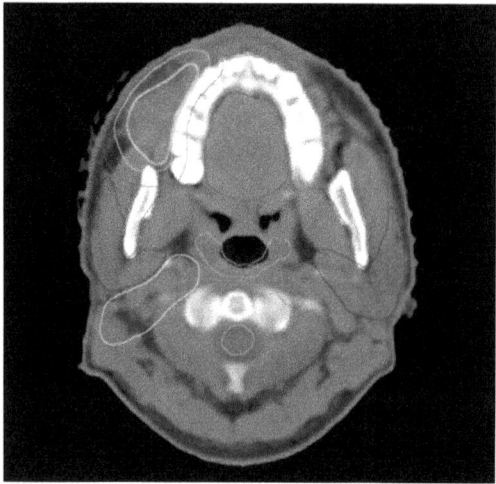

Fig. 9: Various targets and normal surrounding organs delineated on planning CT.

software for contouring. Other imaging modalities such as MRI of neck or PET-CT images are co-registered/fused with planning CT. Then the radiation oncologist delineates the target (primary tumor, involved nodes, and region suspected to have a microscopic disease) and the surrounding normal structures (**Fig. 9**).

This step of IMRT is of utmost importance because any error in delineation can lead to inadequate dose to tumor leading to treatment failure or excessive dose to the surrounding normal structures leading to high toxicity. A standardized nomenclature for targets has been recommended by various reports (ICRU—International Commission on Radiation Units and Measurements reports). Following are the targets which need to be delineated/contoured for radical IMRT for oral cancers:

- *Gross tumor volume (GTV)*: It is the gross visible or palpable disease demonstrated by clinical examination, imaging, or endoscopic examinations. It includes both primary tumor and metastatic lymph nodes. There is no GTV to be contoured if the tumor has been resected.
- *Clinical target volume (CTV)*: It is the region surrounding the GTV which is considered to harbor subclinical or microscopic disease and needs to be eliminated to achieve long-term control. The delineation of CTV requires consideration of factors such as invasive capacity of the tumor, tumor's potential to spread to different regions, and expected regions where the tumor may recur based on the available data from patterns of failure studies. Generally, two or three CTVs are contoured depending upon the risk of harboring disease, e.g., CTV high-risk which requires a high dose enough to have a tumoricidal effect and CTV low-risk which requires a lesser dose enough to cause a subclinical microscopic disease.
- *Planning target volume (PTV)*: It is a three-dimensional geometric margin (3–5 mm) given around CTV to compensate for setup errors while setting the patient on treatment couch and organ and tumor motion. This is the target which ultimately is the prescribed dose.

Following are the various surrounding normal organs which are required to be spared in order to decrease radiation toxicity:
- Spinal cord
- Parotid glands
- Submandibular glands
- Constrictor muscles
- Mandible
- Temporomandibular joints
- Larynx

- Cochlea
- Brainstem
- Optic chiasma
- Optic nerves
- Eyes
- Lens
- Brain

Various dose constraints are set for each organ.

Targets delineation for primary tumor: Following are the regions based on the primary tumor site which need to be included in the primary CTV:

- *Buccal mucosa*: There is a lack of barrier for the submucosal spread for buccal mucosal cancers; hence, CTV extends from just behind the lip commissure anteriorly to the retromolar trigone posteriorly and from the upper gingivobuccal sulcus cranially to the lower gingivobuccal sulcus inferiorly. For locally advanced lesions (T3/T4), especially superiorly located tumors, the infratemporal fossa is also at risk for microscopic tumor infiltration; hence, it needs to be included in CTV. For a posteriorly located lesion such as locally advanced retromolar trigone cancer entire masticator space including masseter, medial pterygoid, lateral pterygoid muscles, ascending ramus of mandible, and temporalis muscle needs to be included.
- *Tongue*: The entire oral tongue is at risk for submicroscopic spread even in early stage lesion, and hence local failures are common in the remaining tongue. CTV should include the entire intrinsic and extrinsic muscles of the tongue, FOM, and base of tongue.
- *Floor of mouth*: Genioglossus and geniohyoid muscles and muscles of root of tongue are to be included in the CTV.

Targets delineation for primary tumor: The nodal levels which need to be included in the nodal CTV are given in **Table 1**.

4. *Treatment planning and optimization*: Once the contouring is done, the plan criteria such as maximum dose, minimum

TABLE 1: Various nodal levels to be included in CTV depending upon the neck staging.

	Nodal levels to be covered	
	Ipsilateral	Contralateral
N0	I, IIa, III IVa for tongue IX for BM	IIa, III Ib for tongue/ant FOM IVa for tongue
N1	I, IIab, III IVa for tongue IX for BM	IIa, III Ib for tongue/ant FOM IVa for tongue
N2a N2b	I, IIab, III, Iva IVb if IVa +ve Vab if III or IV +ve VIIb if bulky upper II	IIa, III Ib for tongue/ant FOM IVa for tongue
N2c	According to N stage on each side	
N3	I, IIab, III, IVab, Vab, VIIb	IIab, III Ib for tongue/ant FOM IVa for tongue

(BM: buccal mucosa; FOM: floor of mouth)

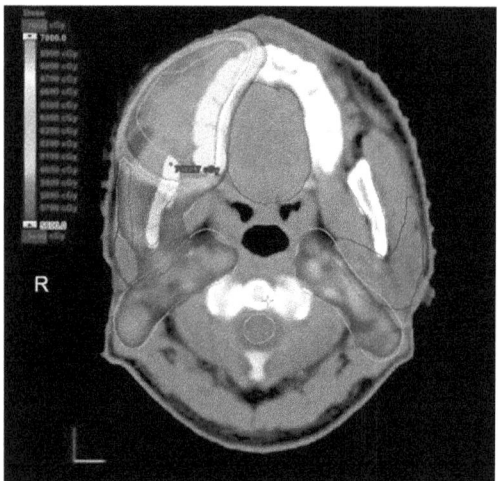

Fig. 10: Intensity-modulated radiation therapy plan showing dose distribution.

dose, desired limiting dose for normal organs, and various other parameters are entered and an optimization process is initiated and run which generates a computer plan which best matches all the input criteria.

5. *Plan evaluation*: In this step, the radiation oncologist evaluates the IMRT plan to check if adequate dose is delivered to the targets and doses to the surrounding normal structures are within the acceptable range **(Fig. 10)**.
6. *IMRT delivery*: This is the final step where the patient is made to lie in the same position and immobilized with the same thermoplastic cast that was used during positioning and immobilization.

RADIOTHERAPY DOSES AND FRACTIONATIONS

Radiotherapy doses vary internationally. However, conventional fractionation schedules utilizing 1.8–2 Gy per fraction, once daily treatment, and 5 days a week treatment are the most common practice. Most centers prescribe different doses to different targets in a single session—a technique called simultaneous integrated boost IMRT.

A common prescription used by most for IMRT for a radical treatment for oral cancers is as follows:
- *PTV high-risk*: 70 Gy in 35 fractions
- *PTV intermediate-risk*: 63 Gy in 35 fractions
- *PTV low-risk*: 56 Gy in 35 fractions.

For postoperative (adjuvant) IMRT:
- *Surgical bed with clear resection*: 60 Gy in 30 fractions
- Surgical bed with a positive resection margin requires a higher dose such as 66 Gy.
- Elective neck nodal irradiation requires 50–54 Gy.

Any deviation from the above fractionation pattern is called altered fractionation. Following are the various such fractionation schedules and their comparison with conventional fractionation:

Hyperfractionation: This schedule provides similar overall treatment to that of the conventional fractionation schedule but a higher total dose, more than 5 fractions per week and a higher dose per fraction (≈1.15 Gy per fraction). This results in increased acute toxicity and reduced late toxicity.

Accelerated fractionation: This schedule provides similar total dose to that of the conventional fractionation schedule but reduction of the overall treatment time by 1–2 weeks, more than 5 fractions per week and ≈1.8–2.0 Gy per fraction. This results in increased acute toxicity with the same/increased late toxicity.

Accelerated hyperfractionation: This schedule provides reduced total dose and reduction of the overall treatment time by 3–4 weeks, more than 10 fractions per week and <1.8 Gy per fraction.

Hypofractionation: This schedule provides reduced total dose as compared to the conventional fractionation schedule and reduced overall treatment time, daily dose >2.2 Gy per fraction. It results in the same acute toxicity and increased late toxicity.

Other altered fractionation schedules are accelerated fractionation with split-course, accelerated fractionation using concomitant boost, etc.

ADVANTAGES OF INTENSITY-MODULATED RADIOTHERAPY OVER CONVENTIONAL TECHNIQUES

- Reduced radiation toxicity by avoiding the surrounding normal structures from a high dose of radiation (**Table 2**):
  - Parotid glands—reducing xerostomia
  - Constrictor muscles—reducing dysphagia
  - Mandible—reducing osteoradionecrosis
  - Cochlea—reducing hearing impairment
- Improved quality of life
- Better survival rates
- Potential for dose escalation—higher doses may be delivered.
- Better shaping of fields and increased conformality
- Better radiation dose distribution
- Rapid dose fall-off beyond target
- Tailored plan for an individual patient

REIRRADIATION FOR ORAL CANCERS

Locoregional recurrence is the most common form of failure for oral cancers. It occurs in approximately 20–50% of patients. Those who survive a recurrence suffer a risk of developing a second primary malignancy, the risk of which varies from 3 to 5% per year. Surgery is the main modality for locally recurrent oral cancers. However, only 15–20% of patients are found to have a resectable disease. Reirradiation (Re-RT) has been the primary standard of care in the last decade for unresectable locally recurrent head and neck cancers, largely due to availability of newer techniques of RT such as IMRT which can deliver a second course of RT with a radical dose. Also, with increasing experience with Re-RT we are able to identify patients suitable for Re-RT. Today, Re-RT has replaced chemotherapy and supportive care as the treatment of choice for unresectable locally recurrent oral cancers.

One of the challenges of Re-RT is the fact that patients have previously received a high dose of irradiation. Therefore, the probabilities of acute and late toxicities are increased, especially in instances where Re-RT is delivered in a short time interval after the first course of RT.

Following are the suitable candidates for Re-RT:
- First course of RT delivered should be at least 1 year ago.

TABLE 2: Adverse effects of external beam radiotherapy.

Acute toxicities	Late toxicities
Mucositis	Dysphagia
Dysphagia	Xerostomia
Dysguesia	Dysguesia
Dermatitis	Trismus
Xerostomia	Skin fibrosis
Pain	Subcutaneous fibrosis
Weight loss	Osteoradionecrosis
Nausea/vomiting	
Anorexia	
Aspiration	

- Good performance status [Eastern Cooperative Oncology Group (ECOG) ≤ 2]
- First course of RT should have been without severe morbidities.
- Patient should have recovered from the morbidities from the first course of RT reasonably well.
- Details about previous RT such as type of techniques, doses delivered to target, and adjacent normal organs are available.
- Small volume and well-defined boundaries of recurrent disease.

The recommended dose for radical Re-RT is 60–66 Gy and for adjuvant Re-RT is 54–60 Gy in conventional fractionation. IMRT should be used for Re-RT if EBRT is being considered. Brachytherapy or stereotactic body radiotherapy (SBRT) should be considered for a very small recurrent lesion.

KEY POINTS

- RT plays a pivotal role in the management of oral cancers of any stage.
- For early stage oral cancer, surgery and RT provide a similar outcome. The choice of one over the other should be discussed in a multidisciplinary meeting.
- Adjuvant RT provides good local control in an adjuvant setting.
- Radical CCRT is the treatment of choice for unresectable oral cancers.
- Brachytherapy provides good disease control, cosmesis, organ preservation, and functional outcomes in suitable early stage cancers.
- IMRT should be the technique of choice for EBRT.
- Acute and long-term RT toxicities can be severe affecting the quality of life; hence, RT needs to be delivered safely, precisely, and accurately so as to achieve the maximum therapeutic ratio.
- For selected candidates with recurrent unresectable oral cancers, Re-RT may provide good outcomes.
- RT is undergoing rapid advancements due to technological improvement and incorporation of imaging, computers, and engineering in RT techniques.
- A multidisciplinary approach is the key for a successful oral cancer management program.

CHAPTER 27

Chemotherapy in Oral Cavity Cancer

Sumit Goyal

INTRODUCTION

At present, the standard of care for resectable locally advanced oral squamous cell carcinoma (OSCC) is the surgical treatment of the primary tumor and neck followed by postoperative radiotherapy (RT) or chemoradiotherapy, depending on the presence of intermediate- or high-risk features. The tentative treatment plan should also take into consideration the likely functional outcome expertise and the infrastructure available.

Stages I and II: Lip and oral cavity cancer
- Primary surgery is the preferred modality of treatment.
- Definitive RT is an alternative. It should be used only as an alternative treatment when primary surgery is not feasible.
- The role of chemotherapy is limited in early stage oral cavity cancer.

Stages III to IVB: Lip and oral cavity cancer
- Locally advanced OSCC are aggressive cancers with high rates of recurrence following single modality; thus, a combined modality treatment is preferred wherever feasible.
- However, a decision about optimal integration of surgery, radiation, or chemotherapy should be taken after multimodality discussion.

Chemotherapy in oral cancers can be used in the following situations:
- Adjuvant chemotherapy
- Chemoradiation:
  - Primary chemoradiation
  - Adjuvant chemoradiation
- Induction chemotherapy followed by definitive treatment
- Palliative chemotherapy

ADJUVANT CHEMOTHERAPY

At present, adjuvant chemotherapy has no established role after definitive treatment. It should not be used outside the context of a clinical trial.

CHEMORADIATION

- Concurrent chemoradiation is used as either definitive therapy or postoperatively depending on risk factors [extranodal extension (ENE)(+); positive margin]
- A meta-analysis of 63 randomized, prospective trials published between 1965 and 1993 showed an 8% absolute survival advantage in the subset of patients receiving concurrent chemotherapy and radiation therapy (MACH NC 2000).

The National Comprehensive Cancer Network (NCCN) lists the following regimens for concurrent chemoradiation:
- Primary definitive therapy (squamous cell cancers—lip, oral cavity)

- Primary systemic therapy + concurrent RT:
  - High-dose cisplatin (preferred) (category 1)
  - Carboplatin/infusional 5-fluorouracil (5-FU) (category 1)
  - Weekly cisplatin 40 mg/m^2 (category 2B)
  - Carboplatin
  - Cetuximab
  - 5-FU/hydroxyurea (category 2B)
  - Carboplatin/paclitaxel (category 2B)
  - Cisplatin/infusional 5-FU (category 2B)
  - Cisplatin/paclitaxel (category 2B)
- *Postoperative chemoradiation*: Cisplatin (category 1 for high-risk nonoropharyngeal cancers)

Of these regimens, the most commonly used are weekly cisplatin, carboplatin, paclitaxel + carboplatin, and 3-weekly cisplatin.

Primary Chemoradiation

When surgery is not feasible, combined chemoradiation is an option. There are other small and single institutional studies which have shown the benefit of chemoradiation. The available data suggest that compared with radiation alone, primary chemoradiation has a definite role in the management of unresectable OSCC and it improves survival and reduces the risk of recurrence. However, this benefit is less with increasing age (>70 years).

Adjuvant Chemoradiation

Chemotherapy is given as a radiation sensitizer and is used with the aim to reduce radiation resistance.

Adjuvant chemoradiation is given if the following high-risk factors are present postsurgery:
- Positive margins and ENE (recommended indications)
- A multiple lower level nodal disease may be considered for adding chemotherapy to RT.

Evidence is based on two large studies, European Organization for Research and Treatment of Cancer (EORTC) 22931 and radiation therapy oncology group (RTOG) 9501; however, both reached a different conclusion, probably due to different inclusion criteria, and used different criteria as high-risk features. Both studies had 25–30% of patients with oral cancer.

CHOICE OF REGIMEN

- There is no consensus as to the optimal chemotherapy regimen.
- The various regimens have not been compared directly with each other.
- The benefit of platinum-based regimens seems to be better than nonplatinum-based regimens.
- In platinum-based regimens, cisplatin is preferred, the other agent being carboplatin alone or in combination with 5-FU.
- The preferred regimen is 3-weekly cisplatin for the fit patients; in patients who are not fit, a weekly cisplatin regimen or alternate regimens can be used. A lower dose weekly cisplatin regimen is better tolerated and is less nephrotoxic.
- The doses of cisplatin (100 mg/m^2) are most effective.
- Cetuximab (for cisplatin in eligible patients), although used in this setting, is not supported by any data in patients with oral cancer in the adjuvant setting and cannot be recommended routinely.

Factors determining the choice of regimen:
- Goal of therapy
- Performance status
- Age and comorbidities
- Expertise available

INDUCTION CHEMOTHERAPY FOR LOCALLY ADVANCED ORAL CAVITY CANCERS (STAGES III–IVB)

The potential advantages of induction chemotherapy are:
- To reduce its size for subsequent surgery or radiation therapy
- To reduce the risk of metastatic disease

The NCCN lists the following regimens for induction/sequential chemotherapy:
- Docetaxel/cisplatin/5-FU (category 1 if induction is chosen)
- Paclitaxel/cisplatin/infusional 5-FU

Induction Chemotherapy

Two trials in patients with *resectable* OSCC failed to demonstrate an improvement in overall survival with preoperative chemotherapy. However, both trials have shown a possible impact on minimizing surgery or postoperative radiation.

In a trial from Italy, in 195 patients with oral cancer, three cycles of preoperative cisplatin plus fluorouracil followed by surgery were compared with surgery followed by postoperative RT for high-risk patients. There was no significant difference in the overall survival (5-year survival, 55% in both arms), although the use of chemotherapy prior to surgery resulted in a decreased requirement for mandibulectomy (31 vs. 52%) and postoperative radiation (33 vs. 46%). An updated report with 11.5 years of median follow-up confirmed the lack of a statistically significant difference in local disease control, rate of distant metastasis, or overall survival.

In a second trial from China, 256 patients were randomly assigned to two cycles of the DCF (docetaxel, cisplatin, 5-FU) regimen followed by surgery and postoperative RT versus surgery followed by RT. This study also showed no significant difference in either overall or disease-free survival [hazard ratios (HRs) 0.98 and 0.97, respectively].

The addition of taxane (docetaxel) to cisplatin plus 5-FU combination (TAX 323 and TAX 324) showed that it improved response rates and survival as compared to cisplatin plus 5-FU alone; however, it remains unknown that induction therapy improves survival as compared to definitive chemoradiation. These studies had about 13–17% of patients with OSCC.

CHEMOTHERAPY FOR METASTATIC OR RECURRENT ORAL CANCERS (STAGE IVC)

- Single-agent or combination chemotherapy is recommended based on intent, PS, and comorbidities.
- If platin eligible, preference should be given to the cisplatin-based regimen.
- Pembrolizumab is approved for use in combination with platinum and 5-FU for all patients with metastatic or unresectable recurrent head and neck squamous cell carcinoma, and as a single agent for patients whose tumors express PD-L1 [combined positive score (CPS) ≥ 1] as determined by a test approved by the Food and Drug Administration (FDA).

PROGNOSTIC FACTORS

- *Disease-related*:
    - Early-stage disease (stages I and II)
    - Positive margins
    - Depth of invasion > 5 mm [incorporated into American Joint Committee on Cancer (AJCC), 8th edition, for staging]
    - Presence of ENE
    - Worst pattern of invasion (WOPI)
    - Perineural invasion (PNI)
    - Lymphovascular invasion (LVI)

- *Other patient-related factors which have an impact on outcome*:
  - Comorbidity
  - Overall health
  - Lifestyle (tobacco and alcohol use)

SURVIVAL

The rate of curability of cancers of the lip and oral cavity varies depending on the stage and specific site. The survival curves are shown in **Figure 1** (as per AJCC).

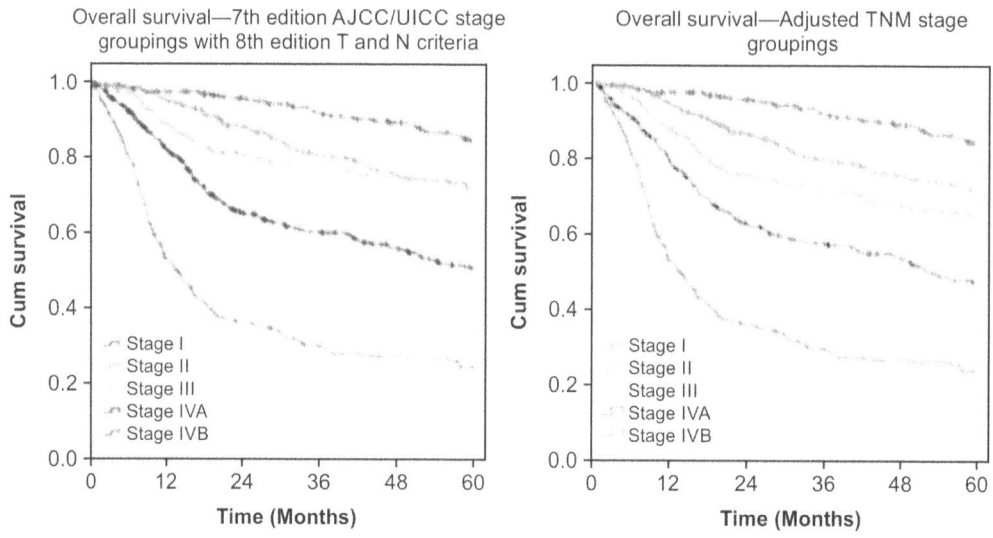

Fig. 1: Survival rates as per the American Joint Committee on Cancer (AJCC).
(TNM: tumor, node, and metastasis; UICC: Union for International Cancer Control)

KEY POINTS

- The role of chemotherapy is limited in early stage oral cavity cancers.
- Adjuvant CT has no established role after definitive treatment.
- Primary CTRT has a definite role in the management of unresectable OSCC.
- In adjuvant CTRT, a lower dose weekly cisplatin regimen is better tolerated and is less nephrotoxic.
- In patients with resectable OSCC, preoperative chemotherapy failed to demonstrate an improvement in overall survival.

Management of Recurrent Head and Neck Carcinoma

Sumit Goyal, Venkata Pradeep Babu Koyyala

INTRODUCTION

- 30% of patients will relapse in the head and neck area without distant metastases.
- Imaging becomes difficult due to the morphological modification of the local tissues induced by previous surgery and/or (chemo) radiation.
- The differential diagnosis includes radionecrosis, infection, and scar from previous treatment(s).
- Effort should be made to obtain pathological confirmation.
- Positron emission tomography-computed tomography (PET-CT) is indicated in a recurrent setting to identify the sites of recurrence. This will also help to assess the efficacy of therapy after starting the systemic therapy.

PROGNOSIS OF RECURRENT HEAD AND NECK CANCER

The most important prognostic factor in recurrent head and neck cancer is the "performance status" of the patient **(Box 1)**.

Box 1: Prognostic factors for poor survival in recurrent head and neck cancers.

- Weight loss > 5%
- ECOG 1 versus 0
- Well and moderate differentiation
- Primary tumor oral cavity or hypopharynx
- Prior radiation therapy

(ECOG: Eastern Cooperative Oncology Group)

A nomogram is used to predict survival in recurrent head and neck cancers.

Based on the analysis of data from randomized trials in head and neck cancer:

- *Patients with 0-2 unfavorable prognostic factors*: Median overall survival (OS) = 1 year
- *Patients with 3-5 unfavorable prognostic factors*: Median OS = 6 months

P16 positivity is a favorable prognostic factor compared to P16 negative disease in both locoregional and distant metastases and even in patients who undergo salvage surgery.

Other prognostic factors are:
- Comorbidity
- Ongoing tobacco and alcohol use
- Hypercalcemia
- Response to prior treatment
- Social support

Salvage Surgery

Salvage surgery is defined as surgery applied for the resection of residual or recurrent disease after failure of primary (chemo) radiation. Any detectable disease within 3 months of initial treatment is named residual or persistent, and any disease emerging after 3 months is called recurrent **(Table 1)**.

Principles of Salvage Surgery

Salvage surgery after primary (chemo) radiation is challenging and should only be

TABLE 1: Definitions of residual and recurrent cancer.

Definition	Time from treatment
Residual cancer: Persisting cancer not eradicated by initial treatment	Within 3 months
Recurrent cancer: Re-occurring cancer at the treatment site after primary eradication	After 3 months

Box 2: Approach to salvage surgery.
- Select patients carefully
- Difficult surgery—needs an experienced surgical team
- Deliberate use of vascularized flaps for reconstruction
- Radical resection with wide margins
- Resection follows at least the extension of the initial tumor
- Consider functional outcome and quality of life

performed in centers and by surgeons with vast experience. Majority of patients will not qualify for a meaningful salvage surgery. Patients have to be selected restrictively (Box 2).

Large bone and soft-tissue defects should be generously reconstructed with well-vascularized, pedicled or free flaps. The local and regional irradiated tissue is prone to wound healing problems and should not be used for reconstruction. Palliative salvage surgery should only be performed with clearly defined aims, e.g., palliation of symptoms, avoidance of complications, and improvement of function.

DIAGNOSIS OF RESIDUAL OR RECURRENT CANCER

There is no accepted consensus on how to perform the follow-up visits. For early cancers, it is our policy to follow the patients with thorough physical examination including transnasal fiber endoscopy and ultrasonography of the neck. Only patients with advanced cancers, with cancers in sites not well amenable to clinical examination, or with flap reconstructions hiding a possible recurrence are evaluated radiologically by either CT, magnetic resonance imaging (MRI), or PET. In patients with a high likelihood of locoregional recurrence, a baseline CT or MRI is obtained 3 months after the end of the radiation therapy. Using this scan as a baseline for comparison to a follow-up scan performed 6 months later, abnormalities can be better interpreted with respect to the possible presence of a tumor.

Oral Cavity and Oropharynx

Cancer of the oral cavity that recurs locally after initial (chemo)radiation presents a difficult management problem. Re-irradiation with an external beam is generally not possible due to the previous high radiation dose and the limited tissue tolerance. In this situation, salvage surgery or interstitial brachytherapy is advocated. The majority present with unresectable disease and undergo palliative care.

For salvage surgery in the oral cavity, the same approaches as for the primary surgery can be used. Due to the wide exposure achieved with a transmandibular lip-splitting access, this approach seems to be preferable over merely transoral procedures or pull-through techniques. To achieve the wide margins needed for a successful salvage surgery, extensive ablative procedures are necessary. For recurrent tongue tumors, this leads to near total or total glossectomy for most patients. With appropriate free flap reconstruction, acceptable speech function and swallowing are possible.

Neck

Regional residual or recurrent disease is probably the most frequent indication for salvage surgery. Mendenhall et al. reviewed a large series of patients with head and neck squamous cell carcinoma (HNSCC) undergoing primary radiation. They concluded that irradiation alone is equally efficient in controlling the neck as combined treatment, for solitary nodes up to a maximum size of 3 cm. As the size and number of nodes increased, there was a higher rate of neck disease control for irradiation followed by neck dissection. They advocated the use of planned neck dissection 4–6 weeks after radiation for patients with extensive neck disease. In summary, the data supporting a planned neck dissection after primary radiation is sparse and based mainly on protocols without concurrent chemotherapy and conventional schedules.

We recommend restaging patients with advanced (N2/3) neck disease 6–8 weeks after termination of radiation. In our hands, ultrasonography with fine needle aspiration cytology seems to be very accurate. The PET scan should be done in all such cases. All five levels have to be dissected. The sternocleidomastoid muscle and the internal jugular vein are deliberately resected. Great efforts are made to preserve the spinal accessory nerve if oncologically sound. The primary site should always be carefully re-evaluated and searched for residual or recurrent cancer.

COMPLICATIONS

There is a general agreement that preoperative radiotherapy increases the risk for postoperative complications, e.g., pharyngocutaneous fistula, wound complications, and carotid rupture. In studies with preoperative radiation with 50 Gy, complication rates of 40–54% have been reported. This is higher than that after primary surgery. Therefore, with the considerably higher doses of primary radiation even higher rates of complications have to be expected.

Treatment of Lung Metastases

The concept of oligometastasis is unclear in head and neck cancers and with limited data available, this is limited to metastasis to lung.

Aggressive treatment of lung metastases may result in increased disease-free survival.

The 5-year survival in surgical metastatectomy in head and neck cancers with the lung being the only site of metastases has been shown to be to the tune of 30%. However, at this point of time, there is no immunohistochemical (IHC) marker or any other test that can differentiate synchronous/metachronous lung primaries (squamous cell) from metastases from head and neck primary.

The increased survival may be due to resection of primary lung cancers in such patients.

- The rate of synchronous pulmonary tumor is around 4%.
- The overall incidence of metachronous second primary cancers is 2% per year.
- The 5-year survival after pulmonary metastatectomy is 26–59%.
- It is reasonable to recommend lung resection for a single cancerous lung nodule.
- For two or more lung metastases, it to be discussed within a multidisciplinary team.

The role of stereotactic ablative radiotherapy in lung metastases is unclear at this point of time.

ROLE OF REIRRADIATION

The patients who are not candidates of salvage surgery can be considered for reirradiation (after 1 year of primary radiation).

Indications for reirradiation may include:
- Patients who undergo salvage surgery but are found to have high-risk features
- Patients who are medically suitable for curative-intent interventions but are not amenable to curative-intent resection
- Patients who are not candidates for curative-intent interventions but may benefit from palliative treatment

The patients whose tumors recur within 6 months and within the radiation field are likely to have radiation resistance and are not considered candidates for reirradiation. Also, the dose delivered [maximum tolerated dose (MTD)] to the adjacent normal tissues (skin, blood vessels, spinal cord) needs to be considered.

The toxicity and morbidity from reirradiation can be substantial.

SYSTEMIC THERAPY

The systemic chemotherapy options and their response rates are given in **Table 2**.

Chemotherapy improves survival over the best supportive care only in fit patients.

TABLE 2: Systemic chemotherapy options and their response rates.

Chemotherapy option	Response rate
Cisplatin	14–41%
Carboplatin	20–30%
Oxaliplatin	10%
Methotrexate	6–10%
5-Fluorouracil	15%
Capecitabine	8%
Docetaxel	21–42%
Paclitaxel	13–40%

- The median survival of patients is 6–8 months.
- Polychemotherapy versus monochemotherapy in a recurrent setting:
  - Higher response rate
  - More toxic
  - No improvement in survival
  - Cisplatin/5-FU
- Taxanes, in addition to platinum chemotherapy, may increase the response rates.

TARGETED THERAPIES IN RECURRENT ORAL CANCERS

Epidermal growth factor receptor (EGFR) is universally expressed in squamous cell cancers of head and neck.

The level of expression of EGFR may result in differences in responses to systemic therapy, prognosis, and rate of recurrence. The more the expression, the worse the prognosis.

Apart from EGFR mutations, other actionable mutations that are under clinical trials are HER-2, FGFR, PI3K pathways, and HRAS mutations.

- *Anti-EGFR first-line palliative treatment*: mAbs (cetuximab)
- *EXTREME regimen*: Cisplatin + 5-FU + Cetuximab improves survival. However, toxicities can be severe. Patient selection is extremely important before opting for multidrug chemotherapy along with targeted therapy, and careful consideration of comorbidities and expected outcomes is pivotal.
- *Anti-EGFR second line*: mAbs and tyrosine kinase inhibitors (TKIs; cetuximab and afatinib, gefitinib).

IMMUNOTHERAPY IN HEAD AND NECK CANCER

- *CheckMate 141 study*: Nivolumab has been approved in recurrent/metastatic head

and neck cancer, particularly oral cavity, pharynx, or larynx, and also in patients who have progressed within 6 months of the last dose of platinum therapy.
- *Pembrolizumab*: Keynote 048—comparison of pembrolizumab alone or with chemotherapy against "extreme regimen."

There is no perfect biomarker to choose immunotherapy alone or in combination with chemotherapy.

In head and neck cancer, PDL-1 is a poor biomarker (expression of PDL-1 on tumor cells).

Combined positive score (CPS) is a relatively better biomarker (combined PDL-1 expression over tumor cells and infiltrating inflammatory cells).

As per the available data from trials:
- In patients with CPS score > 20, pembrolizumab single agent can be used.
- In patients with CPS score < 1, extreme regimen or chemotherapy is preferred.
- In patients with CPS score 1–20, no definite guidelines are there. Immunotherapy alone or in combination with chemotherapy can be used.
- In patients in whom rapid shrinkage is needed, with no CPS score available, pembrolizumab + chemotherapy can be used.

The question of what is the best therapy following progression on immunotherapy in combination with chemotherapy is not yet known.

METRONOMIC THERAPY

In patients with a poor general condition or who are not willing to opt for IV therapy, metronomic therapy is an option.

It is an oral therapy where small regular doses of chemotherapy are given with a predominant effect on the angiogenesis of tumor rather than on the tumor itself.

Some of the available options of metronomic therapy are:
- Erlotinib + Methotrexate + Celecoxib
- Methotrexate + Capecitabine

KEY POINTS
- 30% of patients will relapse in head and neck area without distant metastases.
- Aggressive treatment of lung metastasis may result in increased disease-free survival.
- No IHC marker/test can differentiate between metastasis to lung from head and neck primary and synchronous/metachronous lung primary.
- It is reasonable to recommend surgery for a single malignant lung nodule.
- Chemotherapy improves survival over best supportive care only in fit patients.
- The patient selection is extremely important before opting for multidrug chemotherapy (cisplatin+5 FU) with targeted therapy (cetuximab).
- Metronomic therapy acts on tumor angiogenesis rather than on the tumor itself.
- Toxicity and morbidity from reirradiation may be substantial.

CHAPTER 29

Role of Interventional Radiology in the Management of Oral Cancers

Abhishek Bansal

INTRODUCTION

As personalized medicine becomes more applicable to oncologic practice, interventional radiology procedures are proving to be a valuable asset in the diagnosis, treatment, and surgical management of various oral malignant tumors. Interventional radiology's subset, called *interventional oncology*, is being rapidly recognized as the fourth pillar of oncology after the surgical, medical, and radiation oncology branches. Various applications where interventional radiology plays a key role in oral malignancies are:

- Transarterial embolization for uncontrolled hemorrhage
- Chemoembolization of unresectable tumors
- Percutaneous tracheostomy
- Lymphatic interventions
- Percutaneous radiological gastrostomy
- Lymph node ablation
- Pain management
- Image-guided biopsies

TRANSARTERIAL EMBOLIZATION FOR UNCONTROLLED HEMORRHAGE (FIGS. 1 AND 2)

Oral cavity carcinomas are prone to hemorrhages, some of which could be life threatening, as they occur on a background of medically vulnerable patients and the excessive blood loss can cause hemorrhagic shock or respiratory compromise due to

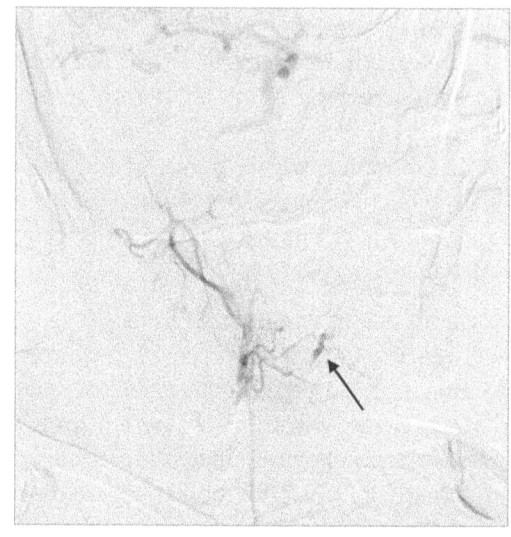

Fig. 1: Right external carotid artery (ECA) angiogram revealing a pseudoaneurysm arising from the right lingual artery in a patient with carcinoma of the tongue who presented with massive oral bleed.

blood occluding the respiratory passage. Most of these patients had already undergone surgical or chemoradiotherapy treatment. Hence, access to bleeding vessels and possibilities of surgical or radiotherapeutic interventions are limited or even impossible. Therefore, endovascular management in the form of transarterial embolization provides an easy, minimally invasive, and effective way of controlling these hemorrhages. With the advancements in hardware, technique and embolic agents, the results of embolization have improved significantly over the last

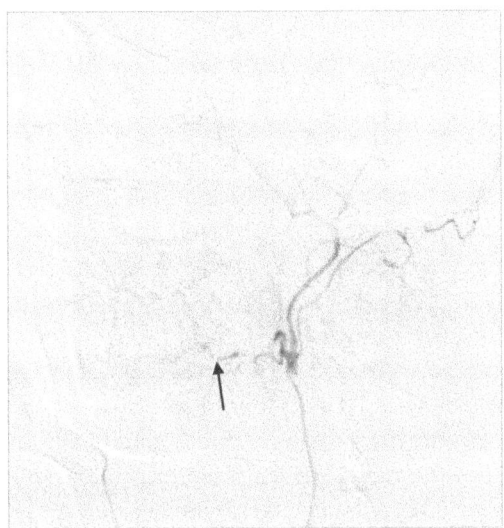

Fig. 2: Left external carotid artery (ECA) angiogram revealing a dilated and tortuous left lingual artery supplying the abnormal tumor blush of tongue mass in the same patient.

few years. Embolization can be done in postoperative or irradiation patients where access to the carotid bulb area may be difficult.

Embolization involves closing the arterial vessel that supplies the tumor as close to the tumor bed as possible, and this leads to more durable results as the occlusion is done on the microcirculation level. This reduces the risk of complications associated with nontarget embolization as well as reduces the re-bleeding risk by decreasing the risk of recanalization of the tumor bed. For the same reason, surgical ligations are associated with rapid development of collateral circulation. Many of the tumors have arterial feeders from both external carotid arterial branches, and embolization allows for occlusion from both sides. Commonly used embolic agents are polyvinyl alcohol particles, gelfoam, embolization coils, and glue (N-butyl cyanoacrylate).

Embolization can also be done preoperatively to reduce intraoperative blood loss, hence giving a blood-less field to the surgeon, shortening the time of surgery, and increasing the chance of total tumor resection by reducing the tumor mass.

The majority of embolizations are not associated with complications. The most common complications include bleeding or hematoma formation at the femoral puncture site or intima dissection of the involved artery and are minor and transient. The most serious complication that may occur involves nontarget embolization caused by reflux of embolization material, especially the ones where reflux occurs into the internal carotid artery causing ischemic strokes. All the above-mentioned complications can be prevented by using the meticulous technique of embolization.

If the patient is stable, then computed tomography (CT) angiography should be done prior to the embolization as it enables planning of the procedure which ultimately reduces the radiographic contrast used and the fluoroscopic times and improves the embolization outcomes. The interventional radiologists practicing embolizations in the head and neck region should be well trained with precise knowledge of the functional anatomy of vessels, specifically with regard to the anastomosis between the intra- and extracranial arteries.

CHEMOEMBOLIZATION OF UNRESECTABLE TUMORS

Transarterial chemotherapy: The basis of this approach is to deliver an extremely high dose of the anticancer drug directly into the artery supplying the tumor. This approach increases the amount of cisplatin delivered to the tumor, thus increasing its cytotoxic effects.

In addition, the cisplatin also acts as a radiosensitization agent, increasing the effectiveness of the concurrent radiation.

Locoregional control response of 57–96% has been quoted at 2–5 years.

PERCUTANEOUS TRACHEOSTOMY

Percutaneous tracheostomy is a commonly performed procedure in critically sick patients which can be safely performed bedside and is generally performed by the surgeons or intensivists. This has become the standard of care in an intensive care unit (ICU) and has resulted in decline in the use of surgical tracheostomy. It involves blunt dissection of pretracheal tissues followed by dilatation of tract and trachea over a guidewire and insertion of a tracheal cannula using the Seldinger technique.

LYMPHATIC INTERVENTIONS (FIGS. 3A AND B)

Oral cavity carcinomas with neck lymphadenopathies frequently undergo surgical resections with neck dissections. Some of these patients may have persistent chyle or lymph leakage from the surgical site. Lymphatic interventions in the form of lipiodol lymphangiography and embolization of thoracic duct or disruption of cistern chyli are effective methods for controlling these leakages. Lipiodol lymphangiography is a minimally invasive method of injecting lipiodol in inguinal lymph nodes which leads to ascent of lipiodol into the lymphatics and further through the cisterna chyli into the thoracic duct. It shows the site of leakage in the neck, and lipiodol itself causes local inflammation at the site of leakage and further seals the leak. Thus, it acts as both a diagnostic and a therapeutic intervention. Furthermore, percutaneous access into the thoracic duct can be obtained and its embolization can be safely performed.

PERCUTANEOUS RADIOLOGICAL GASTROSTOMY

Nutrition is an important concern for oral cavity carcinoma patients, due to the tumor itself or post-treatment changes. Endoscopic gastrostomy tubes were placed traditionally; however, percutaneous radiological gastrostomy is preferred for patients with oral

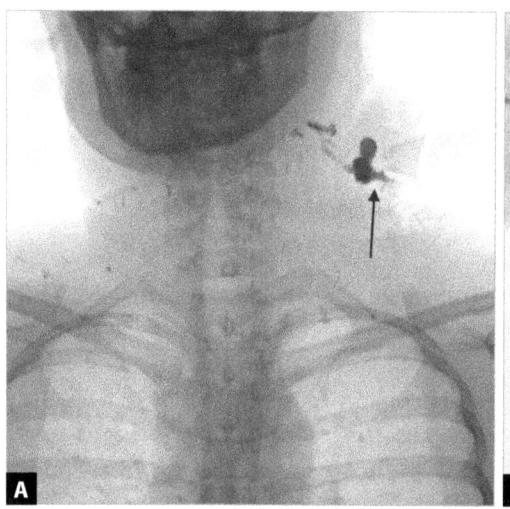
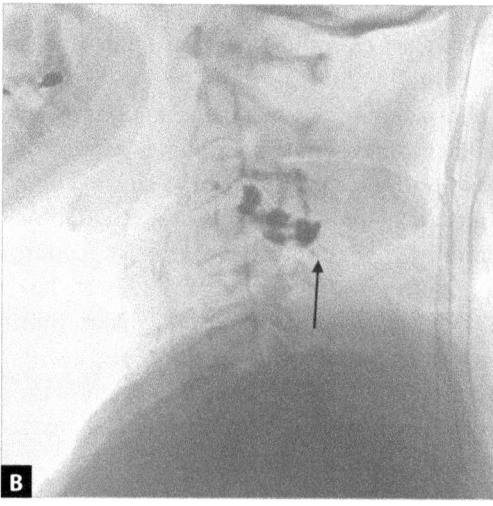

Figs. 3A and B: Anteroposterior and lateral fluoroscopic images demonstrating the site of chyle leak in neck.

malignancies as it obviates the need for passage of endoscope or large tubes from oral cavity to stomach. The radiologically inserted gastrostomy tubes can be placed even for patients in whom a nasogastric tube cannot be inserted. In addition, the usage of gastropexy sutures decreases the risk of peritonitis as it keeps the stomach wall abutted against the anterior abdominal wall.

LYMPH NODAL ABLATION

Surgery remains the gold standard for neck lymph nodes' clearance and along with radiotherapy and chemotherapy, it is the "standard of care" in the management of oral cavity carcinomas with cervical lymph nodal metastases. Image-guided percutaneous ethanol injection or radiofrequency ablation of metastatic cervical lymph nodes can be considered for persistent or recurrent cervical lymph nodal disease and is generally limited to a single lymph node or an N1 disease. There is good data regarding the usage of the above modalities for metastatic lymph nodes from thyroid malignancies; however, the usage can be extrapolated to metastatic lymph nodes to oral cavity carcinoma patients also.

PAIN MANAGEMENT

It has been shown that early use of an interventional nerve block may help in decreasing the requirement of opioids. The ultrasound or CT-guided nerve blocks offer the advantage of greater accuracy, increased safety, and success rate of the block. Trigeminal nerve blocks via the pterygopalatine approach and glossopharyngeal nerve blocks can be performed for orofacial pains. Depending on the site of the pain, the pain block can be performed at various levels of the nerve including ganglions, major divisions, or smaller branches.

IMAGE-GUIDED BIOPSIES

Image-guided biopsies play an important part in the diagnosis and management of deep-seated head and neck lesions. CT scan is the most commonly used technique for image-guided biopsies of these deep-seated lesions; however, ultrasound and interventional magnetic resonance imaging (MRI) systems can also be used. Most of these can be performed using local anesthesia, only with a few requiring conscious sedation. Safe needle trajectories can be planned using the radiological anatomical knowledge.

KEY POINTS

- Commonly used embolic agents are polyvinyl alcohol particles, gelfoam, embolization coils, and glue (N-butyl cyanoacrylate).
- *Transarterial embolization*:
  - Occlusion is done on the microcirculation level.
  - Reduces the re-bleeding risk by decreasing the risk of recanalization of the tumor bed.
  - Most common complications include bleeding or hematoma formation at the femoral puncture site.
- *Transarterial chemotherapy*: The basis of this approach is to deliver an extremely high dose of the anticancer drug directly into the artery supplying the tumor.
- Lipiodol lymphangiography is a minimally invasive method of injecting lipiodol in inguinal lymph nodes. It acts as both a diagnostic and a therapeutic intervention.
- Percutaneous thoracic duct embolization can be safely performed.
- *Percutaneous radiological gastrostomy is preferred in*:
  - Severe trismus
  - Large proliferative growth in the oral cavity
- Image-guided percutaneous ethanol injection for recurrent metastatic lymph nodes from thyroid malignancies can be done in patients who are medically unfit or unwilling for surgery.
- Image-guided (USG/CT) biopsies play an important part in the diagnosis and management of deep-seated head and neck lesions.

Dental Management in Oral Cancer Patients

Sheetal Bhalla

INTRODUCTION

Head and neck cancers (HNC) are treated with surgery and radiation therapy (RT)/chemotherapy. Patients undergoing multimodal treatment for oral cancers are prone to a range of dental complications. Oral complications occur because of the damage of cells of the mucous membrane, underlying soft tissue, tooth, periosteum, bone, glands, and vasculature.

- Early effects include fungal infections, xerostomia and dysgeusia from salivary gland damage, mucositis from epithelial damage, radiation caries, reduced mouth opening from changes in collagen structure, and osteoradionecrosis (ORN) of the jaw in some cases.
- Xerostomia may affect up to 90% of patients undergoing radiotherapy, mucositis > 60%, candidiasis > 40%, postradiotherapy dental decay > 50%, and ORN up to 15%.
- As oral complications are common, potentially preventable, and have iatrogenic factors, it is important to be aware of the prevention and management of radiotherapy- and chemotherapy-related oral complications.

PRE-RADIOTHERAPY DENTAL ASSESSMENT

The benefits of pre-radiotherapy dental evaluation are to assess, diagnose, and manage oral and dental implications that are related to treatment.

At our center, every patient receives a thorough pre-radiotherapy assessment by an experienced general dentist who gives preventive advice and performs dental procedures.

- Oral rehabilitation should be considered at the beginning of treatment. The assessment includes consideration of the diagnosis, prognosis, proposed treatment, individual patient factors, and pre-existing oral health.
- Immediate management involves extractions of unrestorable teeth or those with gross periodontal disease prior to treatment, irrespective of fields. All healthy teeth as well as deeply impacted teeth without pathology are left in situ.
- Extractions are undertaken with as little trauma as possible and minimal flap surgery.
- In general, we advise routine 3-monthly check-ups, daily fluoride and bicarbonate mouth rinses, and restorations as required.
- Important treatment factors affecting dental health include the anticipated radiation dose, field size, and location. Specific areas receiving doses over 60 Gy should be flagged as higher risk for complications, especially if the major salivary glands are included. The use of surgery or chemotherapy should be known.

- A complete dental history should be taken. Factors likely to increase the risk of oral complications should be noted. Smoking and alcohol cessation should be advised.
- Oral cavity should be examined, and relevant radiographic images obtained, such as bitewings and periapical X-rays if indicated.
- Assessment should be recorded. If the patient wears dentures, he/she should be advised to avoid using them until treatment is completed.

Before head and neck radiation therapy
- Conduct a pretreatment oral examination and prophylaxis.
- Schedule dental treatment in consultation with the radiation oncologist.
- Extract teeth in the proposed radiation field that may be a problem in the future.
- Prevent tooth demineralization and radiation caries:
  - Fabricate custom gel-applicator trays for the patient.
  - Prescribe a 1.1% neutral pH sodium fluoride gel or a 0.4% stannous, unflavored fluoride toothpaste (not fluoride rinses).
  - Be sure that the trays cover all tooth structures without irritating the gingival or mucosal tissues.
  - Have patients brush with a fluoride gel if using trays is difficult.
- Allow at least 14 days of healing for any oral surgical procedures.
- Conduct prosthetic surgery before treatment, since elective surgical procedures are contraindicated on irradiated bone.

Pre-radiation treatment
Oral health examination
Objectives
- Conduct evaluation 1 month, if possible, before cancer treatment begins.
- Establish a schedule for dental treatment.
  - Complete invasive procedures at least 14 days before head/neck radiation therapy starts
  - Postpone elective oral surgical procedures until cancer treatment is completed.

Contd...

Contd...
- Identify and treat sites of low-grade and acute oral infections:
  - Caries
  - Periodontal disease
  - Endodontic disease
  - Mucosal lesions
- Identify and eliminate sources of oral trauma and irritation such as ill-fitting dentures, orthodontic bands, and other appliances.
- Identify and treat potential oral problems within the proposed radiation field before radiation treatment begins.
- Instruct patients about oral hygiene.
- Educate patients on preventing demineralization and dental caries.

PRE-RADIOTHERAPY DENTAL MANAGEMENT
Restorations
- The goals of dental care are to become functional and to get an aesthetic dentition.
- Scaling, prophylaxis, and fluoride application should be performed and where simple restorations are required, these should be carried out before radiotherapy begins.
- If time does not permit definitive restoration, temporary restoration with glass ionomer cement (GIC) is often appropriate.
- As amalgam may cause backscatter and subsequent local mucositis, they are therefore generally avoided.
- The presence of sharp cusps or restorations is an important issue for the HNC patient, as these may cause considerable trauma to the vulnerable irradiated soft tissues.
- If the patient wears dentures, these should be checked to ensure that they are well fitting and not at risk of causing ulceration.

Extractions
The extraction of teeth preradiotherapy is controversial. The criteria used by Ben David

are a useful guide for extractions: "Teeth with nonrestorable caries, or caries that extend to the gum line, teeth with large, compromised restorations with significant periodontal attachment loss (pocketing > 5 mm), and those with severe erosion or abrasion are extracted if they are in parts of the jaws expected to receive a high dose. Teeth residing in the anterior mandible are not considered for extraction unless the primary tumor was anteriorly in the oral cavity."

If extractions are performed, it is important to allow sufficient healing time prior to the commencement of radiotherapy but not to unduly delay it. An accepted interval between extractions and radiotherapy is 10 days to 3 weeks.

DENTAL MANAGEMENT DURING RADIOTHERAPY (FIGS. 1 TO 3)

Mucositis

In HNC patients receiving RT, up to 80% of patients may develop mucositis usually occurring after 7–10 days of treatment and potentially lasting for months.

- The soft palate is affected most severely, followed by floor of mouth (FOM), cheeks, tongue, and lips. Grading scales such as the World Health Organization oral toxicity scale adapted for oral mucositis are useful. Grade 0 is no oral mucositis and Grade 4 is where the patient has ulcers and alimentation is not possible.
- Methods used to prevent and treat mucositis include good dental hygiene such as frequent brushing with a super soft, regularly replaced toothbrush, regular flossing, 4-hourly alcohol-free oral rinses, adequate hydration, and the avoidance of oral irritants such as alcohol, tobacco, and spices.
- Symptomatic treatment includes tooth mousse and topical barrier gels. The International Society of Oral Oncology (ISOO) guidelines recommend that sucralfate, chlorhexidine, and antimicrobial lozenges not be used for the prevention of radiotherapy-induced oral mucositis but do state that benzydamine has a role for a patient receiving moderate-dose RT.
- Other agents that have been investigated include aloe vera gels and honey products, which may be beneficial for some patients.

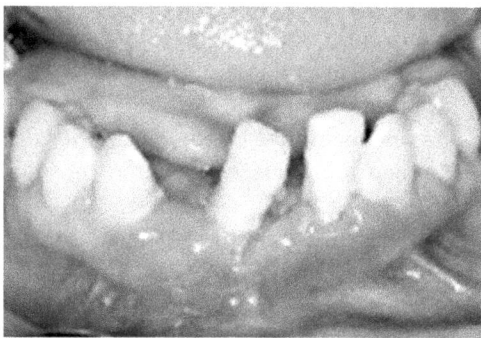

Fig. 1: Loose, periodontally compromised tooth.

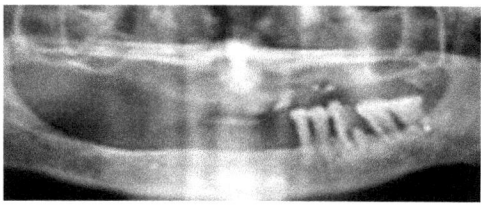

Fig. 2: Carious tooth, which cannot be restored.

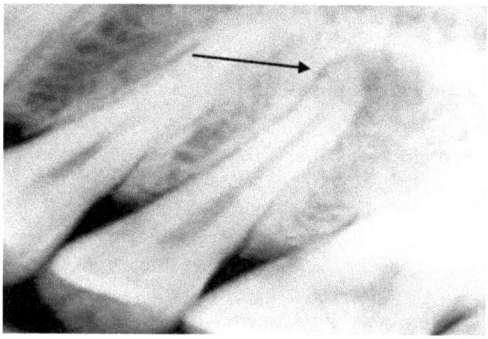

Fig. 3: Tooth having periapical abscess.

Candidiasis

- Candidiasis is caused by both candida albicans (>80%) and nonalbicans species and is a frequent infection after RT to the head and neck. Radiotherapy-related hyposalivation alters the oral environment and significantly increases the risk of colonization and infection.
- Candidiasis typically affects the tongue and labial commissure and presents in three forms: (1) pseudomembranous, (2) erythematous/atrophic, and (3) cheilitis.
- The usual appearance is that of removable white lesions overlying an erythematous and atrophic patch.
- Symptoms may be absent or include burning pain, difficulty swallowing, dysgeusia, and halitosis.
- It is treated when symptomatic and focuses on local therapy unless the presentation is severe, disseminated candidiasis is suspected, and the patient is at high risk (immunosuppressed) or fails to respond to local methods. Prevention is through regular dental hygiene, salivary substitutes, and smoking and alcohol cessation. First-line treatment includes topical miconazole, fluconazole or nystatin, available in several forms such as creams, suspensions, or lozenges. When systemic therapy is indicated, the first-line drug is oral fluconazole.

Xerostomia

- Xerostomia affects speech and taste as well as chewing and swallowing difficulties. Furthermore, hyposalivation increases the risk of oral infections such as candidiasis, gingivitis, and acute suppurative sialadenitis and risk of caries.
- Salivary substitutes should be used as well as regular nonmedicated oral rinses.
- Sialogogues such as chewing gum and the cholinergic agonist pilocarpine can also be used for the relief of symptoms.

Hygiene and Radiation Caries (Fig. 4)

- The incidence of radiation caries is related to radiotherapy dose, with an odds increase of two to three times at 30–60 Gy and ten times at over 60 Gy.
- The proposed mechanism is that the salivary glands withstand doses up to 30 Gy and sustain maximal damage between 30 and 60 Gy. The additional risk is due to direct radiation effects on the tooth structure, which weakens dentine–enamel bonds and results in shear fracturing.
- The sites that are most affected post-radiotherapy are the labial surfaces of the cervical, cuspal, and incisor areas. These areas receive compression, torsion, and shearing forces and are the regions that are most resistant to caries in nonirradiated patients.
- Use of fluoride-based toothpaste or fluoride varnish application reduces the risk of radiation caries/decay.
- Rinses should be either nonacidic fluoride preparations or bicarbonate preparations, and brushing and flossing should be gentle and thorough.

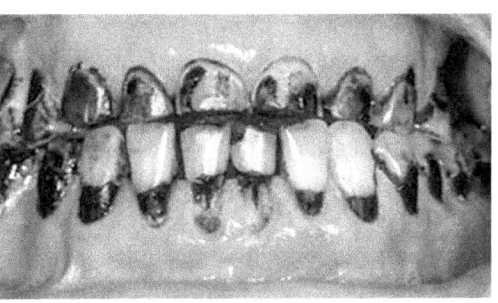

Fig. 4: Teeth having radiation caries.

Restorative Considerations

- Restorative management of radiation caries can be challenging and may be compounded by limited access due to trismus and poor salivation as a result of marginal gingivitis. The restorative material should have ideal properties that would include resistance to recurrent caries, adhesion to tooth structure, durability, acceptable aesthetics, and ease of handling.
- Radiation-induced changes in enamel and dentine may compromise bonding of adhesive materials.
- GICs lack strength, however, they have simpler bonding procedures and chemical adhesion as well as fluoride release and reuptake, which may reduce recurrent caries, even if the material is subsequently lost. Evidence suggests that where the caries risk is high or patient compliance is poor, GICs (conventional or resin modified) are the materials of choice. Extensive caries increases the risk of pulpal involvement. Irradiation may alter pulp vascularity and therefore its capacity for repair. Within radiation fields, where caries involves the pulp, endodontic treatment is generally preferred to extraction. Generally, removable prostheses should be avoided in irradiated partially dentate patients unless they are essential for aesthetics or function.
- Conventionally, denture wearing should be avoided for 1 year or more after completion of radiation to allow healing and ridge remodeling.

Dental Implants

- Dental implants may facilitate effective oral rehabilitation following cancer treatment (including radiotherapy). They can be used to support fixed or removable prostheses.
- Implants' placement should be done at least 1-2 years after radiotherapy gets completed.
- Osteoradionecrosis is an acknowledged risk of implant placement in irradiated bone.

Extractions and Osteoradionecrosis

- Osteoradionecrosis is a serious and typically late complication following RT to the head and neck, whereby the irradiated bone is exposed and undergoes necrosis.
- The exact pathophysiology is unclear.
- A great number of staging systems exist for ORN **(Table 1 and Fig. 5)**. One of the first methods was Marx's system where the stage was based on response to the Wilford Hall hyperbaric oxygen (HBO) protocol, with the potential to directly enter a higher stage if the initial presentation was severe. More contemporary systems such as Kagan and Schwartz's three stages classify ORN based on clinical presentation, and then treatment is decided according to the stage.
- A simple system is presented by Notani et al. based on clinical presentation. Staging systems have focused on the mandible, as the maxilla is unlikely to develop ORN.

Preventive measures are taken to avoid the need for dental intervention such as extractions to reduce the risk of ORN. Dental extraction with minimal trauma is indicated in the irradiated patient. In addition to that, the number of teeth removed in a single session should be limited.

Treatment of Osteoradionecrosis

- In order to further reduce the risk of ORN, the dentist uses prophylactic

TABLE 1: Selected staging systems for osteoradionecrosis.

Marx, 1983

I	Initial cases of ORN and those responding to 30 HBO treatments
II	Failure to respond to initial 30 HBO treatments and/or response to alveolar sequestrectomy
III	Failure to respond to 60 HBO treatments and sequestrectomy, or initial presentation either with pathologic fracture, orocutaneous fistula, or radiographic evidence of resorption to the inferior border

Kagan and Schwartz, 2002

I	Superficial involvement of the mandibular cortex only with minimal soft-tissue ulceration
II	Localized involvement of the mandibular cortex and underlying medullary bone
IIa	As for II, with minimal soft-tissue ulceration
IIb	As for II, with soft-tissue necrosis, including an orocutaneous fistula
III	Diffuse involvement of the mandible. Full-thickness necrosis including the lower border
IIIa	As for III, with minimal soft-tissue ulceration
IIIb	As for III, with soft-tissue necrosis, including an orocutaneous fistula

Notani et al., 2003

I	ORN confined to the alveolar bone
II	ORN confined to the alveolar bone and/or the mandible above the mandibular alveolar canal
III	ORN extended to the mandible under the level of the mandibular alveolar canal and ORN with a skin fistula and/or pathological fracture

(HBO: hyperbaric oxygen; ORN: osteoradionecrosis)

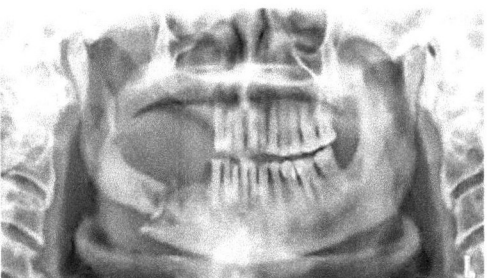

Fig. 5: Osteoradionecrosis of mandible.

antibiotics, platelet-rich plasma (PRP), and steroids. The use of prophylactic and therapeutic HBO for ORN is controversial. The theoretical benefit of HBO links with one of the proposed mechanisms of ORN, where ORN is the result of "hypoxia, hypocellularity and hypovascularity." HBO promotes angiogenesis and therefore should reduce ORN. The standard Marx 30/10 HBO protocol consists of 30 treatments at 2.4 atmospheres for 90 minutes prior to extraction, followed by 10 treatments of 90 minutes post-extraction.

- Conservative methods, such as saline rinses through to debridement, sequestrectomy, resection and free flaps, with or without the use of adjuncts such as HBO or pentoxifylline, tocopherol, and clodronate should be administered.
- In general, we advise to consider endodontic treatment first, to avoid extractions. Should this fail or if extractions become necessary, dentists can safely extract teeth out of field or in fields with primary closure of the socket.

PRE-CHEMOTHERAPY DENTAL ASSESSMENT

Patients undergoing chemotherapy are at a risk of fungal as well as bacterial infection. Thrush is the most common mouth infection during chemotherapy. It is advised to eliminate any area of infection or irritation, such as teeth with fractured cusps, fractured restorations, carious lesions, pulpal or periapical involvement, periodontal inflammation, or ill-fitted prosthesis.

Oral prophylaxis should be performed, if indicated, to maintain adequate oral hygiene. Dental procedures should be done at least 7–10 days before chemotherapy begins.

DENTAL MANAGEMENT DURING CHEMOTHERAPY

During chemotherapy, patients are at a risk of thrombocytopenia and neutropenia. It is advised to maintain optimum oral hygiene during that period. Oral prophylaxis and restorative dental treatment can usually be scheduled within a few days of the next proposed round or course of therapy when a patient's blood counts get recovered from the toxicity of the previous course of drugs. Blood counts, however, should be monitored the day before dental treatment to document hematologic status.

POSTCHEMOTHERAPY DENTAL MANAGEMENT: BISPHOSPHONATE-RELATED OSTEONECROSIS OF JAW

Bisphosphonate-related osteonecrosis of jaw (BRONJ) is an area of exposed bone in the maxillofacial region for >8 weeks in patients who were receiving or have received a bisphosphonate therapy. It can be related to any dental treatment or trauma. The diagnosis of BRONJ is based on the medical history of bisphosphonate treatment and clinical evaluation (pain, bone exposure, purulent secretion, or swelling).

POSTSURGERY: DENTAL MANAGEMENT AND REHABILITATION

Rehabilitation is an essential phase of cancer care and should be considered from the time of diagnosis in a complete and comprehensive plan. Surgical resections often create large defects accompanied by dysfunction and disfigurement. The primary objective of rehabilitation is the restoration of appearance and function.

- *Maxillary defects*: Most tumors of the paranasal sinus, palatal epithelium, or minor salivary glands require surgical removal of a portion of the upper jaw, which may produce a variety of problems.
- *Hypernasality* could make speech unintelligible; chewing may be difficult and swallowing likely will become awkward since food and liquid may be forced up into the nasal cavity and nose.
- A *temporary prosthesis*, known as "obturator," is placed. This will provide closure of the surgical defect. The purpose of obturator prosthesis is to restore the physical separation between the oral and nasal cavities, thereby restoring speech and swallowing to normal, and to provide support to the lip and cheek **(Figs. 6A and B)**.
- *Obturators are of three types*:
    1. *Temporary*: Placed immediately after surgery
    2. *Intermediate*: Placed after 3 months post-radiotherapy or 6–9 months post-surgery
    3. *Permanent*: Placed after 1 year post-surgery/post-radiotherapy
- *Mandibular guiding prosthesis*: It can be made in patients who have undergone surgical resection of the mandible, either segmental, hemi or total mandibulectomy, that can cause mandible deviation **(Figs. 7 and 8)**.
- The *prosthesis* helps the patient to move the mandible normally without deviation during functions such as speech and mastication. It is molded in wax and processed in clear acrylic resin where wire loops may be used for the support.

The guide flange is extended into the maxillary mucobuccal fold superiorly and diagonally on the nondefect side.
- *Dental implants*: Prosthetic rehabilitation with fixed dental implants is preferred as removable prosthesis may be difficult to adapt due to the postsurgical alteration of the anatomy. Implants can be placed during the surgery in the avascular free fibular bone graft in order to give cosmetic and functional outcome to the patient **(Figs. 9 and 10)**.

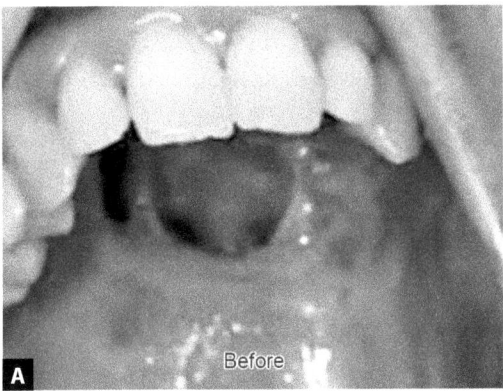
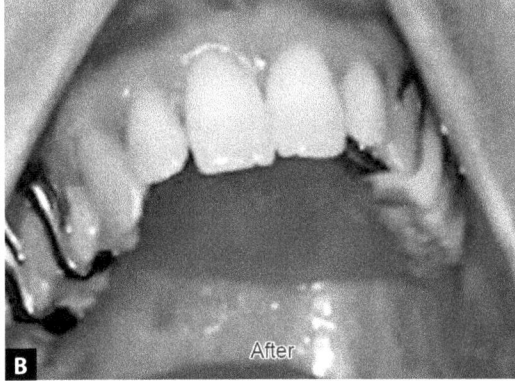

Figs. 6A and B: Before and after obturator placement.

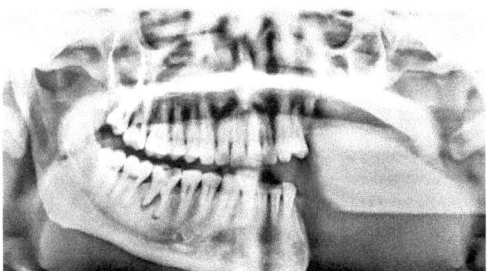

Fig. 7: Post-mandibular resection.

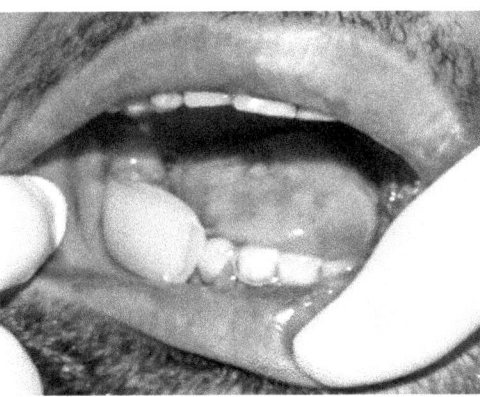

Fig. 8: Placement of mandibular guiding prosthesis.

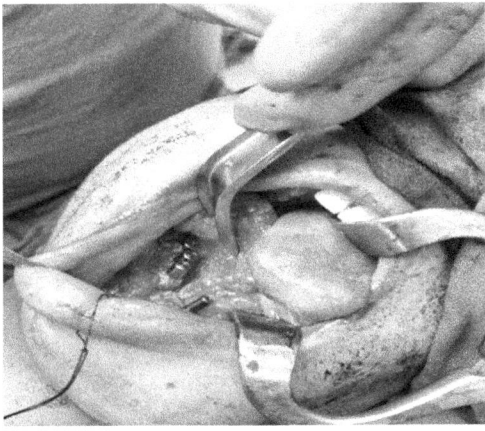

Fig. 9: Dental implants in free fibular bone graft during surgery.

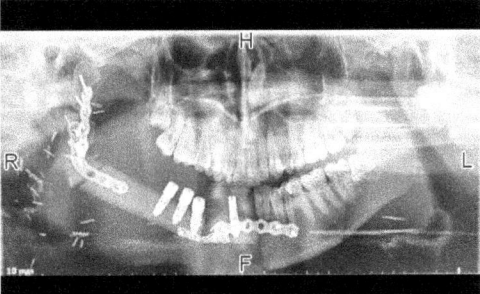

Fig. 10: Orthopantomography showing dental implants.

KEY POINTS

- The benefits of preradiotherapy dental evaluation are to assess, diagnose, and manage oral and dental implications that are related to treatment.
- Immediate management involves extractions of unrestorable teeth or those with gross periodontal disease prior to treatment, irrespective of fields. All healthy teeth as well as deeply impacted teeth without pathology are left in situ.
- Where simple restorations are required, these should be carried out before radiotherapy begins.
- If time does not permit definitive restoration, temporary restoration with GIC is often appropriate.
- The presence of sharp cusps or restorations is an important issue for the HNC patient, as these may cause considerable trauma to the vulnerable irradiated soft tissues.
- Dental management during radiotherapy includes that for mucositis, candidiasis, xerostomia, and radiation caries.
- Implants' placement should be done at least 1–2 years after RT gets completed.
- ORN is a late complication following RT to the head and neck, whereby the irradiated bone is exposed and undergoes necrosis.
- In order to reduce the risk of ORN, dentists use prophylactic antibiotics, PRP, and steroids.
- *Mandibular guiding prosthesis*: It can be made in patients who have undergone surgical resection of the mandible that can cause mandible deviation.

CHAPTER 31

Swallowing and Speech Therapy in Oral Cancer

Navneet Singh

INTRODUCTION

Patients with cancers of the oral cavity may be treated with surgical removal of the tumor, radiotherapy, chemotherapy, or a combination of these procedures. Each type of cancer treatment may result in some degree of swallowing problem. The type and severity of dysphagia will depend upon the size and location of the original tumor, the structures involved, and the treatment modality used for cure.

There are various modalities—including postures, maneuvers, modifications to bolus volume and viscosity, range of motion exercises, and strengthening exercises, which are helpful in dealing with swallowing problems in these patients.

NORMAL SWALLOWING FUNCTION

Swallowing is a complex series of sequential neuromuscular events that are integrated into a smooth and continuous process. Generally, the process is divided into four phases **(Figs. 1A to D)**:

1. *Oral phase*: The oral phase is completely voluntary and involves the entry of food into the oral cavity and preparation for swallowing; this includes mixing with saliva, mastication, and formation into a cohesive bolus in preparation for the swallow. It requires coordination of the lips, tongue, teeth, mandible, and soft palate.
2. *Oral transit phase*: It is a voluntary phase that begins with the posterior propulsion

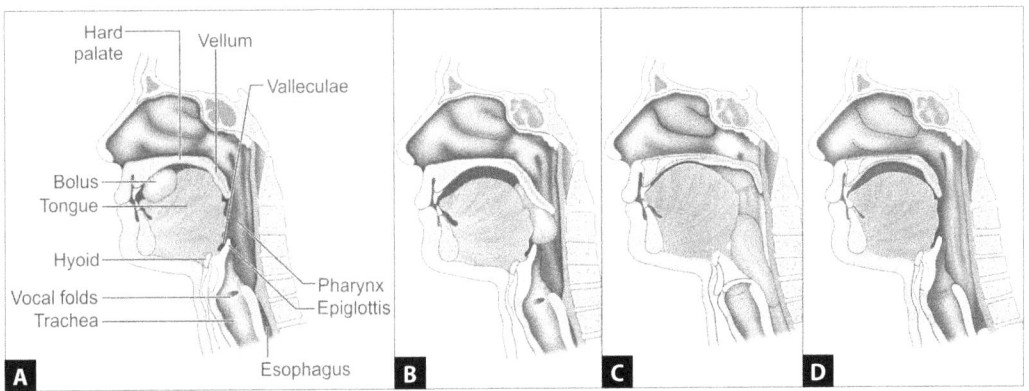

Figs. 1A to D: Phases of swallowing: (A) Oral phase; (B) Oral transit phase; (C) Pharyngeal phase; (D) Esophageal phase.

of the bolus by the tongue and ends with initiation of the pharyngeal swallow.
3. *Pharyngeal phase*: The pharyngeal phase is initiated as the tongue propels the bolus posteriorly and the base of tongue contacts the posterior pharyngeal wall eliciting a reflexive action that begins a complex series of events. The soft palate elevates to prevent nasal reflux. The pharyngeal constrictor musculature contracts to push the bolus through the pharynx. The epiglottis inverts to cover the larynx and prevents aspiration of contents into the airway. The vocal folds adduct to further prevent aspiration. The hyolaryngeal complex moves anteriorly and superiorly, which, in combination with the pressure generated by a bolus, provides anterior traction and intrabolus pressure to open the cricopharyngeus muscle.
4. *Esophageal phase*: The esophageal phase is completely involuntary and consists of peristaltic waves that propel the bolus to the stomach. Total swallow time from oral cavity to stomach is no more than 20 seconds.

CAUSES OF DYSPHASIA IN ORAL CANCER

The causes of dysphasia in oral cancer are given in **Box 1**.

IMPORTANCE OF SWALLOWING THERAPY IN ORAL CANCERS

Patients who have a portion of the oral tongue removed exhibit worsened swallowing function characterized by prolonged oral preparatory time, slowed oral transit time, increased oral residue, and increased pharyngeal residue. Oral stage swallowing disorders tend to worsen for these patients as bolus viscosity increases. As the extent of resection of the oral tongue increases, swallowing function also worsens.

Box 1: Causes of dysphasia associated with surgical treatment.

- *Causes associated with surgical treatment*:
  - *Structural changes*:
    - *Changes of soft tissue and hard tissue*: Anatomic deficit, postoperative swelling, scar formation, and contracture in the lips, maxilla, palate, tongue, floor of the mouth, mandible, and oropharynx
    - *Changes of muscles*: Anatomic deficits, postoperative swelling, scar formation, and contracture in the facial muscles, tongue muscles, suprahyoid muscles, masticatory muscles, palatine muscles, and pharyngeal muscles
    - *Reconstruction*: Morphological change and reduction of movements in remained tissues
  - *Impaired motor and sensory function*: Damage to the trigeminal nerve/7th/9th/10th/12th nerve
  - *Complications after tracheostomy*:
    - Restricted laryngeal movement
    - Compression of the esophagus
    - Excess tracheal secretion and pooling of the secretion
    - Reduced subglottic pressure
    - Reduced laryngeal sensitivity and delayed glottic closure reflex
- *Dysphagia associated with radiotherapy*:
  - Mucositis
  - Neuropathy
  - Fibrosis
  - Xerostomia
- Chemotherapy-induced stomatitis and mucositis resulting in eating problems

With the resection of the floor of mouth (FOM) muscles, patients may experience problems with hyolaryngeal elevation, resulting in residue in the pyriform sinuses that may be aspirated after swallowing. A marginal resection of mandible does not disrupt the continuity of the mandibular arch and has little impact on swallowing function. After segmental mandibular resection, swallowing becomes difficult postoperatively.

Diagnosis and Treatment Planning

A thorough examination begins with a clinical swallow assessment that includes a detailed history of subjective complaints and medical status, clinical observations, and a physical examination. Swallowing trials can be initiated with a range of food textures. An oromotor examination assesses the function of the oral structures for swallowing. Blue dye testing can be utilized with patients who are tracheostomized to accurately determine the relative risk of aspiration. Cervical auscultation using a stethoscope on the larynx can be used to detect the sounds of swallowing and respiration.

The most useful imaging techniques for diagnosing swallowing disorders are the modified barium swallow (MBS) procedure with videofluorography (VFG) and fiberoptic endoscopic evaluation of swallowing (FEES).

During the MBS, patients are administered calibrated boluses of radiopaque material of varying consistency. The patient's swallow is viewed in the lateral plane with VFG, so that disorders of the swallowing during oral preparation, the oral propulsive stage of swallowing, and the pharyngeal stage of swallowing may be observed and documented.

FEES visualizes the pharynx from above by placing an endoscopic tube transnasally such that the end of the tube is suspended over the end of the soft palate. This procedure gives a different view of the pharynx that seen videofluoroscopically and permits observation of true cord closure; however, FEES does not provide information concerning the oral stage of swallow, which may be the most problematic for oral cavity tumors **(Box 2)**.

> **Box 2:** Functional oral intake scale.
> - *Level 1*: Nothing by mouth
> - *Level 2*: Tube dependent with minimal attempts of food or liquid
> - *Level 3*: Tube dependent with consistent oral intake of food or liquid
> - *Level 4*: Total oral diet of a single consistency
> - *Level 5*: Total oral diet with multiple consistencies, but requiring special preparation or compensations
> - *Level 6*: Total oral diet with multiple consistencies without special preparation, but with specific food limitations
> - *Level 7*: Total oral diet with no restrictions

Goals of Swallowing Rehabilitation

- To prevent malnutrition and dehydration
- Reduce the risk of aspiration
- Re-establishment of safe and efficient oral intake
- Prevention of dysphagia prior to medical treatment
- Patient education regarding the specifics of their disorder

Swallowing Interventions

- *Postures*: Postures are used to control the flow of the bolus and to reduce or eliminate aspiration **(Table 1)**. There are a number of postures that are effective in oral cancer patients. The efficacy of postures will vary depending upon the swallowing disorder identified causing the aspiration.

TABLE 1: Postures which help in better swallowing.	
Postures	Significance
Chin down	The chin-down posture is useful for patients who have a delayed pharyngeal swallow, reduced tongue base retraction, or reduced laryngeal elevation
Head back	The head-back posture uses gravity to clear the bolus from the oral cavity in patients who have difficulty with oral transit of the bolus
Head rotation	Head rotation toward the weak or damaged side of the pharynx or larynx closes the damaged side, so that the bolus flows down the more nearly normal side. This posture is useful for patients with unilateral pharyngeal wall impairment or unilateral vocal fold weakness
Lateral head tilt	The lateral head tilt posture may be used for a patient who has both unilateral oral and pharyngeal impairment on the same side. The patient tilts the head to the stronger side, so that gravity drains the bolus along the stronger side and avoids the weaker side

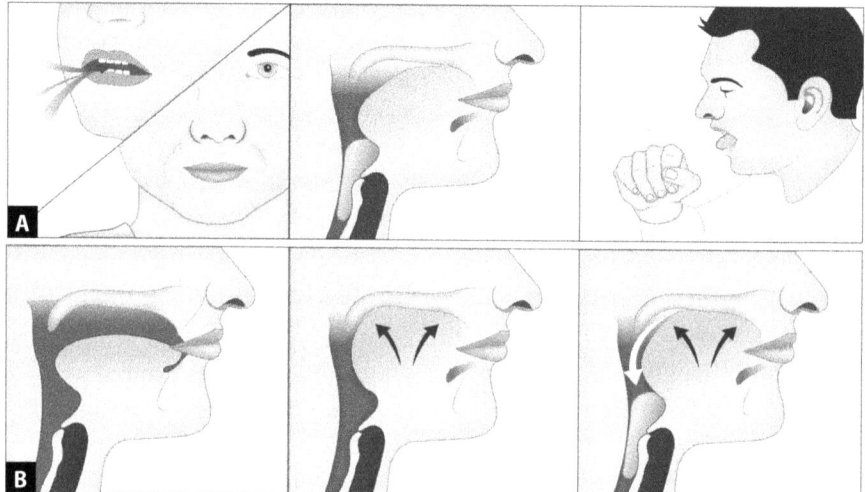

Figs. 2A and B: (A) Supraglottic swallow; (B) Effortful swallow.

- *Swallowing maneuvers*: Swallowing maneuvers are designed to place specific aspects of the oropharyngeal swallowing under voluntary control. These are supraglottic swallow and super supraglottic swallow maneuver/effortful swallow maneuver/Mendelsohn maneuver/tongue-hold maneuver **(Figs. 2A and B)**.
- *Active exercises*:
  Range of motion (ROM) exercises **(Table 2)**: In the first 3 months after surgery, patients practicing significantly better swallowing function than those who do not perform these exercises. ROM exercises can be used for the lips, jaw, tongue, and hyoid-related musculature.
- Jaw mobilization, tongue mobilization, and hold-relax techniques
- Neuromuscular electrical stimulation (NMES) for pharyngeal dysphagia
- *Tongue isometric or strengthening exercises*: Resistance or strengthening exercises are used to build or maintain strength in the oral tongue.

TABLE 2: Range of motion (ROM) exercises.

ROM exercises	Methods
Jaw ROM exercises	Finger-assisted stretching exercises, TheraBite **(Fig. 3)**
Oral tongue ROM exercises	*Tongue ROM exercises*: Extension, lateralization, elevation, and retraction
Bolus manipulation exercises	Strip of gauze soaked in water or beverage, a flexible licorice stick or similar candy, or a small lollipop on a stick. • Tongue cupping • Tongue side-to-side movement • Tongue posterior movement
Tongue base ROM exercises	Retraction of the tongue as far back as possible in the oral cavity will exercise the tongue base (pretending to gargle and pretending to yawn)

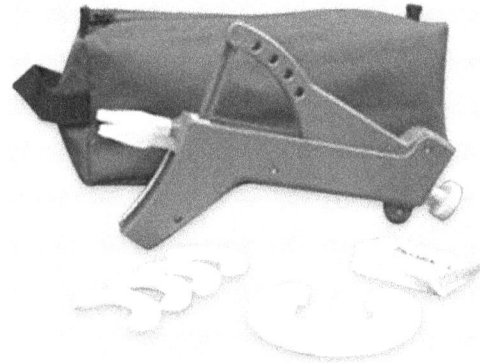

Fig. 3: TheraBite.

- *Thermal/Tactile stimulation*: It is designed to sensitize or stimulate the area of the oral cavity where the swallow reflex is thought to trigger.

Swallowing Exercise

Why it is Important to Avoid Swallowing Problems?

Swallowing problems can affect your ability to eat solid food and drink liquids of swallow own saliva (spit). Eating and drinking well are important during and after your radiation treatment to help you heal.

Swallowing problems can become lifelong (chronic). They can also cause the following:
- Chest infection
- Weight loss
- Dehydration
- Needing a feeding tube

What can I do to Reduce my Risk of having Swallowing Problems?

It is important to continue to swallow through the course of your radiation treatment, even it is just sips of water several times a day.

How to do your Swallowing Exercise?

- Do each exercise 5–10 times in a row every hour that you are awake.
- Do these exercises before you start your treatment, during your treatment, and after your treatment is finished.
- Do not have any food or drink in your mouth while doing these exercises.
- You may feel very tired and be in pain during your radiation treatment, but try to continue with the exercise as best as you can. Your healthcare team is here to support you, so ask for help when you need it **(Fig. 4)**.

Key Points in Swallowing
- Speech and swallowing outcomes are critical survivorship endpoints.
- Pretreatment functional assessment is essential to plan rehabilitation and supportive care, to predict functional outcomes, and to select the modality of therapy, most likely to maximize functional outcomes.
- Refinements in surgical reconstruction, conformal radiotherapy techniques, and preventive therapy can be used to reduce functional problems after treatment.
- Post-treatment rehabilitation requires individualized planning on the basis of standardized, instrumental assessments.

Swallowing and Speech Therapy in Oral Cancer

Remember to keep swallowing:
- It is important to continue to swallow through the course of your radiation treatment, even if it is just sips of water several times a day.
- You may feel very tired and be in pain during your radiation treatment, but try to continue with the exercises as best as you can. Your healthcare team is here to support you, so ask for help when you need it.

Useful tips:

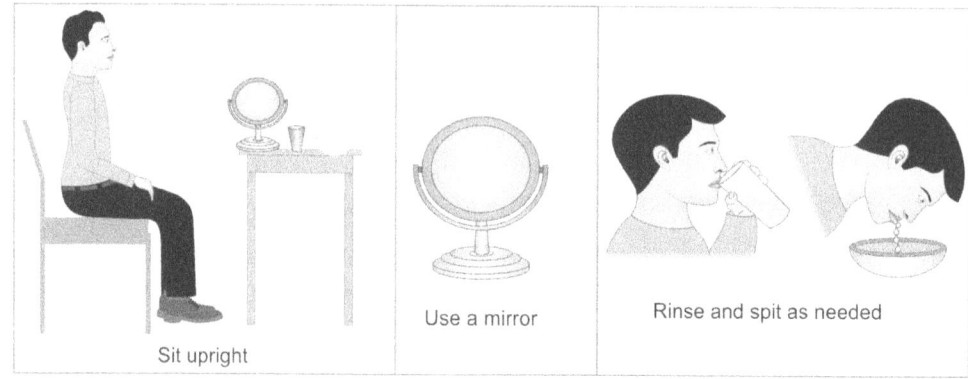

Sit upright   Use a mirror   Rinse and spit as needed

How to make your swallow stronger?
Repeat these exercises 5–10 times. Remember to keep your mouth wet!

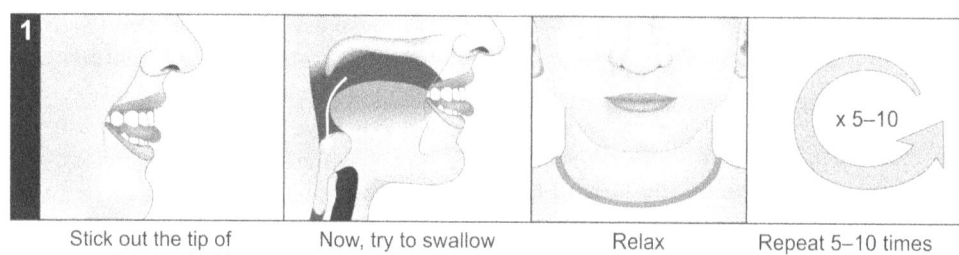

1. Stick out the tip of your tongue. Hold it between your teeth or lips | Now, try to swallow your spit with your tongue in that position | Relax | Repeat 5–10 times

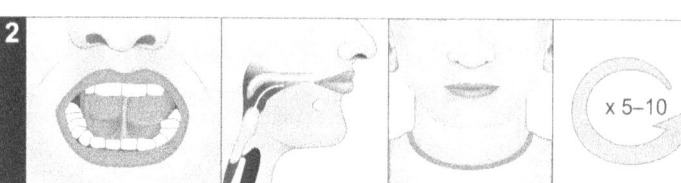 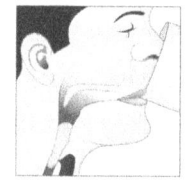

2. Press your tongue against the roof of your mouth as hard as you can | With your mouth closed, swallow your spit (saliva) as hard as you can | Relax | Repeat 5–10 times | **Try swallowing some water now** Take a small sip of water and swallow it. You may need to swallow it a few times to get it all down. Clear your throat or cough if you need to

Contd...

Contd...

Keep the muscles in your mouth moving

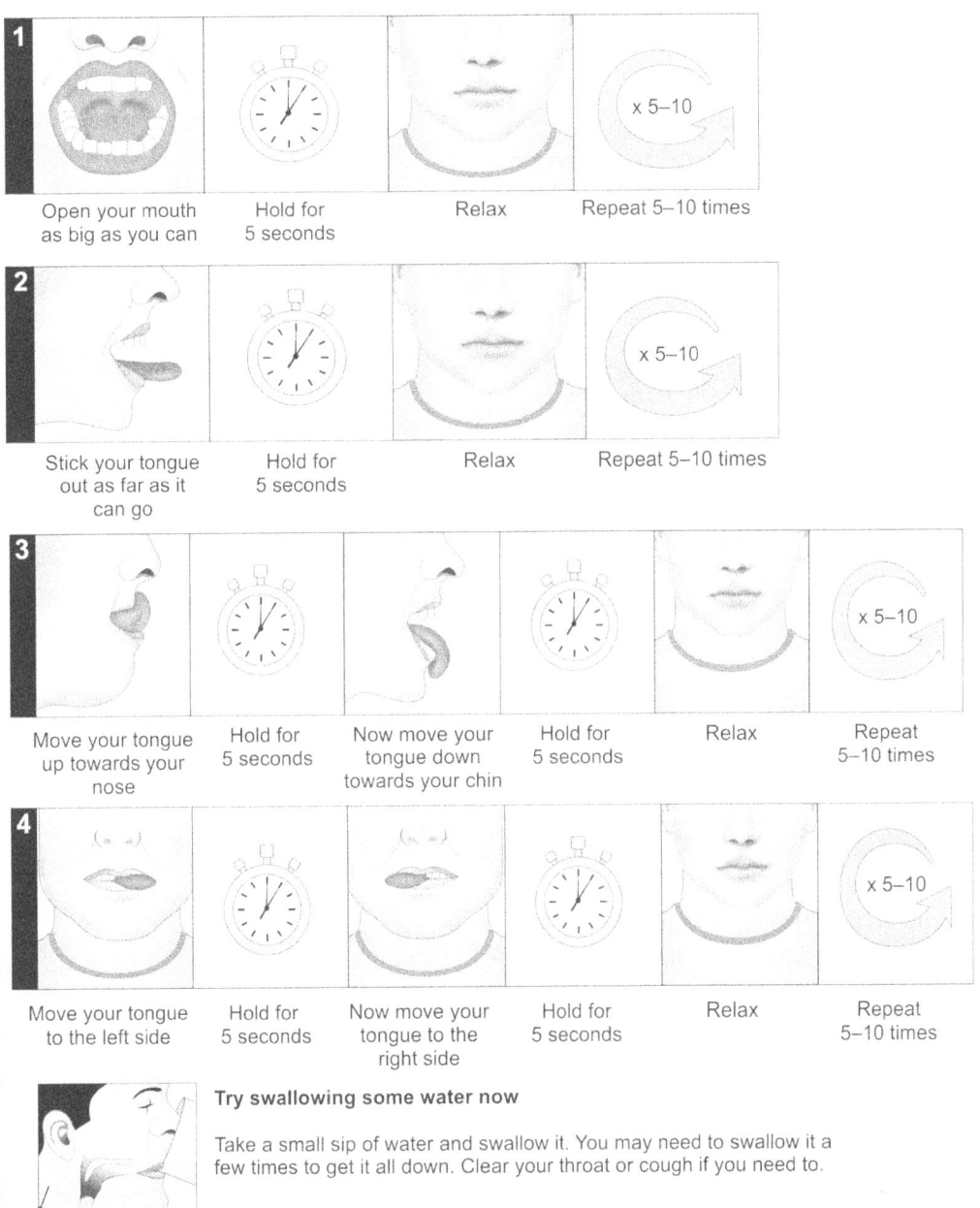

Fig. 4: Swallowing exercise procedure.

SPEECH THERAPY IN ORAL CANCER

The primary goal of speech rehabilitation in oral cancer patients is to optimize the potential for communication as soon as possible. Changes in the ability to produce intelligible speech are common after ablative surgery and reconstruction of the oral structures. In addition, complication from reconstruction may adversely affect articulation and resonance. Trismus may diminish vocal quality. However, the quality of articulation is not greatly influenced by trismus.

Xerostomia is also a common side effect of radiation treatment secondary to inadequate salivation. Xerostomia may affect the resonance of sound through dry vocal tract and articulation produced by dry oral structures.

Components of Speech

- *Respiration*: Normally during respiration, the inhalations and expirations are of equal interval. But during speech, the inhalation phase is shortened and expiration phase is prolonged. In laryngeal, pharyngeal, oral, and nasal components of the respiratory tract, the stream of air is modified in its course from lungs by maxillofacial structures and gives rise to the symbols, which are recognized as speech.
- *Phonation*: When air leaves the lungs, it passes through the larynx whose true vocal folds or vocal cords modify the stream and setup a sequence of laryngeal sound waves with characteristic pitch and intensity. These laryngeal sounds provide the basis for organization of speech.
- *Resonation*: The sound waves produced by the vocal folds are still far from being the finished product that we hear in speech. It is the resonators that give the characteristic quality to voice. The resonating structures are the air sinuses, organ surfaces, and cavities such as the pharynx, oral cavity, nasal cavity, and chest wall. The resonating structures do not contribute any energy to the stream of air.
- *Articulation*: It is the function of articulatory mechanism to break up, to modify the laryngeal tones, and to create new sounds itself within the oral cavity. The articulatory mechanism involves the lips, teeth, palate, and tongue. The final action of articulatory apparatus is to articulate in a fluid sequence all the sounds, which have been synthesized into symbols. Amplified, resonated sound is formulated into meaningful speech by the articulators, namely, the lips, tongue, cheek, teeth, and palate, by changing the relative spatial relationship of these structures. The tongue is considered to be the single most important articulator of speech because of its ability to affect rapid changes in movement and shape.
- *Neural integration*: Speech is integrated by the central nervous system both at the peripheral and central levels.

Importance of Speech Therapy in Oral Cancer

After resection of oral carcinomas, patients experience verbalization issues due to tissue loss structure modification or tongue mobility impairment. Target sounds may be misshaped, substituted, or discarded, prompting diminished comprehensibility, air stream cannot escape through the nose, and the nasal consonants are denasalized.

Sufficient control of lips, tongue, and soft palate is important for the production of speech. Any impairment in the range of movement, strength, and adaptability of these dynamic articulators might influence the capacity to make exact individual speech movements and coarticulations required in connected speech.

The impacts of cancer on speech rely on the area and size of the growth. For instance, a sore or lump on the lips might restrict movement. This could bring about unclear production of speech sounds made with the lips, e.g., p, b, and m. Cancer of the tongue can bring about issues with many sounds, e.g., if lesion is in the anterior portion of the tongue or in the posterior aspect of the tongue, articulation is affected.

The outcomes after surgical treatment depend on the site and size of the cancerous growth, extent of resection, and type of reconstruction.

Evaluation of Speech in Oral Cancer

- *Oral examination*:
  - Structural integrity including oral mucosa and dentition
  - Functional integrity including strength, speed, and ROM of oral musculature
  - Symmetry and movement of structures of the face, oral cavity, and respiratory system while at rest and while speaking
  - Sensation of oral and facial structures
  - Sensation (i.e., taste and smell)
- *Respiration*:
  - Respiratory pattern (abdominal, thoracic, and clavicular)
  - Coordination of respiration with phonation
  - Presence of tracheostomy tube, type, and size of tube
- *Voice and resonance*:
  - Voice quality—including roughness, breathiness, strain, pitch, and loudness
  - Resonance—normal, hyponasal, and hypernasal
- Articulation and speech intelligibility assessment
- Cognitive—communication
  Evaluate memory, attention, problem-solving, and executive skills in the context of functional communication.

SPEECH THERAPY INTERVENTIONS (BOX 3)

- *Oral facilitative exercise*: These exercises increase strength, ROM, and flexibility of the oral articulators. These exercises also improve swallowing function. Muscular strength and endurance can be improved through three basic types of exercises: (1) isometric, (2) isotonic, and (3) isokinetic.
- *Directed articulation therapy*: This therapy is frequently indicated to improve production of specific phonemes and phonemes groups. Patients who have undergone anterior or lateral tongue resections may have difficulty with sounds requiring tongue elevation and/or protrusion. Patients with lip incompetence following lip resections may experience difficulties with bilabial sounds and developing adequate lip plosion. Articulation therapy with lip

Box 3: Speech therapy in oral cancers.

- Articulation:
  - Oral facilitative exercises
  - Directed articulation therapy
  - Compensatory techniques
  - Surgical procedures
- Resonance
- Speech quality

closure exercise may improve the production of these groups of sounds.
- *Compensatory technique*: Compensatory technique is considered when the patient does not have the potential for correct placement of a targeted sound or group of sounds. Compensatory patterns differ between patients who have undergone total glossectomy versus those that have had a partial glossectomy. Partial glossectomies have been found to make use of the residual tongue stump in adaptive movements approximating the normal movements, whereas total glossectomies use true compensatory strategies. The primary purpose of the compensatory strategy is to improve the intelligibility of speech in the most inconspicuous manner possible; some compensatory strategies are developed unconsciously by the patient.
- *Surgical procedures*: Although complete tumor removal remains the prime objective during major oral cancer surgery, the emphasis is also on immediate functional restoration through primary reconstruction.
- *Resonance*: The primary function of the palate is to separate the oral and nasal cavities during swallowing to prevent nasal regurgitation and aerate and equalize pressure in the middle ear. The secondary objective of velopharyngeal mechanism is for speech purposes; velopharyngeal closure is produced by sphincteric actions of the levator veli palatini and the superior pharyngeal constrictor muscles. Closure is selective during production for all vowels and consonants, except for the nasal consonants.

Velopharyngeal insufficiency (VPI), even in small degree, can lead to the perception of hypernasality. This may result from surgical resection of lesions extending to the palate with remaining insufficient bulk, secondary scarring, and inadequate tissue mobility. In addition, neurological denervation (cranial nerve 9 and 10) may temporarily or permanently interfere with palatal motion. This may result from direct tumor invasion, from radiation fibrosis, or from surgical resection. VPI may result in nasal regurgitation of the bolus during swallow.

Hyponasality is typically perceived when there is blockage of nasal airflow during production of the nasal consonants. Nasal airflow can be impeded due to a space-occupying lesion in the nasopharynx, severe obstruction of the nasal cavities, or overcorrection of VPI.

Velopharyngeal closure is best assessed through videonasendoscopy in which dynamic images of the nasopharynx during production of specific speech tasks are viewed. Small gap with minimal bubbling of secretions may be managed with speech therapy alone. More significant VPI may require a combined approach of prosthetics, surgical reconstruction, and speech intervention.

Prosthetic management of VPI includes the use of palatal obturators, bulbs, and lifts.

KEY POINTS

- Patients treated surgically can begin with speech and swallowing therapy when the suture lines are healed, whereas those receiving radiotherapy can begin with rehabilitation prior to, during, or after treatment.
- It is important for patients undergoing oral cancer surgery to receive rehabilitation team follow-up and adequate intervention as soon as possible to treat the sequelae caused by resection/or irradiation of the oral structures.

Pain and Palliative Care in Oral Cavity Cancers

CHAPTER 32

Bablesh Mahawar

Don't just be there, do something rather
Don't just do something, be there

INTRODUCTION

The incidence of cancer is increasing worldwide. The GLOBOCAN 2018 estimated 1,157,294 number of new cancer cases in India with 10.4% incidence of oral cavity cancer. Oral cavity cancer is most predominant among Indian males. A number of factors appear to be driving this increase, particularly a growing and aging global population and an increase in exposure to cancer risk factors linked to social and economic development.

The most worried and disabling symptom of cancer is pain. Up to 80% of patients suffering from oral cavity cancer have pain. Pain is the first symptom on presentation in 50–55% of patients. Cancer pain dramatically affects not only patients and their families rather the entire society. That is why, effective control of cancer pain has long been one of the most important and pressing issues in oncology. Despite its importance, chronic cancer-related pain and its symptoms are inadequately managed most of the times; as a result, many patients spend the last days of their lives suffering in great discomfort and disability.

In oral cancers, patient needs not *only* pain relief but also *relief support* from other symptoms such as dry mouth, bad breath, limited mouth opening, stiffness, fatigue, nausea, shortness of breath, deglutition problems, communication problems, and wound problems as social taboo is attached to disfigured face and feeding tube. All these factors further behave as constant pain triggers causing emotional distress and psychological and functional challenges. Thus, oral cavity cancer has a catastrophic impact on quality of patient's lives.

The term cancer pain is not synonym with pain in a cancer patient or pain in a cancer survivor. The current International Classification of Diseases-11 (ICD-11) describes chronic cancer-related pain as chronic pain caused by primary cancer itself, metastasis, or its treatment. It is distinct from pain caused by comorbid conditions.

CAUSES OF OROFACIAL PAIN (TABLE 1)

Orofacial pain management is particularly challenging due to its rich sensory innervations causing nociceptive, neuropathic, and mixed type of pain (93% of patients).

MECHANISM OF PAIN

Due to Local Spread

Pain among oral cavity cancer patients can be nociceptive, inflammatory, or neuropathic in nature. In oral cancers,

TABLE 1: Causes of pain in oral cancer.

	Acute	Chronic

Primary disease	Mucosal damage, invasion of bone, nerve, muscle, tumor pressure, and inflammation	• *Nociceptive:*
		  – Soft tissue and muscle
		  – Bony involvement
		• *Neuropathic:* Cranial neuropathy

Treatment related (surgery, chemotherapy, and radiotherapy)	Mucositis, infection, dental pain, and neuropathy	• Mucosal atrophy/xerostomia • Dental caries • Mucosal infection • Osteoradionecrosis • Temporomandibular joint disorders • Neuropathy • Postherpetic neuralgia • Lymphedema and fibrosis • Dysphagia and esophageal toxicity
Unrelated causes	Myofascial pain/trauma	–

inflammation is the major cause of pain initiated by reactive oxygen species (ROS). Inflammatory mechanisms can be activated by both tumor cells and cancer therapies and include release of cytokines and other analgesic molecules that induce pain in the pre-existing tumor environment of hypoxia and low pH. ROS may cause endothelial cell damage and increase vascular permeability, whereas nitric oxide (NO) may induce second messenger mechanism within the neurons that may cause neuropathic pain.

Due to Chemotherapy/Radiotherapy

Oral cavity has rich sensory innervations. Peripheral neurotoxicity is associated with a number of chemotherapeutic agents, e.g., vinca alkaloids and taxanes that may lead to damage or loss of large myelinated fibers. Other noncytostatic drugs such as interferon and amphotericin B used in supportive care may also induce sensory neuropathy. So far, no established agents are recommended for the prevention of chemotherapy-induced peripheral neuropathy (CIPN). There is consistent evidence that patients receiving vinca alkaloids, taxanes, etc., should not be offered agents such as:

- Acetyl-L-carnitine (ALC)
- Amifostine
- Amitriptyline
- Glutathione (GSH) for patients receiving paclitaxel/carboplatin chemotherapy
- Glutamine
- Vitamin E
- Alpha-lipoic acid
- Tablet duloxetine has a positive recommendation only in platinum-based CIPN.

Due to Surgery

Surgery on the neck is associated with fibrosis and stiffness. Recent studies demonstrated that more extensive neck dissections are associated with higher shoulder-related disability. This has a negative impact on quality of life and health status. Attention should be given in the preservation of cervical sensory nerves as well as spinal accessory nerves.

ASSESSMENT OF PAIN

Patients may be unable or unwilling to complete lengthy questionnaires, particularly when their pain is at its worst. Mostly, Visual Analog Scale (VAS) or Numerical Rating Scale (NRS) is used to assess pain.

No	Pain	Worst Pain
	0–10 Numerical Rating Scale	
0		10

Palliative care catch:
- Ask more frequently on initial contact and at regular intervals
- Whenever there is a change in existing pain
- When patients report a new pain

PAIN AND SUPPORTIVE MANAGEMENT IN ORAL CAVITY CANCERS

Orofacial Pain

Pain control by the World Health Organization (WHO) ladder, which is efficacious in almost 70–85% of patients. Goal is to reduce pain to allow adequate quality of life.

Multimodal approach is required. There is a need for individualized analgesia.

Two-step ladder approach is more preferred nowadays from nonopoids to directly low-dose strong opioids **(Flowchart 1)**.

CRANIAL NEURALGIA/NEUROPATHY

The route of spread of oral cavity squamous cell carcinoma (SCC) is not only direct or through lymphatic pathway, but there is also extension along the neurovascular bundle leading to different types of neuropathic pain.

Sometimes, patient presents with painful trigeminal and glossopharyngeal neuropathy.

Painful Trigeminal Neuropathy

Painful trigeminal neuropathy (PTN) is the term reserved for patients in which tumor,

Flowchart 1: Treatment algorithm for opioid therapy.

multiple sclerosis, and neuroma have been demonstrated as the causative lesion other than vascular compression. 5-10% of reported trigeminal neuralgia are PTN secondary to brain, head, and neck tumors.

Usual presentation is the facial pain, unilateral or bilateral, in one or more divisions of trigeminal nerve. It is the first symptom of a tumor extension in Meckel's cave (**Fig. 1**) in >65% of patients. Patient often complaints of constant dull, background pain in one or more divisions of trigeminal nerve with sudden brief episodes of intolerable burning and stabbing type of pain several times a day usually lasting for 30-40 seconds. On examination, neurological deficit is common such as palsies, numbness, or ptosis. Advanced imaging and expedient workup are necessary to confirm PTN. Usually, such tumors are inoperable due to intracranial and cavernous sinus extension. Gasserian ganglion block (**Fig. 2**) at the level of foramen ovale at the base of the skull usually benefits them from facial pain. Interventional Gasserian ganglion block can be performed under fluoroscopic or computed tomography guidance for precise percutaneous techniques in advanced oral cavity cancers.

Glossopharyngeal Neuralgia

In 1921, Harris coined the term glossopharyngeal neuralgia. He suggested that blockade of the glossopharyngeal nerve (GPN) might be useful in palliating cancer pain. Destruction of the GPN is indicated in the palliation of cancer pain including invasive tumors of the tongue, hypopharynx, and tonsils. This technique is useful in the management of the pain of glossopharyngeal neuralgia for those patients who have failed to respond to medical management or for acute painful emergencies. Diagnostic block can be performed as an outpatient department (OPD) procedure followed by radiofrequency ablation of GPN using landmark technique or under fluoroscopic guidance.

The landmarks (**Fig. 3**) are ipsilateral mastoid process and the angle of the mandible, anteriorly, and the styloid process of the temporal bone. An imaginary line is drawn running from the mastoid process to the angle of mandible. Needle entry point should be in the middle of the two landmarks in a plane perpendicular to the skin. Usually, styloid process is encountered within 3 cm. After contact is made, the needle walked off the styloid process posteriorly. As soon as bony contact is lost and careful aspiration reveals

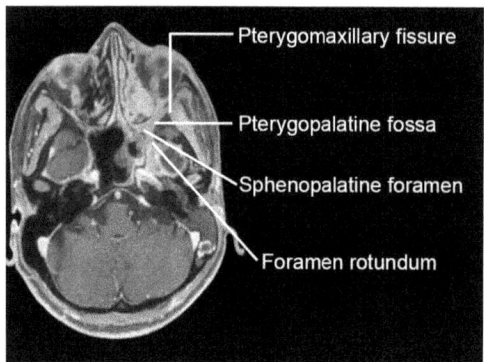

Fig. 1: MRI revealed lesion in Meckel's cave.

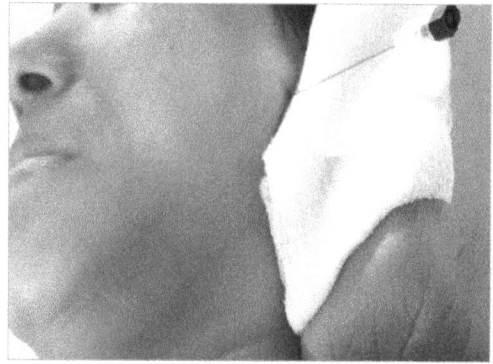

Fig. 2: Needle directed through subzygomatic area.

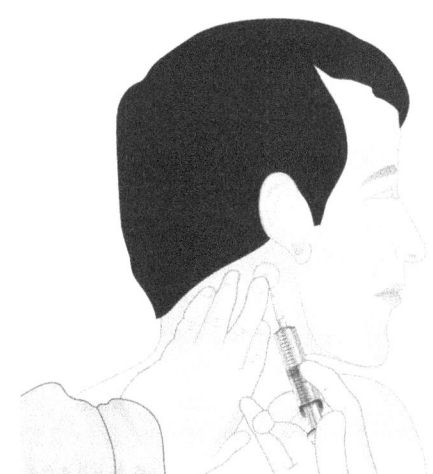

Fig. 3: The landmark for a glossopharyngeal nerve block is between mastoid process and the angle of the mandible. Contact over the styloid process is made in <3 cm.

no blood or cerebrospinal fluid (CSF), 7 mL of 0.5% preservative-free lidocaine combined with 8 mg of dexamethasone is injected. If pain is relieved >50%, radiofrequency ablation of GPN will be done in next setting.

Stellate Ganglion Block

Stellate ganglion block can be performed in painful conditions of oral cavity cancers and posttraumatic syndrome accompanied by swelling and cold sweat. Stellate ganglion block is useful to treat the autonomic component in facial pain.

ORAL MUCOSITIS (TABLE 2)

Incidence of oral mucositis is almost 100% in patients undergoing chemoradiation for oral cavity cancer. Usually, it begins a few days after the start of treatment and peaks in 2 or 3 weeks with the formation of ulceration **(Fig. 4)** and white plaques. Pain is the usual presentation, which becomes worse, if accompanied with superadded fungal, bacterial, or viral infection in neutropenic patients.

TABLE 2: Grades of mucositis.

Grades	Description
0 (none)	None
I (mild)	Erythema and soreness
II (moderate)	Erythema, ulcers, and tolerate solid food
III (severe)	Oral ulcers and tolerate liquids only
IV (life-threatening)	Oral intake impossible

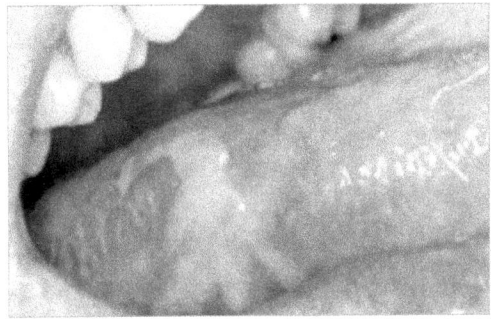

Fig. 4: Ulceration with pseudomembrane on the lateral border of tongue.

Treatment

- Maintain a good oral hygiene
- Maintain hydration adequately
- *Topical analgesia*:
  - Lidocaine viscous 10–15 mL 6 hourly
  - Magic mouthwash 15 mL every 4 hourly
  - Doxepin 0.5%
- Systemic opioids remain the mainstay of treatment.
- Infections such as candidiasis and herpes simplex virus (HSV) should be treated as appropriate.

SALIVARY GLAND DAMAGE AND XEROSTOMIA

Salivary gland has both an acute and late response after the initiation of RT, which is mostly dose dependent. Decreased oral intake due to mucositis and certain medications also further contribute to decreased saliva production. Xerostomia later increases the risk of dental caries and nutritional deficiencies.

Treatment

- Nonpharmacological stimuli such as bitter sweet and sour substances and chewing sugarless gum can increase salivary flow
- Amifostine—in patients receiving RT in head and neck
- Pilocarpine and cevimeline (acetylcholine analog) stimulate saliva production from residual salivary gland, but has no role in prevention of xerostomia.

DENTAL ISSUES

Dental status has a significant impact on quality of life of patients. A comprehensive detailed dental examination prior to the treatment is recommended. Sometimes, long time follow-up too is required, if pain and dental symptoms persist. *Trismus* is characterized by limited jaw opening secondary to mucositis and pain caused by the combination of spasm, fibrosis, and contraction of muscles responsible for temporomandibular joint movement. Trismus results in poor oral hygiene leading to halitosis. Smelling one's own breath odor is often difficult, limiting patient's sociocultural interactions with long-term detrimental effects on psychosocial relationships. Passive motion devices with lifelong stretching exercise are beneficial.

OSTEORADIONECROSIS

Exposure of irradiated bone in the absence of recurrent or residual tumor is termed as osteoradionecrosis. It is important to discuss about osteoradionecrosis because of its symptoms such as pain, bad breath, problems in swallowing and chewing, and communication problems, sometimes leading to pathological fracture. Radiotherapy (RT) in oral cavity cancers generally administers higher doses of radiation in a wider area of mandible and the vascular supply of mandible is not as rich as maxilla. This predisposes mandible for more risk of osteoradionecrosis. Bisphosphonate therapy used for skeletal-related events, hypercalcemia, and reducing cancer-associated metastatic bone pain increases the risk of bisphosphonate-associated osteonecrosis (BON) with vague mandible pain, which later can spread to involve nerve bundles.

Treatment

- Always consider a comprehensive evaluation of disease recurrence
- Conservative debridement with antibiotics and reconstruction in extensive cases are usually successful.

WOUND CARE

Malignant wounds **(Fig. 5)** occur when cancerous cells invade the underlying epithelium and infiltrate adjacent vessels.

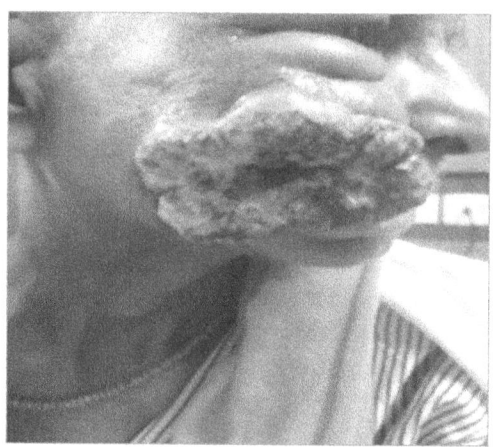

Fig. 5: Malignant wound in submandibular area.

TABLE 3: Problems of malignant wounds.	
Physical problems	Psychosocial problems
Infection	Fear and anxiety
Pain	Depression
Exudate	Body image alteration
Itching	Sexual issues
Bleeding	Social isolation
Nausea	Agitation and guilt
Malodor	Embarrassment and shame

This causes loss of vascularity leading to tissue death and necrosis. Problems of malignant wounds are described in **Table 3**.

Treatment

- Wound assessment—adherent, necrotic, presence of exudates, superficial or deep, odor, bleeding, and painful with or without fistula formation.
- Wound cleaning—shower the wound with water warmed to at least room temperature.
- Malodor—one of the most distressing symptom associated with fungating malignant wounds.

Domiciliary wound care by caregivers:
- Crush 10 tablets of metronidazole (according to the size of wound) into powder form, sprinkle on a gauze piece, add charcoal or newspaper (absorb malodor) is sandwiched between two layers of gauze, and place directly on the wound.
- Pieces of charcoal under the four corners of bed in patients room also help in absorption of malodor.

- Exudate care—use of silicone polymers, zinc oxide, hydrocolloid, or adhesive film dressing may be done.
- Pain—managed using lignocaine- or bupivacaine-soaked gauze pieces covering the wound 15–20 minutes prior to dressing.
- Always maintain a moist environment by avoiding trauma secondary to dryness and crusting.
- Bleeding—local pressure, adrenaline-soaked dressing, bleeding secondary to the infiltration of large vessels, and use of red or green towels should be promoted to reduce the fear and anxiety of the patient and family.
- Maggots—turpentine-soaked gauze close to the wound helps in removing the maggots easily.

KEY POINTS

- Oral cavity cancers affect patient's ability to breathe, speak, and to accept adequate oral intake leading to severely impaired nutrition, disfigurement, and fear of change in self causing a major impact on patient's quality of life.
- A coordinated team involving surgeons, radiologists, medical oncologists, radiation oncologists, dentists, pathologists, supportive care specialists, occupational therapists, speech therapists, nutritionists, and skilled nurses are required for multimodal team-based approach.
- Supportive care team educates the patients about emotional stress-coping strategies and guide families.
- Do not abandon patients, if their disease is no longer curable because there may be a limit to cure, but no limit to care.
- Postradical neck dissection, e.g., where sternocleidomastoid muscle has been removed, makes identification of styloid process much easier, almost in the subcutaneous plane; this block can be performed in a much easier way.

Quality of Life of Oral Cancer Patients

Kinshuki Jain

INTRODUCTION

Oral cancers constitute 10% of all cancers in India. It is estimated that more than 70,000 people in India died of oral cancer in 2018. A diagnosis of cancer is usually associated with significant anxiety and its treatment has implications not only on physical being, but also on psychological well-being. Cancers involving head and neck have a huge impact on every aspect of quality of life (QOL) of patients due to the anatomical structures involved with vital functions such as eating, swallowing, speaking, and also the physical appearance. Many patients suffering from oral cancer in India are from poor socioeconomic status, who already have limited resources and lack awareness. This leads to late presentations of the patients with advanced disease and poor QOL.

The World Health Organization (WHO) defines QOL as an individual's perception of his/her position in life in the context of the culture and value systems in which he/she lives and in relation to his/her goals, expectations, standards, and concerns. The patient's QOL is increasingly being recognized as a major objective of cancer treatment.

Even though a highly subjective and multidimensional issue, various scales and instruments have been formulated to record the QOL.

The various scales for QOL assessment can be broadly classified into the following categories **(Table 1)**:

- *Performance instruments*: To assess the performance status of the patient, e.g., Karnofsky performance scale and Eastern Cooperative Oncology Group (ECOG).
- *Global or generic instruments*: These include simple indicators, health profiles, and utility measures. They are applicable to health status in general and best suited for population and comparative studies, e.g., Medical Outcomes Study SF-36 health survey, Duke health profile, and WHOQOL-100.
- *Disease-specific instruments*: These concentrate on a particular disease or symptoms. These have higher specificity for a particular disease state. They are best suited for evaluative purposes, e.g., EORTC QLQ-30 (European Organization for the Research and Treatment of Cancer Quality of Life Questionnaire) and cancer-specific modules, FACT-cancer-specific modules, chronic respiratory disease questionnaire, and adult asthma QOL questionnaire. For purposes of use in head and neck cancer patients, it can be divided into general cancer instruments and those specific for head and neck cancer **(Table 2)**.
- *Function-specific instruments*: Designed for detailed assessment of a particular

TABLE 1: QOL assessment scales specific for head and neck cancers.

Scales	Questions	
UW-QOLR4	15	12 single questions + 3 global questions
EORTC QLQ-H&N35	35	• 7—pain, swallowing, senses, speech, social eating, social contact, and sexuality • Includes 10 single items
LORQ	25	• 25 items about oral function and denture satisfaction • A four-point Likert scale is used
FACT-H&N	39	FACT-G + 12 items
NCCN-FACT FHNSI-22	22	3—DRS, TSE, FWB
HNCI	30	4—speech (10), eating (11), aesthetics (2), and social disruption (7)
HNQOL	20	• 4—pain, emotion, communication, and eating • Includes single item on overall disturbance of both
PSS-HN	3	3—understandability of speech, normalcy of diet, and eating in public
N	39	39 questions marked on Likert scale of 10

(DRS: disease-related subscale; EORTC QLQ-H&N35: European Organization for Research and Treatment of Cancer Quality of Life Questionnaire Head and Neck Module; FACT-H&N: Functional Assessment of Cancer Therapy—Head and Neck; FWB: functional well-being subscale; HNCI: head and neck cancer inventory; HNQOL: University of Michigan Head and Neck Quality of Life Survey; LORQ: Liverpool Oral Rehabilitation; NCCN-FACT FHNSI-22: NCCN-Functional Assessment of Cancer Therapy-Head and Neck Cancer Symptom Index-22; PSS-HN: Performance Status Scale-Head and Neck; QOL: quality of life; QOL-RTI/H&N: Quality of Life Radiation Therapy Instrument/Head and Neck Module; TSE: treatment side-effect subscale; UW-QOL-R: University of Washington Quality of Life Head and Neck Questionnaire Revised)

symptom, e.g., xerostomia, swallowing, voice, and sleep, for head and neck cancer patients.

- *Preference-based (utility measures)*: Used for determination of quality-adjusted life-years (QALYs) as a unit of effectiveness in cost-effectiveness analysis of medical interventions, e.g., Health Utilities Index-3 (HUI-3) and SF-6D.

There is still no ideal questionnaire encompassing every aspect. Thus, open interview, semi-structured interview, and even customized simple questionnaires may be utilized for better patient care. The choice should be guided by patient condition, patient and clinician preferences, required outcomes in focus, and available resources. The QOL questionnaire may be completed over telephonic interview, in-clinic interview, through mail, or handed to the patient to be filled at home and brought on the next follow-up visit. Computer-adaptive tests (CATs) utilize a technology for logical presentation of questionnaires to reduce respondent burden by producing high reliability and validity with fewer questions. This type is also known as *dynamic questionnaires*.

The QOL instruments intend to improve a patient's QOL by not only improving health outcomes but also serving as one of the two primary endpoints (survival benefit and improvement in QOL) that could be considered for approval of new anticancer drugs.

TABLE 2: Other specific scales of use in head and neck cancer patients.

Care impact	Care satisfaction	Voice and speech	Mucositis and xerostomia	Swallowing and mastication
Caregiver Quality of Life Index-Cancer (CQOLC)	EORTC InPatient SATisfaction with care questionnaire 32 (IN-PATSAT 32)	Vocal Handicap Index (VHI)	Oral Mucositis Weekly Questionnaire—Head and Neck Cancer (OMWQ-HN)	MD Anderson Dysphagia Inventory (MDADI)
Neck Dissection Impairment Index (NDII)	OutPatient SATisfaction with care questionnaire (OUT-PATSAT 35)	Speech Handicap Index (SHI)	Oral Mucositis Daily Questionnaire (OMDQ)	Subjective Chewing Ability
Head and Neck Radiotherapy Questionnaire (HNRQ)		University of Michigan Voice-related Quality of Life (V-RQOL)	Oropharyngeal Mucositis Quality of Life Scale (OMQOL)	Sydney Swallow Questionnaire (SSQ)
Quality of Life Radiation Therapy Instrument with Head and Neck Companion Module (QOL-RTI/H&N)		Voice Prosthesis Questionnaire (VPQ)	Swallowing Quality of Life Questionnaire (SWAL-QOL)	
Quality of Life—Enteral Feeding (QOL-EF) questionnaire			Xerostomia Questionnaire (XQOL)	Swallowing Quality of Care Questionnaire (SWAL-CARE)
			Xerostomia Questionnaire VAS	
			Xerostomia-related Quality of Life Scale (XeQOLs)	

(EORTC: European Organization for Research and Treatment of Cancer)

DOMAINS OF IMPACT OF ORAL CANCER ON QOL

- Physical
- Psychosocial
- Financial

Physical Impact

Oral cancer and its treatments affect the face, voice, speech, and swallowing physically **(Boxes 1 and 2)**. The functional impairment in these domains leads to significant psychological impact related to each of the domains. QOL assessment tools should assess both of these components. Functional end points measure the degree to which the patient can carry out the activity. Psychosocial impact refers to the effect caused by the functional impairment on the patient's psychological and social well-being.

Aesthetics Impact

Oral cancer itself and its treatment (both during and after) disfigure the face and affect the cosmetic appearance leading to multitude of physical and psychosocial issues associated with it. The functional outcomes after oral cancer resection depend upon the

> **Box 1:** Challenges associated with quality of life (QOL) assessment.
> - Difficulty to maintain uniformity due to subjective issue
> - Lack of inclination of practicing clinicians to give importance to QOL
> - Lack of awareness amongst patients to take informed decisions to maintain their QOL
> - Time constraints
> - Lack of resources
> - Responder burden
> - Deciphering what research findings mean and their significance for a particular patient

> **Box 2:** Psychosocial impact.
> - Physical disfigurement
> - Social stigmatization
> - Pain
> - Skin changes due to radiotherapy
> - Alopecia due to chemotherapy
> - Speech and voice problems
> - Eating problems
> - Depression or anxiety due to disease and its sequelae
> - Weakness due to nutritional issues
> - Halitosis

size and location of tumor and the extent of resection. Reconstructive surgery is often warranted to help restore functions to a certain extent.

Voice and Speech Impact

Speech is affected in most of the patients of oral cancer both due to the tumor itself and as sequelae of chemotherapy and radiotherapy. These treatments lead to mucositis, xerostomia, pain as well as oral ulcerations which lead to altered speech due to difficulty in articulation. Articulation problems are most common in patients with tongue cancer in comparison to those with buccal cancer. The voice may also be severely affected due to several reasons—altered anatomy of tongue or larynx or oral mucosal edema or xerostomia, impairment of vocal cord mobility, and pain or extreme weakness. Resonance may also be altered due to anatomical changes. Some of these effects decrease with time (e.g., due to mucositis) but may also increase with passing time (e.g., due to increase in tumor size).

Swallowing Impact

Swallowing is commonly affected in oral cancer. Many causes include improper mastication post-surgery (e.g., mandibulectomy), dental problems, distorted tongue anatomy, postradiation fibrosis, mucositis, etc. Impaired swallowing is associated with an increased risk of aspiration and its sequelae. Swallowing dysfunction is managed by teaching the patient different postures (head turn or chin tuck), certain maneuvers (e.g., breath-hold before swallow), or tongue exercises under specialist guidance. Diet modifications, use of intraoral prosthetics, or insertion of enteral tubes may also be required.

Psychosocial Impact

Oral cancer patients experience low self-esteem and social alienation due to multiple reasons **(Box 2)**.

A multidisciplinary approach involving a comprehensive rehabilitation plan, including dentist, psychotherapist, and occupational and physical therapist may help improve the patient's QOL. Group therapy with survivors is also very beneficial.

The family or the caregiver burden is often an ignored aspect in cancer care. Family is integral in patient care, and its reactions and opinions during patient care can have a positive or negative impact on the patient and disease management. There are various issues associated with family which have a direct impact on patient management, e.g., collusion, abandonment of patient, or pathological grief. Involvement of a psychiatrist or support groups helps improve QOL for the family and in turn the patient.

Financial Impact

Cancer treatment is costly and most patients report a significant impact on finances due to treatment. The patients consider the cost as a major burden on their families. Loss of work by both the patient and the caregiver compound the situation. These financial struggles lead to materialistic as well as emotionally and psychologically poor QOL. The guilt of not being able to provide "best" treatment to their loved one due to financial constraints is one of the most common guilts that persists for a prolonged duration in the caregivers. Social workers, support groups, government aids, or community resources usually extend help in such cases.

KEY POINTS

- QOL considerations are increasingly attaining priority position in the management of oral cancers. Thus, a clinician must be aware of various instruments to assess, record, and plan for improving QOL of the patient.
- Active patient participation in treatment planning should be encouraged. The clinician should pay attention to not just the clinical effects of treatment but also the impact on QOL as a primary endpoint.
- The complex interplay of various symptoms and their impact on physical, psychosocial, emotional, and financial aspects should be assessed and addressed through a multidisciplinary team approach.

CHAPTER 34

Case Presentation for Postgraduate Students

Vikas Arora

INTRODUCTION

Case presentation should be done in chronological order and discussion goes in following order.
- History taking
- Physical examination
- Clinical diagnosis
- Special investigation
- Treatment—both medical and surgical
- Progress during postoperative period
- Follow-up

It is a good practice to observe each patient when he walks into the room, observe any facial asymmetry, obvious swelling, and whether the patient is wheelchair-bound or cachectic. Is he moving with hanky in his hand (due excessive to salivation) or a water bottle in hand (postradiation)?

HISTORY TAKING

It starts with particulars of the patient.
- *Name*: It is important for identification of the patient, data record, and to make personal rapport with the patient. Addressing the patient with first name initiates trust relationship between doctor and patient.
- *Age*: The highest incidence of oral cancer is usually seen in 50–59 years of age group. The lowest incidence is noted among young patients age < 40 years.
- *Sex*: Prevalence of tobacco use in the ages of 13–15 years among boys is 19% and girls is 8.3% according to the Global Youth Tobacco Survey, which was done in 2009. According to the recent National Family Health Survey for the study in the year 2015–2016, there were 38.9% of men who used tobacco (any form) in urban areas while 48% of men who used tobacco in rural areas of India. On the other hand, 4.4% of women in urban and 8.1% of women in rural use any kind of tobacco. Tobacco and alcohol-related oral cancer is much more common in men, while sharp tooth or ill-fitted dentures-related oral squamous cell carcinoma (OSCC) is equally prevalent among men and women.
- *Residence and socioeconomic status*: The prevalence of oral cancer is more common in lower socioeconomic strata related to tobacco use.
- *Occupation*: Tobacco use has a strong association with outdoor occupation, mainly farmers and laborers. The lower lip is subjected to intense and chronic sun exposure and, thus ultraviolet (UV) radiation, which may contribute to it being the most common site for OSCC in males and in population of fair skin.

CHIEF COMPLAINTS

Patients suspicious of oral malignancy usually present with following symptoms:
- *Ulcer or swelling in mouth*: In spite of conservative treatment, the lesions of lip, cheek, tongue, and floor of mouth (FOM)

may present as a nonhealing ulcer. Enquire about the onset, duration, and progress of the lesion.
- *Pain in mouth*: Careful history must be taken about its site, radiation, or referred pain, which is not relieved with medications. If a patient presents with ulcer of the tongue without pain, it is an ominous sign of malignancy.
  Site of pain is important. For example, local site of pain over the tongue suggests a dental ulcer due to sharp tooth. Late cases of carcinoma of tongue may present as referred pain to ear (it is usually observed in lateral tongue lesions more specifically at the base of tongue).
- *Excessive salivation*: It is a very common specific complaint of carcinoma of tongue. If a patient is seen in outdoor patient department, holding handkerchief in his mouth, he is probably suffering from carcinoma of tongue. This is partly due to irritation of nerves of taste and partly due to difficulty in swallowing due to ankyloglossia.
- *Difficulty in speech*: It is also one of the complaints of carcinoma of tongue, especially if the lesion involves either tip of tongue or posterior one-third of tongue.
- *Deviation of tip of tongue*: When protruded outward toward the side of lesion is a sign of carcinoma of tongue.
- *Trismus*: Difficulty in opening mouth.
- *Ankyloglossia*: Difficulty in protruding tongue and also named as tongue-tie. This indicates that the carcinomatous process has infiltrated the lingual musculature and even FOM.
- *Fetor oris*: History of offensive smell usually indicates fungating malignant lesion in the oral cavity.
- *Erythroleukoplakia*: A white or red patch on the gums, tongue, or cheek of mucosa.
- *Dysphagia*: Difficulty in swallowing or chewing (FOM lesions and jaw lesions).
- Pain in the teeth or jaw and loosening of one or more teeth without obvious reason (*ill-fitted dentures*).
- Numbness of the tongue or teeth or lips.
- Bleeding from gums or cheek lesions.
- History of neck swelling persisting >3 weeks.

HISTORY OF RISK FACTORS/ LIFESTYLE BEHAVIORS OR HABITS

- *Tobacco consumption*: To be asked in detail for smoking pack years.
- *Alcohol intake*: There is a higher incidence of oral cancer in people who are heavy smokers and heavy drinkers. The reason for the increased cancer risk may be due to the carcinogenic effect of the metabolites of ethanol and acetaldehyde. Women who drink heavily and smoke have a higher incidence of oral cancer.
- Sun exposure is the primary risk factor for lip cancer, but pipe smoking also is a risk factor.
- Repeated trauma by sharp tooth
- Lower socioeconomic status
- Unhealthy diet with low fruit and vegetable intake
- Lack of physical activity
- History of drug abuse

TREATMENT HISTORY

- History of any treatment taken before first presentation should be noted such as chemotherapy, radiotherapy, and any symptomatic treatment for sore mouth or throat.
- Koch's treatment
- Medication for diabetes, hypertension, hypo- or hyperthyroidism, and for other

long-term illnesses such as chronic obstructive pulmonary disease (COPD), arthritis, and psychiatric illness.
- History of allergic reaction to any medication.
- Any history of anesthesia in past and any difficulties during or after (previous) anesthesia.

FAMILY HISTORY

History of cancer in immediate or close relatives.

PERSONAL HISTORY

- Marital status and number of children
- History of extramarital sexual activity

PAST HISTORY

- History of any treatment for cancer in form of surgery, radiotherapy, or chemotherapy in past (this may interfere or need modification in current treatment plan). *Also, modification in reconstructive plan, if needed in the present malignancy.*
- History of any major surgery in the recent past.
- History of any cerebrovascular accident (CVA) episode, seizures, or comorbidities such as diabetes mellitus (DM) and hypertension (HTN).

EXAMINATION

A thorough oral, head, and neck cancer examination can easily be completed in <5 minutes. It primarily consists of inspection and palpation.

General Examination

- Once good rapport has been established with the patient, the clinician is ready to begin the examination.
- It is important to explain to the patient exactly what you are doing before doing it.
- Not only will this help put the patient at ease, but it also gives you the opportunity to educate your patient about the signs and symptoms of head and neck cancers and how to detect it at an early stage.
- The initial physical evaluation of a patient actually begins as soon as you meet the patient.
- Note the level of consciousness, posture, vitals, pallor, jaundice, pedal edema, nails, and jugular venous pressure (JVP).
- While taking the patient's history, it is helpful to note any facial asymmetry, swelling on face, neck, skin lesions, facial paralysis, swelling or temporal wasting, and watering of eyes.
- Inspection of the lips, both moving and at rest, can also be performed while first meeting the patient. Again, look for any asymmetry or gross lesions on the lips.
- Commonly changes noticed in a person's face and body pertaining to weight loss, anorexia, and/or fatigue may be the first sign of a malignancy.
- *Listening is an important part of this examination.* The sound of one's voice and speech are important in consideration of the location of tumors as a "hot potato" voice that may signal the presence of an oropharyngeal tumor whereas a raspy, hoarse voice could be the first sign of a laryngeal neoplasm.

Listen → Look → Feel

Inspection

- The entire face should be examined with an external light source (overhead light or headlight) to evaluate for pigmented (red, brown, and black), raised, ulcerated, or firm areas of the skin including the

hair-bearing regions of the face and scalp. Note any satellite nodules and obliteration of nasolabial fold.
- The facial bones, skeleton, and soft tissue should be inspected particularly noting asymmetry or masses.
- Outer surface of lips is to be examined and retract the lips to see the mucosal surface of the lips.
- Mouth opening to be evaluated—*look for trismus*.
- Finding which gets noticed first—*look for oral submucous fibrosis* (OSMF).
- Observe the condition of tooth near any ulcerated area and also note orodental hygiene and dentition.
- Lips:
  - Cracked lips are usually observed when exposed to cold lips and also observed near the angle of mouth.
  - Ectopic salivary neoplasms are usually seen in the upper lip as slow-growing lobulated tumors.
  - Carcinoma of the lip is seen in old individuals and presents as erosion in the early stage—as red granular appearance with whitish flecks followed by yellowish crusting in the middle of the erosion. Gradually, the center becomes ulcerated and the margin becomes everted.
- *Tongue*:
  - Ask the patient to open the mouth wide while relaxing the tongue. Note any ulcerations, swellings, or other abnormalities. Then have the patient stick out his or her tongue and move it from side to side. Make a note of factor breath as soon as patient opens mouth.
  - Any ulcerated area over tongue, look for shape, surface, margins, and color.
  - It should move easily and completely toward both sides without spasm or asymmetry. *Look for ankyloglossia.*
  - Observe the dorsum of the tongue and noting any discolorations, irregularities, or limitations to movement, all of which may be a sign of cancer.
  - One of the most common sites of oral cancer is on the lateral aspect of the tongue and it must be evaluated completely. This often requires using gauze to pull the tongue out and roll it from side to side while retracting the cheek with a tongue blade or stick.
  - Involvement of FOM, midline, and base of tongue. See surrounding mucosa around the index lesion.
  - Look for any other lesion or patch in mouth, such as *leukoplakia*, which is a white patch, often present as chronic superficial glossitis and sometimes present as thickened plaque.
  - Certain tongue lesions, which need attention and are kept in differential diagnosis:
    - *Red-glazed tongue* when the leukoplakia plaques are desquamated.
    - Blue color of *venous hemangioma*
    - *Black hairy tongue*, due to hyperkeratosis of the mucous membrane in heavy smokers or caused by a fungus called *Aspergillus niger*, are characteristic.
    - *Lingual thyroid*—angioma-like swelling in the region of the foramen cecum.
  - Other nonspecific lesions of tongue—crack or fissure is noted over tongue. Note the direction of the fissures. Congenital fissures are mainly transverse, whereas syphilitic fissures are usually longitudinal.

- *Palate*:
  - Note for congenital cleft, perforation, ulceration, or swelling over palate.
  - Patients with reverse smoking may present with ulcerated area over hard palate. Map the lesion. Extent of lesion, particularly upper buccogingival sulcus involvement, soft palate, retromolar trigone (RMT), and midline extension.
  - Condition of teeth
- *Gums*:
  - One needs to evert the lips or retract cheek to look for gums in entirety with the help of spatula. Healthy looking gums are bright pink in color.
  - The earliest sign of pyorrhea alveolaris is deep red line along the free edge of the gum.
  - Vincent's stomatitis is an inflammatory condition of the gingivae.
  - Any ulcerated area of gums can be seen as proliferative or infiltrative lesion, and can sometimes bleed, is suspicious of carcinoma of lower alveolus.
  - See condition of teeth, tanning, and caries.
- *Floor of mouth*:
  - FOM lesion can be observed by asking the patient to keep the tongue upward to touch the palate. Note for any swelling or ulcer.
  - A *ranula* appears as a unilateral bluish translucent cyst over which Wharton's duct can often be seen.
  - An ulcerated lesion in FOM usually presents as infiltrative lesion. It can be an extension of carcinoma of ventral tongue.
  - Ask the patient to protrude his tongue (Note any ankyloglossia).
  - Adjacent mucosa around index lesion.
  - Condition of teeth and gingival thickness (GT) of sulcus.
- *Cheek*:
  - The inner surface of cheek is to be examined carefully for any ulcer, patch, mucous cyst, lipoma, mixed salivary tumor, or pigmented lesion.
  - People sometimes present with dental impression (as interdentate line) over buccal mucosa, which is a normal finding. Mention about surrounding mucosa.
  - Special mention of buccogingival sulci (upper and lower), RMT, angle of mouth, extension to palate or alveoli and overlying skin.

Palpation

- Palpate the dorsum and lateral margins of the tongue, paying special attention to any masses or firm/fixated areas. Being careful not to gag the patient and palpate the lingual tonsils.
- Palpate third dimension of the lesion between two fingers and also look whether the lesion is crossing midline or involving base of tongue. This may change the treatment plan or modify reconstructive plan, if needed.

The patient has touched the roof of their mouth with the tip of their tongue. This will allow the examiner to inspect the ventral surface of tongue.

- FOM should be examined thoroughly and also bimanual palpation is to be done.
- Examine temporomandibular (TM) joint movement. Palpate obvious swelling on face, neck, and nape of neck.
- *Lips*: Any lesion of the lip should be carefully palpated. While benign neoplasms are firm and lobulated, whereas carcinoma of the lip is hard in consistency.

- *Tongue*:
  - While palpating for induration of the base of an ulcer, it is desirable that the tongue should be relaxed and at rest within the mouth. If it is kept protruded, the contracted muscles may give a false impression of induration and lead to error in diagnosis.
  - On palpation, the ulcer may bleed, usually suggestive of malignant ulcer. Also, palpate sharp tooth or tooth plate against an ulcer in the tongue.
  - Palpate the back of the tongue for any ulcer or swelling. The patient sits on a stool. The examiner stands on his right side.
- *Palate*: Mixed tumor of minor salivary gland (such as adenoid cystic carcinoma or acinic cell carcinoma) may be felt in the palate, as smooth bulge with no ulceration.
- *Gums*:
  - Epulis is a swelling of the alveolar margin of the gum. The margin, consistency, surface, and mobility are to be noted.
  - Pyogenic granuloma over gums may also sometimes mimic malignancy of alveolar process.
- *Floor of mouth*:
  - A *ranula* is a fluctuating swelling with positive translucency. To know its extent, bimanual palpation of the FOM on one side and submandibular triangle on the other hand are necessary.
  - Carcinoma of the FOM may be revealed by its indurated base and probable fixation to the underlying structures.
  - Bimanual examination of tongue and FOM is extremely important.
- *Cheek*:
  - Mucous cyst has a smooth surface and is movable over the deeper structures. Fluctuation can be elicited by pressing on the top of the cyst, while the sides are palpated by other two fingers. Carcinoma is fixed and indurated.
  - In case of trismus, finger palpation may not be feasible, a spatula may be useful.

EXAMINATION OF NECK (FIGS. 1A AND B)

The patient sits, so that his face is at your eye level; support the head with a headrest. Palpate the neck comparing both sides for signs of enlargement.

- Palpate carefully for enlarged lymph nodes. Examine the submental and submandibular region carefully.
- The anterior deep cervical lymph nodes are palpated with the patient's head hyperextended and turned to relax sternocleidomastoid muscle.
- Using two hands, the fingertips of one gently retract the sternocleidomastoid muscle backward, while the fingertips of the other hand, hooked around the front of the neck, palpate the region of the carotid sheath.
- This examination also can be performed with one-hand palpation by placing aligned fingertips along the posterior border of the sternocleidomastoid muscle, while the thumb provides counterpressure from the anterior aspect of the muscle.
- The fingertips are gradually moved inferiorly along the sternocleidomastoid muscle.
- The preauricular and posterior auricular lymph nodes are examined next using

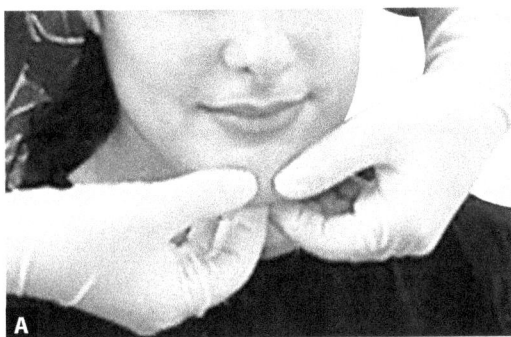 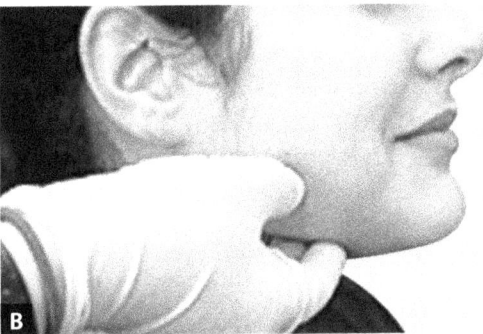

Figs. 1A and B: Examination of neck.

bilateral placement of both hands. The preauricular lymph nodes are located in front of the ear and the postauricular nodes are located behind the ear.
- The supraclavicular nodes are located on the inferior part of the front of neck, superior to the clavicle.
- The occipital lymph nodes are located at the base of the skull.
- The auricular lymph nodes are palpated by the bilateral placement of both hands on the skin surface with the fingertips arranged to cover a large surface area.
- Note the size, location and number, fixity of nodes, and involvement of skin. Any signs of inflammation and satellite nodules in neck and upper chest should be mentioned.
- Palpate other sites of lymph node enlargement, e.g., axilla.

DIFFERENTIAL DIAGNOSIS OF CARCINOMA OF TONGUE

- *Leukoplakia*: This presents as white-colored thickened patches of epithelium, which have lost their papillae and cover the dorsal surface of the tongue. If the superficial epithelium shed over a considerable area, a "red-glazed tongue" may develop. It has been observed that 30% of cases of carcinoma of the mouth are preceded by leukoplakia.

Five stages are recognizable in this condition:
1. *Stage I*—mild thickening of the surface with hypertrophy of the papillae and hyperkeratosis
2. *Stage II*—stage of leukoplakia—the tongue is covered with smooth paint
3. *Stage III*—the surface becomes irregular such as dried paint
4. *Stage IV*—warty projections appear with cracks and fissures (precancerous stage)
5. *Stage V*—desquamation of the abnormal mucosa leading to "red-glazed tongue." This condition may gradually lead to carcinoma.

- *Macroglossia*: This means chronic painless enlargement of the tongue. The causes are lymphangioma, hemangioma (which may be associated with congenital arteriovenous fistula), plexiform neurofibroma, muscular macroglossia (is often a feature of cretinism), and amyloid infiltration.
- *Ulcers of the tongue*: Various types of ulcers may be found in the tongue. Of these, the important ulcers are described below:
  - *Aphthous (dyspeptic) ulcer*: It is a small painful ulcer seen on the tip, undersurface, and sides of the tongue in its anterior part. The ulcer is small and superficial, with white floor and

yellowish border, and surrounded by a hyperemic zone.
- *Dental ulcer*: It is caused by mechanical irritation either by a jagged tooth or denture. These ulcers occur at the periphery or on the undersurface of the tongue at the sides. This ulcer is elongated, often presents a slough at its base, and surrounded by a zone of erythema and induration. This ulcer is quite painful.
- *Chronic nonspecific ulcer*: This usually occurs in the anterior two-thirds of the tongue. No etiological factor can be found out. It is moderately indurated and not very painful.
- *Carcinomatous ulcer*: This is painless to start with and only becomes painful in late cases. Pain may be referred to the ear. The ulcer has a raised and everted edge with indurated base. Lymph node involvement is also quite early.
- *Carcinoma of the tongue*: It can be—(a) Warty or proliferative type, (b) Ulcerating or excavating type, (c) Fissure or crack type following chronic superficial glossitis, (d) Nodular type, (e) Frozen type, when the tongue is transformed into indurated mass or infiltrative, and (f) Verrucous/bush like.
- *Spread of tongue carcinoma*:
  - *Local*—the tumor may locally spread into the FOM and mandible when the growth is situated on the anterior two-thirds of tongue.
  - *Lymphatic*—spread takes place into the submental, submandibular, jugulodigastric, and jugulo-omohyoid group of lymph nodes of the same side as well as opposite side.
  - *Blood spread*—lung
- *Cause of death*:
  - Inhalation bronchopneumonia due to aspiration
  - Cancer cachexia and starvation
  - Hemorrhage from primary growth
  - Asphyxia

COMMONLY ASKED QUESTIONS

1. What are the causes of otalgia? Discuss neural pathways of otalgia.
2. What are the causes of recent-onset trismus?
3. What are the causes of ankyloglossia? Enumerate muscles of tongue.
4. What are the morphological types of tongue cancer?
5. Discuss the approach to nonhealing ulcer of tongue.
6. How do you counsel a patient for tongue cancer surgery? What functional deficits can occur?
7. How do you decide about type of reconstruction?
8. What are the indications of postoperative radiotherapy?
9. When do you add chemotherapy? Which trials support addition of CT to RT?
10. What salient features do you expect that your pathologist should report?
11. What is the role of immunotherapy in recurrent tongue cancer?
12. What are the side effects of cisplatin? Enumerate the details of DCF regimen, dose, indications, and trials.

CHAPTER 35

Cancer of the Oral Cavity (NCCN Guidelines)

Swarupa Mitra, Abhinav Dewan

BUCCAL MUCOSA, FLOOR OF MOUTH, ANTERIOR MOUTH, ALVEOLAR RIDGE, RETROMOLAR TRIGONE, HARD PALATE

Workup

- H&P including a complete head and neck examination; mirror and fiberoptic examination as clinically indicated
- Biopsy
- *As clinically indicated:*
  - Chest CT (with or without contrast)
  - CT with contrast and/or MRI with contrast of primary and neck
  - Consider FDG PET/CT
  - Examination under anesthesia (EUA) with endoscopy
  - Pre-anesthesia studies
  - Dental/prosthodontic evaluation, including Panorex or dental CT without contrast
  - Nutrition, speech, and swallowing evaluation/therapy
  - Smoking cessation counseling
  - Fertility/reproductive counseling
- Multidisciplinary consultation as indicated

Clinical staging

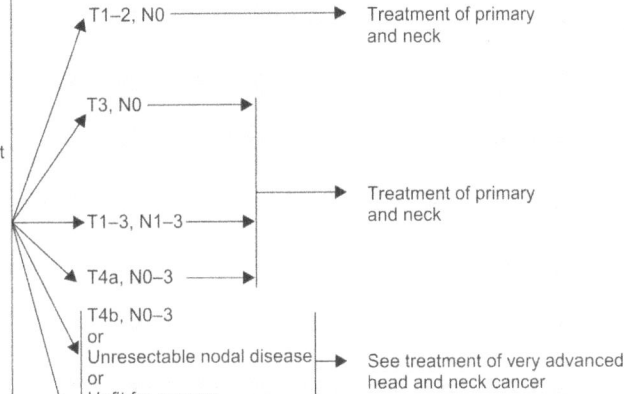

T1–2, N0 → Treatment of primary and neck

T3, N0

T1–3, N1–3 → Treatment of primary and neck

T4a, N0–3

T4b, N0–3 or Unresectable nodal disease or Unfit for surgery → See treatment of very advanced head and neck cancer

Metastatic (M1) disease at initial presentation → See treatment of very advanced head and neck cancer

- H&P should include documentation and quantification (pack years smoked) of tobacco use history. All current smokers should be advised to quit smoking, and former smoker should be advised to remain abstinent from smoking.
- Image-guided (US or CT) needle biopsy of cystic neck nodes may offer better diagnostic yield than FNA by palpation alone for initial diagnosis.

Cancer of the Oral Cavity (NCCN Guidelines)

PRIMARY TREATMENT OF ORAL CANCER

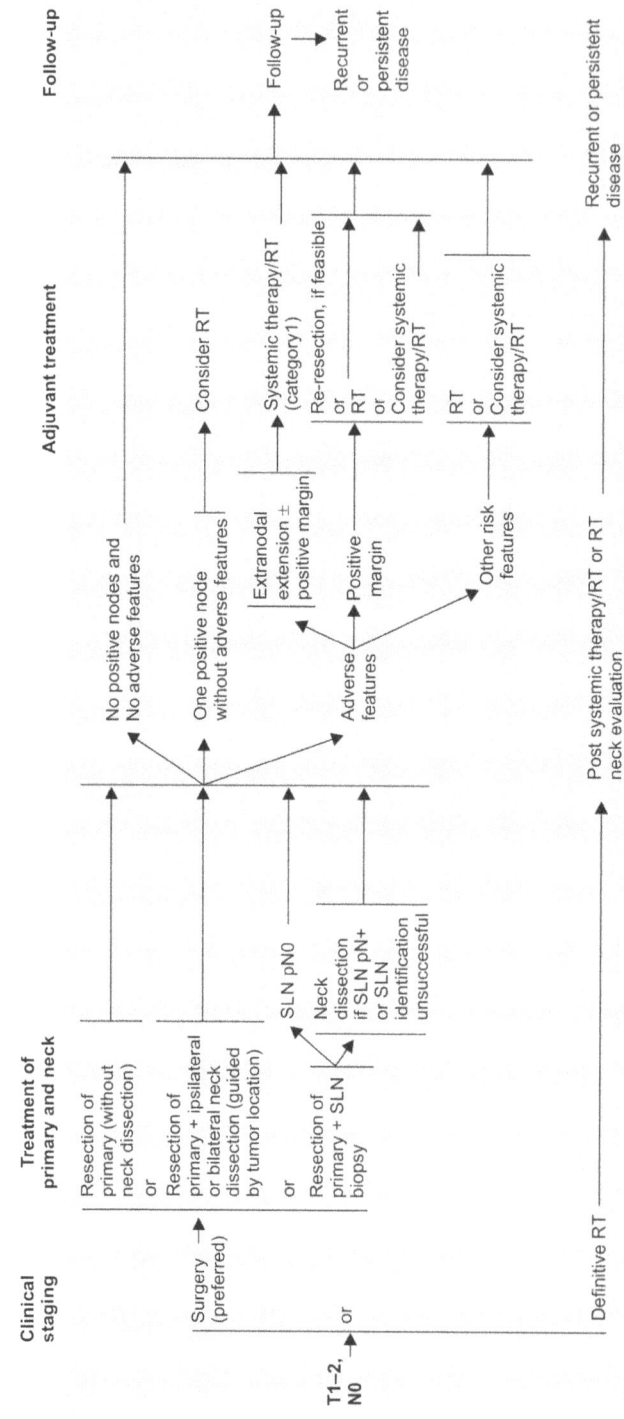

Adverse features: Extranodal extension, positive, close margins, pT3 or pT4 primary, nodal disease in levels IV or V, LVI, PNI.

Cancer of the Oral Cavity (NCCN Guidelines)

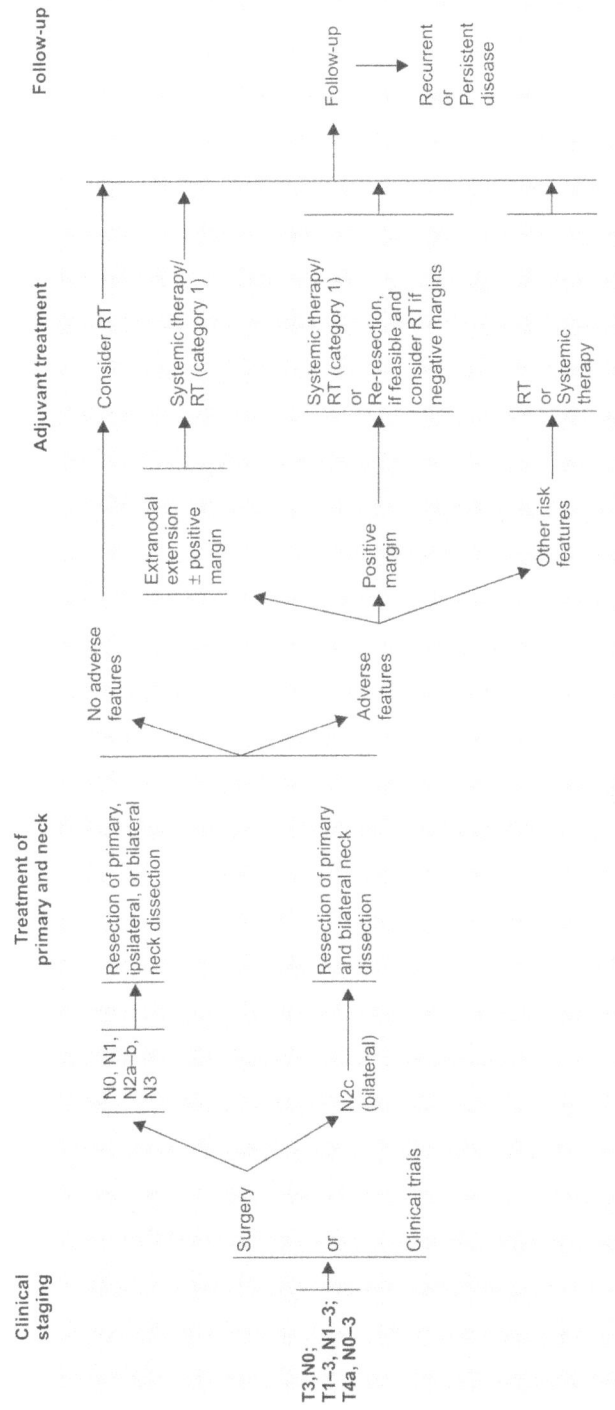

VERY ADVANCED ORAL CANCER (T4b)

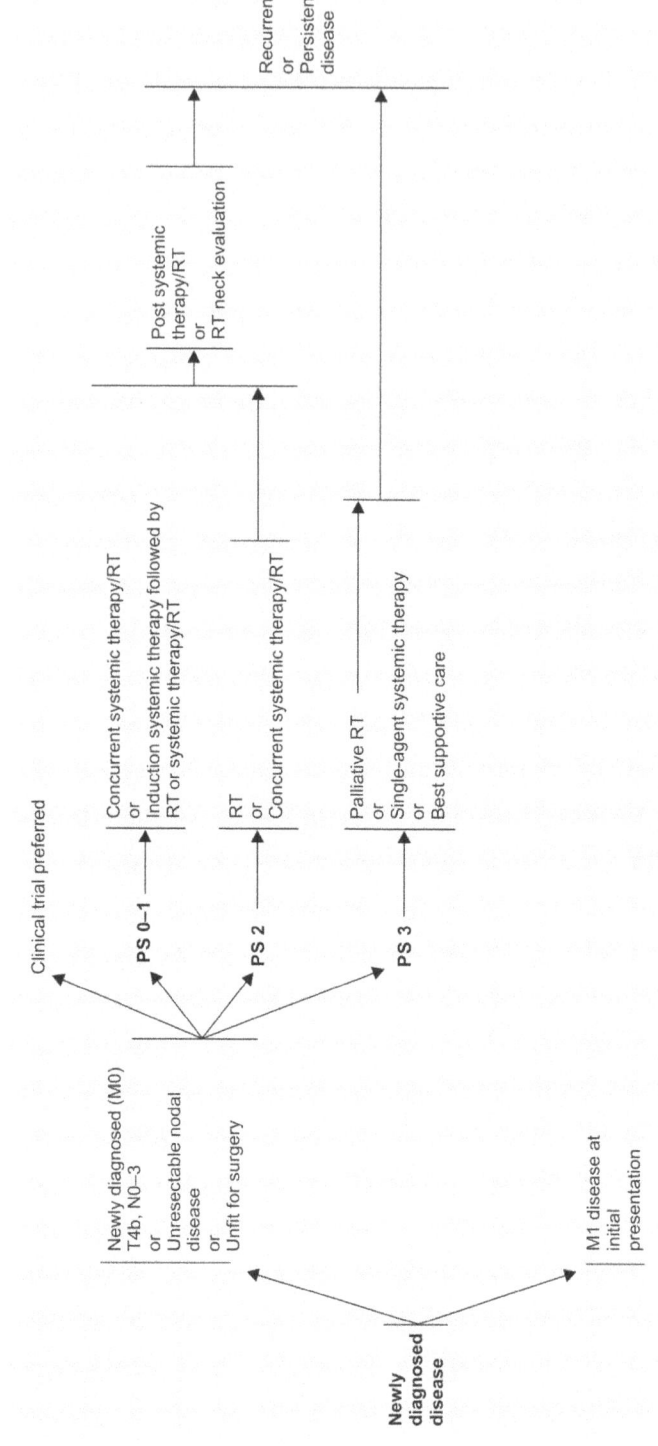

- When using concurrent systemic therapy = RT, the preferred agent is cisplatin (category 1).
- PS = Performance status (ECOG)

Cancer of the Oral Cavity (NCCN Guidelines)

VERY ADVANCED ORAL CANCER (METASTATIC)

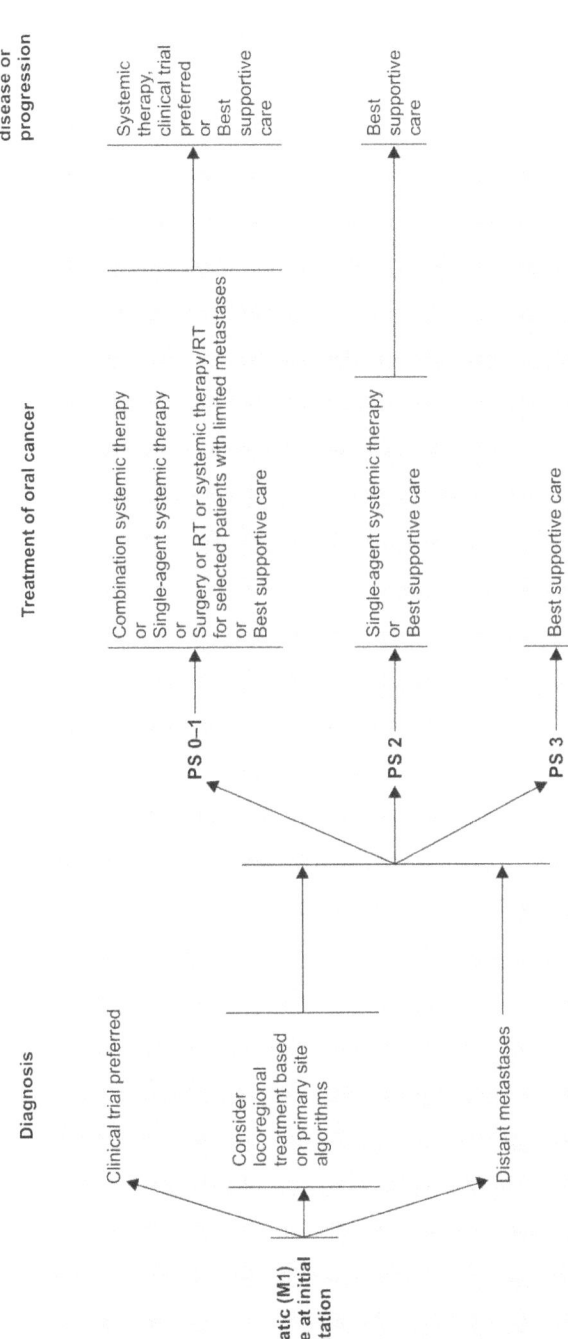

Cancer of the Oral Cavity (NCCN Guidelines)

VERY ADVANCED ORAL CANCER (RECURRENT OR PERSISTENT)

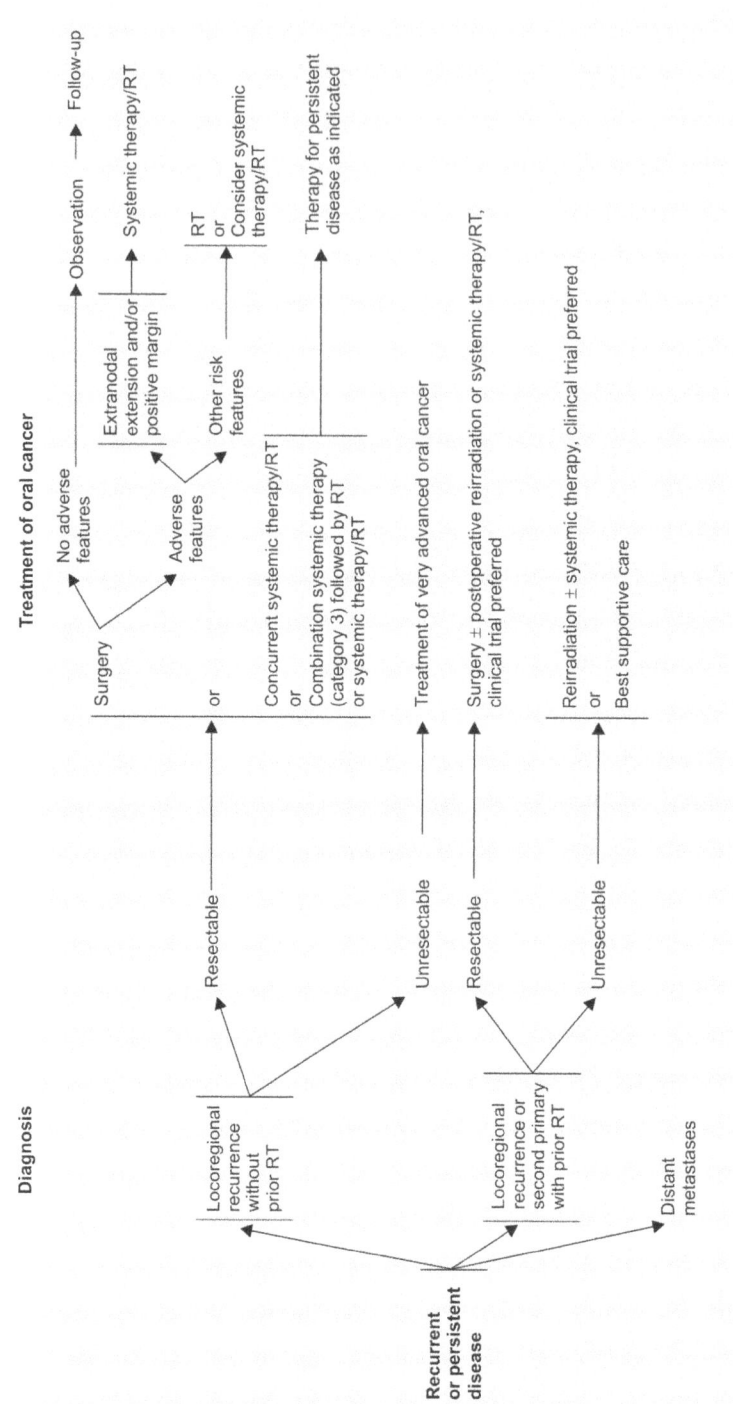

Very Advanced Oral Cancer

Concurrent systemic therapy + RT (preferred for patients eligible for chemotherapy)

Planning target volume (PTV):
- High risk: Typically 70 Gy (2.0 Gy/fraction)
- Low-to-intermediate risk: Sites of suspected subclinical spread:
  - 44–50 Gy (2.0 Gy/fraction) to 54–63 Gy (1.6–1.8 Gy/fraction)

Systemic Therapy + RT

Based on published data, concurrent systemic therapy/RT most commonly uses conventional fractionation at 2.0 Gy/fraction to a typical dose of 70 Gy in 7 weeks with single-agent cisplatin given every 3 weeks at 100 mg/m^2; 2–3 cycles of chemotherapy are used depending on the radiation fractionation scheme (RTOG 0129) When carboplatin and 5-FU are used, then the recommended regimen is standard fractionation plus 3 cycles of chemotherapy. Other fraction sizes (e.g., 1.8 Gy, conventional), multiagent chemotherapy, other dosing schedules of cisplatin, or altered fractionation with chemotherapy are efficacious, and there is no consensus on the optimal approach. Data indicate that accelerated fractionation does not offer improved efficacy over conventional fractionation. In general, the use of concurrent systemic therapy + RT carries a high toxicity burden; altered fractionation or multiagent chemotherapy will likely further increase the toxicity burden.

When the goal of treatment is curative and surgery is not an option, reirradiation strategies can be considered for patients who: develop locoregional failures or second primaries at ≥6 months after the initial radiotherapy; can receive additional doses of radiotherapy of at least 60 Gy; and can tolerate concurrent chemotherapy. Organs at risk for toxicity should be carefully analyzed through review of dose-volume histograms, and consideration for acceptable doses should be made on the basis of time interval since original radiotherapy, anticipated volumes to be included, and patient's life expectancy.

Proton therapy can be considered when normal tissue constraints cannot be met by photon-based therapy.

RERADIATION

- Reirradiation with 3D conformal RT, SBRT, PBT, or IMRT:
  - If the area in consideration overlaps with the previously radiated volume, the prior radiotherapy should have been more than 6 months.
  - In certain rare circumstances, reirradiation with intraoperative RT (IORT) or brachy therapy may be considered.
  - Before reirradiation, the patient should have are asonable ECOG performance status of 0–1. Patients who are more than 2 years from prior radiation, who have surgery to remove gross disease prior to reirradiation, and who are free of organ dysfunction (feeding tube) have better outcomes.
  - The incidence of myelopathy is thought to increase after a cumulative biologic effective dose (BED) of 120 Gy, but this risk is increased if large fraction sizes (≥2.5 Gy/fraction) are used.
  - Radiation volumes should include known disease only to minimize the volume of tissue receiving very high doses in regions of overlap.

Prophylactic treatment of subclinical disease (e.g., elective nodal irradiation) is therefore not routinely indicated.
- When using SBRT techniques for reirradiation, careful selection of patients is advised. The best outcomes are seen in patients with small tumors and no skin involvement. Caution should be exercised in cases of circumferential carotid artery involvement.
- Reirradiation dosing:
  - *Conventional fractionation*:
    - *Postoperative*: 56-60 Gy at 1.8-2 Gy/fraction
    - *Definitive*: 66-70 Gy at 1.8-2 Gy/fraction
  - *Accelerated fractionated*: 60-70 Gy at 1.2-1.5 Gy/fraction twice daily
  - Current SBRT schedules being used or investigated are in the range of 35-44 Gy using 5 fractions.
  - Clinical trials should be strongly considered for patients receiving reirradiation.
- Palliative 3D conformal RT, IMRT, and stereotactic body RT (SBRT):
  - Palliative radiation should be considered in the advanced cancer setting when curative-intent treatment is not appropriate.
  - No general consensus exists for appropriate palliative RT regimens in head and neck cancer. For those who are either medically unsuitable for standard RT or who have widely metastatic disease, palliative RT should be considered. RT regimens should be tailored individually; severe RT toxicities should be avoided when treatment is for palliation.
  - Some recommended RT regimens include:
    - 50 Gy in 20 fractions;
    - 37.5 Gy in 15 fractions (if well tolerated, consider adding 5 additional fractions to 50Gy);
    - 30 Gy in 10 fractions;
    - *30 Gy in 5 fractions:*** give 2 fractions/week with ≥3 days between the 2 treatments.
  - Carefully evaluate the patient's performance status, treatment tolerance, tumor response, and/or any systemic progression. Other palliative/supportive care measures include analgesics, nutrition support, targeted therapy, immunotherapy if indicated.

PRINCIPLES OF SYSTEMIC THERAPY IN ORAL CANCER

- The choice of systemic therapy should be individualized based on patient characteristics (e.g., PS, goals of therapy).
- The preferred chemoradiotherapy approach for fit patients with locally advanced disease remains concurrent cisplatin and radiotherapy.
- Cisplatin-based induction chemotherapy can be used, followed by radiation-based locoregional treatment (i.e., sequential chemoradiotherapy). However, an improvement in overall survival with the incorporation of induction chemotherapy compared to proceeding directly to state-of-the-art concurrent chemoRT (cisplatin preferred) has not been established in randomized studies.

Cancer of the Oral Cavity (NCCN Guidelines)

Primary Systemic Therapy + Concurrent RT

Preferred regimens

- High-dose cisplatin (category 1)
- Carboplatin/infusional 5-FU (category 1)

Other recommended regimens

- 5-FU/hydroxyurea
- Carboplatin/paclitaxel
- Cetuximab
- Cisplatin/infusional 5-FU
- Cisplatin/paclitaxel
- Weekly cisplatin 40 mg/m^2

Useful in certain circumstances

- Carbplatin/etoposide ± concurrent RT
- Cisplatin/etoposide ± concurrent RT
- Cyclophosphamide/doxorubicin/vincristine (followed by RT)

Postoperative Systemic Therapy/RT

Preferred regimens

Cisplatin (category 1 for high-risk)

Other recommended regimens

None

Useful in certain circumstances

Docetaxel/cetuximab (if cisplatin ineligible and positive margins and/or extranodal extension)

Induction Sequential Systemic Therapy

Preferred regimens

Docetaxel/cisplatin/5-FU (category 1 if induction is chosen)

Other recommended regimens

Paclitaxel/cisplatin/infusional 5-FU

Systemic Therapy/RT Following Induction Therapy, or Combination Chemotherapy for Recurrent/Persistent Disease

Preferred regimens

- Weekly carboplatin + concurrent RT
- Weekly cisplatin (category 2B) + concurrent RT

Other recommended regimens

Weekly cetuximab + concurrent RT

Adverse features: Extranodal extension and/or positive margins or close margins.

MUCOSAL MELANOMA

Presentation	Workup	

Biopsy to confirm diagnosis of mucosal malignant melanoma	• H&P including complete head and neck examination; mirror and fiberoptic examination.
	• Verification of pathology using appropriate staining (HMB-45, S-100, Melan-A)
	• CT with contrast and/or MRI extent of disease, particularly for sinus disease
	• As clinically indicated:
	  – Chest CT (with or without contrast)
	  – Consider FDG PET/CT or chest/abdominal/pelvic CT with contrast, and brain MRI (with and without contrast) to rule out metastatic disease
	  – Dental/prosthodontic evaluation
	  – Nutrition, speech, and swallowing evaluation
	  – Smoking cessation counseling
	  – Fertility/reproductive counseling
	• Multidisciplinary consultation as clinically indicated
		→ Oral mucosal melanoma

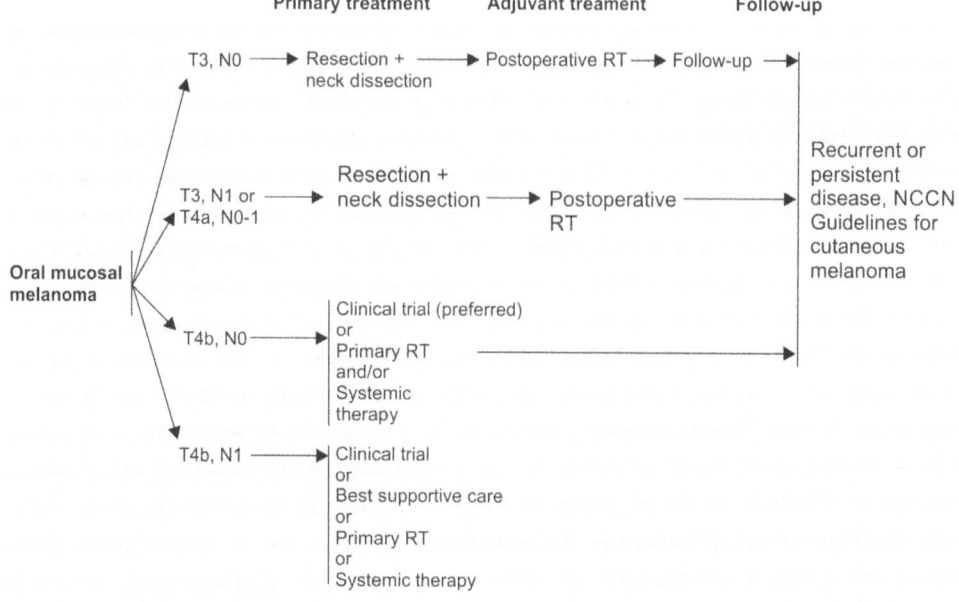

- Nodal basin→Nodal dissection→ ± RT to nodal basin or high-risk features→ ± Adjuvant systemic therapy.
- Recent studies suggest that increased toxicity may occur when RT is used in combination with BRAF inhibitors.
- Optional dose schedules include 48–50 Gy (2.4–3.0 Gy/fraction) and 30–36 Gy (6 Gy/fraction).

ORAL CANCER-FOLLOW-UP RECOMMENDATIONS

Based on risk of relapse, second primaries, treatment sequelae, and toxicities:

- History and physical (H&P) examination (including a complete head and neck examination; and mirror and fiberoptic examination):
  - Year 1, every 1–3 months
  - Year 2, every 2–6 months
  - Years 3–5, every 4–8 months
  - >5 years, every 12 months
- Imaging depending on clinical suspicion.
- Thyroid-stimulating hormone (TSH) every 6–12 months if neck irradiated.
- Dental evaluation for oral cavity and sites exposed to significant intraoral radiation treatment.
- *Supportive care and rehabilitation*:
  - Speech/hearing and swallowing evaluation and rehabilitation
  - Nutritional evaluation and rehabilitation
  - Ongoing surveillance for depression
  - Smoking cessation and alcohol counseling
- Integration of survivorship care and care plan within 1 year.

Cancer of the Oral Cavity (NCCN Guidelines)

FOLLOW-UP RECOMMENDATIONS POST SYSTEMIC THERAPY/RT

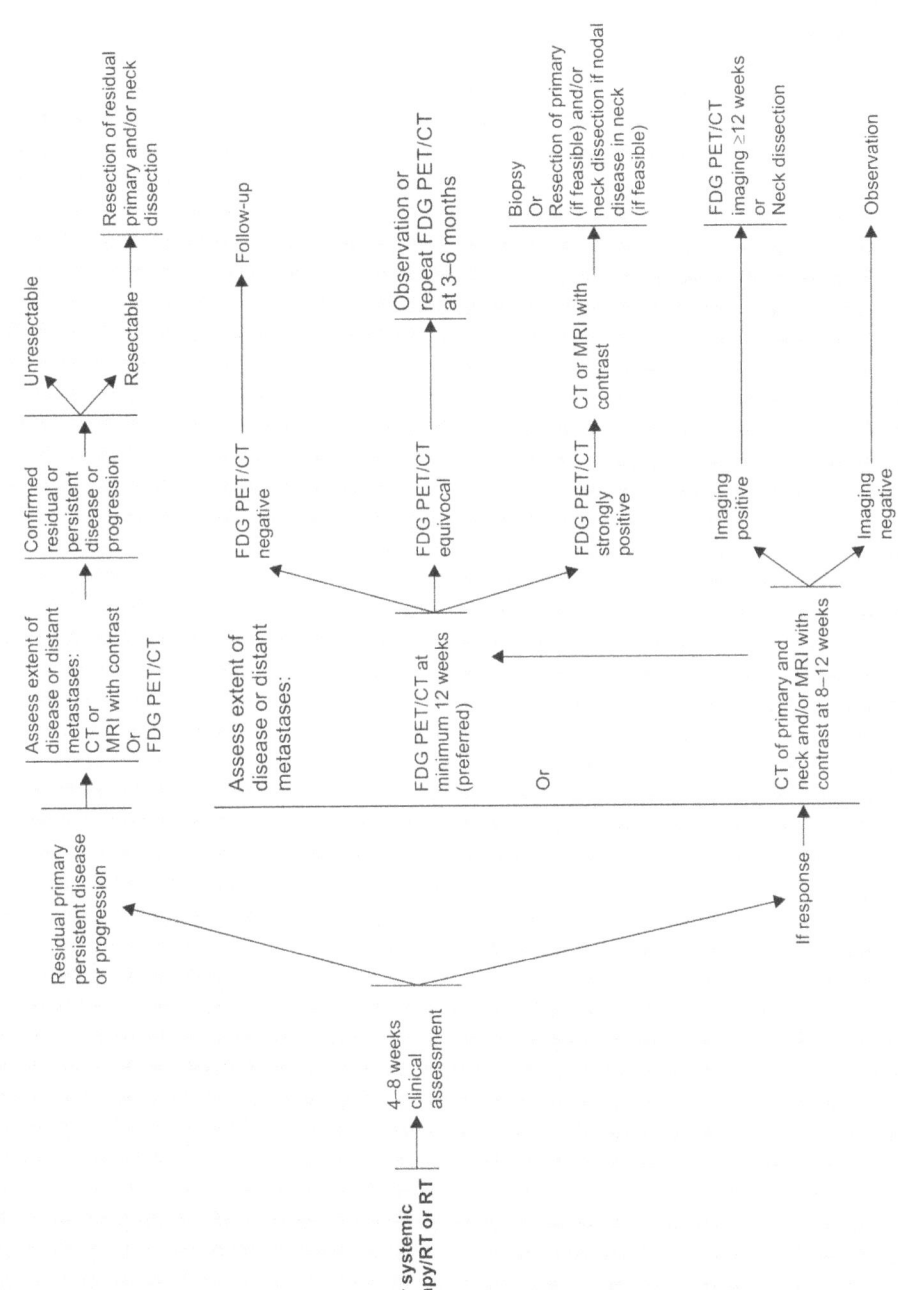

CHAPTER 36

Oral Cancer–2021

Ullas Batra

Oral Cancer-2021 recapitulates the salient features of oral cancer management and incorporates the latest developments in the last 2 years.

INTRODUCTION

In 2020, it was estimated that about 80,000 new oral cancer cases have occurred, constituting 6% of all cancer cases in India. Tobacco abuse is one of the most common etiologic factors in causation of oral cancer. The diagnosis stage predicts survival and guides management in oral cancers. The initial evaluation and development of a plan for treating a patient with oral cancer require a multidisciplinary team (MDT) of health care professionals.

The objective of any treatment strategy for squamous cell carcinoma of the head and neck (SCCHN) is to achieve the highest possible cure rate with the lowest risk of morbidity **(Fig. 1)**. As such, treatment proposals should integrate both objective tumor parameters (e.g., tumor location, tumor histology, T stage, N stage) and patient parameters (e.g., physiological age, comorbidities, previous history of cancer, occupation, expected functional outcome, personal preference). In addition to locoregional staging, every patient should undergo evaluation of his/her nutritional status, comorbidities, cardiopulmonary and renal functions, frailty index (for geriatric patients), psychological and social status, and dental status.

APPROACH TO AN ORAL CANCER PATIENT

- Clinical examination and pathological confirmation are mandatory.
- Head and neck endoscopy, head and neck contrast-enhanced CT (CECT), and/or MRI and chest imaging [with CT and/or fluorodeoxyglucose-positron emission tomography (FDG-PET)] are strongly recommended in locally advanced cases.
- For recurrent and/or metastatic SCCHN, tumor programmed death-ligand 1(PD-L1) expression should be evaluated.

For recurrent and/or metastatic SCCHN, tumor PD-L1 expression should be evaluated by an approved PD-L1 test within the framework of quality assurance. PD-L1 expression is assessed either by the tumor proportion score (TPS), defined as the percentage of tumor cells with membranous PD-L1 staining, or by the combined positive score (CPS), defined as the number of PD-L1-positive cells (tumor cells, lymphocytes, and macrophages) divided by the total number of tumor cells multiplied by 100. The CPS can help to define the first-line treatment strategy for recurrent/metastatic SCCHN. For human papillomavirus (HPV)-negative SCCHN, the two most frequent genomic alterations are p53 (83%) and CDKN2A (57%), respectively, according to The Cancer Genome Atlas (TCGA) data.

cT1-2 cN0 cM0	cT3-4a cN0-3 cM0 cT1-4a cN1-3 cM0	cT4b and/or unresectable lymph nodes cM0
Standard: Surgery (T and N[a]) followed by postoperative RT or CRT if indicated [IV, A] *Options:* • Radical RT (T and N) [IV, B] • Brachytherapy for primary (selected T1) [III, B]	*Standard:* Surgery (T and N) followed by postoperative RT or CRT if indicated [IV, A] *Option:* Definitive CRT (T and N) (contraindications to surgery, including functional unresectability) [IV, B]	*Options:* • Concomitant CRT (T and N) [III or IV, B] • Induction ChT followed by RT or CRT for responders (T and N) [IV, B] • *Palliative treatment:* Systemic ChT/immunotherapy and/or palliative RT and/or BSC [IV, B]

Fig. 1: Management of oral cavity cancer (stage level IV, B) excluding lip carcinoma [European Society for Medical Oncology (ESMO)-2020].
[a]if DOI < 10 mm: Sentinel lymph node biopsy is a valid option; if DOI <5 mm and cT1N0, active surveillance of the neck is a valid option.
(BSC: best supportive care; ChT: chemotherapy; CRT: chemoradiotherapy; DOI: depth of invasion; M: metastasis; N: node; RT: radiotherapy; T: tumor)

- *Unresectable and inoperable*: Unresectable means the disease cannot be removed grossly or local control cannot be achieved even with addition of radiotherapy (RT). Unresectable is different from inoperable where a patient's constitutional state precludes on operation (even if cancer can be easily resected with few sequelae). A subgroup of patients who are declined surgery but are potentially resectable should not be labeled unresectable. When reconstructive expertise is lacking, the patient's disease is considered functionally unresectable, e.g., mandibular resections with extensive soft-tissue and skin removal requiring bone replacement and bipaddled flap for cover and lining.
- *Comorbidity*: It refers to the presence of a concomitant disease that may affect diagnosis, treatment, and prognosis. Comorbidity is a strong independent predictor of mortality. ACE-27 (Adult Comorbidity Evaluation) is a validated instrument for assessing comorbidity in various cancer types.
- *Quality of life (QOL)*: Oral cancer affects basic physiologic function (ability to chew, swallow, breath), senses (taste, smell, hearing), and human characteristics such as appearance and voice. The health status describes an individual's physical, emotional, and social capabilities and limitation. Function and performance refer to how well a patient is able to perform important roles, tasks, or activities. QOL focusses on values (determined by the patient alone) that the patient places on his/her health status and function.

AMERICAN JOINT COMMITTEE ON CANCER (AJCC)-TNM (8TH EDITION, 2017)

Oral Mucosal Melanoma

The staging classification of melanoma is different from that of squamous cell carcinoma:
- *Primary tumor*:
  - T3—tumor limited to mucosa or underlying soft tissue regardless of thickening or greatest dimension
  - T4—moderately advanced or very advanced
  - Same for squamous cell carcinoma—T4a, T4b

- *Regional nodes*:
  - Nx: Regional nodes cannot be assessed
  - N0: No nodal metastasis
  - N1: Regional nodes present
- *Distant metastasis*:
  - M0: No distant metastasis
  - M1: Distant metastasis

Grading: There is no histological grading system at present.

IMAGING

Appropriate selection and utilization of imaging studies are important in managing oral cancer patients:
- MRI is preferred over CT when there is a need to evaluate tongue lesions, the extent of bone marrow invasion, or a patient with extensive dental amalgam that may obscure the anatomy on CT.
- CT is complementary to MRI for evaluation of cortical bone erosion or periosteal invasion.
- Panoramic dental X-ray is recommended for oral cancer patients requiring mandibulotomy/mandibulectomy. When postoperative RT is anticipated, preradiation dental evaluation should be done to assess the health of dentition and to determine if any dental procedure or extraction is required before RT.
- FDG-PET scan:
  - For patients with multistation or lower neck node involvement or high-grade tumor histology, consider FDG-PET for mediastinal nodes or distant metastases.
  - PET scan for malignancies approaching midline to determine the surgical approach to contralateral neck.
  - For patients with T3, T4, >N1 disease, FDG-PET scan is preferred to evaluate distant metastases, thoracic metastases in particular.
  - PET scan cannot rule out brain metastasis, high-risk cancers such as melanoma, high-grade neuroendocrine carcinoma, and adenocarcinoma; hence, contrast MRI of brain should be done.
  - If FDG-PET scan is not performed, CT scan of chest should be done to assess the presence of pulmonary metastasis as well as mediastinal nodes. A low-dose CT scan of chest is enough to screen for lung parenchymal metastasis. The role of annual CT chest screening is controversial. For heavy smokers who are at risk for lung cancer (second primary) or metastasis, an annual CT scan of chest can be considered.
  - PET may complement or replace other imaging modalities when staging recurrent/refractory disease to detect distant metastases or second primaries that may impact the choice of therapy.

Short term: <6-month post treatment evaluation:
- Imaging is recommended before starting postoperative adjuvant therapy when surgery has been performed in patients with locoregionally advanced cancer and are at risk of early recurrence.
- CT/MRI should be performed within 3-4 months of completing definitive treatment of locoregionally advanced disease or in patients with altered anatomy (due to surgery) causing difficult clinical assessment.
- CT/MRI may be done at 4-8 weeks of completing RT/CT in cases of clinical partial/incomplete response. Ultrasound (US) of

neck and guided fine needle aspiration cytology (FNAC) may be helpful.
- PET scan may be performed within 3–6 months of definitive RT + CT for treatment response evaluation.
- Early PET scan within 3 months of RT + CT may be associated with significant false-positive rates and should be avoided in absence of signs of recurrence/residue/progression.
- In case of borderline resectability, when neoadjuvant chemotherapy (NACT) is given, CT/MRI is usually done before definite treatment (RT/surgery). The PET scan may be done if there is a concern for locoregional or distant disease progression.

Long term: >6 months to 5 years post-treatment evaluation:
- Majority of recurrences after treatment of oral cancer occur within the first 2 years. Surveillance can be challenging due to altered signal of fibrosis from surgery/RT. There is no consensus on the frequency and modality of imaging in an asymptomatic patient.
- All imaging modalities have advantages and disadvantages. A 12-month PET scan may reveal a recurrent disease or second primary in 10% of treated patients. Most cases of asymptomatic PET-detected lesions are localized at distant sites. Whether earlier detection leads to improved disease-specific survival or not is not established.
- If PET scan at 3 months (post-treatment) is negative, there is no data to suggest benefit for further routine imaging in asymptomatic patients with negative clinical examination.
- US of neck is useful for detecting nodal recurrence.
- Additional post-treatment imaging is indicated in apprehensive patients or equivocal signs/symptoms.

INTERVENTIONAL RADIOLOGY
- When a PET scan picks up any suspicious residual or recurrent disease, FNAC or core biopsy may be required under US or CT guidance (especially nonpalpable nodes and inaccessible recurrent disease sites).
- Embolization of bleeding vessels
- Insertion of percutaneous endoscopic gastrostomy (PEG) under imaging
- Insertion of chemo port for CT

SURGERY
- Patient should be evaluated by the head and neck oncologist to: (1) ensure confirmation of diagnosis and review of biopsy material, (2) review staging and imaging, (3) exclude metastatic disease/second primary, (4) assess performance status and nutritional status, and (5) evaluate and discuss nonsurgical options also.
- Pretreatment evaluation should include consultation with the medical oncologist, radiation oncologist, reconstruction surgery team, maxillofacial surgeon, speech therapist, and nutritionist.
- Participate in MDT discussion with the aim of maximizing survival with preservation for form and function.
- Develop a prospective plan which includes dental, nutritional, health behavior evaluation, and rehabilitation plan.
- Surgical procedure should not be modified based on any response to prior neoadjuvant therapy. In cases of tumor progression, a more extensive procedure may be required.

- Once the MDT formalizes a treatment plan, the head and neck oncologist should discuss the recommendation, risk, benefits, and potential outcomes with patient + relation (shared decision-making).
- *Unresectability T4b* is based on the inability to obtain a clear margin:
  - Infiltration of pterygoid muscles with pterygopalatine fossa and cranial neuropathy
  - Skull base involvement (pterygoid plate, sphenoid bone erosion, widening of foramen ovale)
  - Direct extension to superior nasopharynx and lateral nasopharyngeal wall
  - Encasement of common carotid artery (CCA)/internal carotid artery (ICA)
  - Direct extension of neck disease (skin involvement)
  - Prevertebral fascial/cervical vertebra involvement
  - Subdermal metastasis
- For oral cancer, as the depth of invasion (DOI) increases, the risk of regional metastasis and need for elective neck dissection also increase.
- Perineural invasion should be suspected when tumors are adjacent to motor or sensory nerves. The aim is total cancer removal. When the nerve is grossly involved, it should be resected both proximally and distally to get clear margins (frozen section helpful to check clearance).
- Adequate resection of bone may require partial, horizontal, or sagittal resection of the mandible for tumors involving or adherent to mandibular periosteum. In an edentulous patient, due to mandibular atrophy, marginal mandibulectomy may not be feasible. Medullary invasion mandates segmental resection. Frozen section of marrow will guide the extent of resection of mandible.
- *Margin*:
  - The goal of cancer surgery is complete resection with histologic verification of tumor-free margin. When there is a cut through the invasive tumor, obtaining additional adjacent margins may be associated with a higher incidence of local recurrence and should be mentioned in operative notes. Obtaining additional margins is subject to ambiguity about whether tissue taken from the surgical bed corresponds to the actual site of margin positivity or not. When positive margins are reported, reresection/adjuvant RT + CT should be considered.
  - Adequate resection is defined as clear margins from gross tumor to obtain 1–1.5 cm of visible or palpable mucosa. A clear margin means that the distance from an invasive tumor is >5 mm. A positive margin is defined as carcinoma in situ or invasive carcinoma at resected margins.
- The *neck dissection* should be oriented in order to identify the level of nodes encompassed in the dissection:
  - Elective neck dissection should be based on occult metastasis in the appropriate nodal basin. For oral cancer, supraclavicular lymph node (SCLN) biopsy or DOI of primary currently are the best predictors of occult metastasis. For tumor depth > 3 mm, elective lymph node dissection (ELND) should be considered if RT is not already planned. For depth of 2–4 mm, clinical judgment

(as reliability of follow-up, clinically suspicious, etc.) determines the appropriateness of ELND. Elective dissections are generally selective, preserving all major structures (levels I-III).

- *N1-N2a-c*: Selective or comprehensive neck dissection.
- *N3*: Comprehensive neck dissection:
  - *SCLN biopsy*: It is an alternative to ELND for identifying occult cervical metastasis in early (T1, T2) oral cancers. Technical expertise and judgment are needed for execution of sentinel lymph node (SLN) mapping. It can pick up suspicious nodes in 95% cases. SLN positive should undergo completion neck dissection.
  Sentinel lymph node biopsy is a technically demanding procedure. The accuracy of sentinel node biopsy for floor of mouth is lower than that for tongue. Upper alveolus and hard palate are not technically suitable sites for SLN biopsy.
  - *Neck dissection*: Cervical lymph node dissections are classified as either comprehensive or selective. A comprehensive neck dissection is one that removes all lymph node groups that would be included in a classical radical neck dissection. Whether the sternocleidomastoid muscle, jugular vein, or spinal accessory nerve is preserved or not does not get affected by the type of dissection. Head and neck squamous cell cancers with no clinical nodal involvement rarely present with nodal metastasis beyond the confines of an appropriate selective neck dissection (<10% of the time).
  - *Basis of postoperative adjuvant treatment*: A combined analysis of prognostic factors and outcome from the Radiation Therapy Oncology Group (RTOG) 9501 and and European Organization for Research and Treatment of Cancer (EORTC) 22931 trials was performed. This analysis showed that patients with extranodal extension had survival benefit with cisplatin added to postoperative RT. For those with multiple involved regional nodes without extranodal extension, there was no survival advantage. In the randomized phase II RTOG-0234 trial, two regimens in patients with stages III and IV SCCHN were compared: (1) adjuvant chemoradiotherapy with cetuximab and docetaxel and (2) adjuvant chemoradiotherapy with cetuximab and weekly cisplatin (N = 238). The randomized phase II/III RTOG 1216 trial continues to investigate docetaxel/cetuximab with postoperative RT in comparison to cisplatin or docetaxel with postoperative RT (NCT01810913). For patients with high-risk adverse features following surgery (i.e., extranodal extension and/or positive margins) who are ineligible for platinum therapy, docetaxel/cetuximab is a category 2B option for postoperative systemic therapy/RT.

Surgery for Relapsed/Refractory Disease

For patients who do not have a complete clinical response to systemic therapy/RT, surgery including neck dissection is recommended (as indicated). However, it may be difficult to detect local or regional recurrence due to radiation-related tissue changes, and this may result in a delayed diagnosis of persistent or recurrent disease. There is an increased risk of complications when surgery in patients with relapsed/refractory disease is attempted.

RADIOTHERAPY

- Standards for target definition, dose specification, fractionation (with or without CT), and normal tissue constraints are still evolving.
  Intensity-modulated radiotherapy (IMRT), three-dimensional conformal radiation therapy (3DCRT), helical tomotherapy, volumetric modulated arc therapy, and proton therapy may be used depending on stage, site of tumor, physician experience, and availability of a medical physicist.
- Proton beam therapy (PBT) is recommended in patients with tumors in periocular area, skull base + cavernous sinus who may still be treated with curative intent. PBT is useful for recurrent tumors.
- Altered fractionation has not proven to be useful in the context of concurrent chemotherapy (ChT).
- These are no consensus guidelines for appropriate palliative RT regimens. Some recommended RT regimens are:
  - 50 Gy/20 Fraction (Fr)
  - 30 Gy/10 Fr
  - 30 Gy/5 Fr (2 Fr/wk with >3 days' gap between the Fraction)
- *Re-radiation*: If the area in consideration overlaps with previously related volume, the prior RT should here be >6 months from the appearance of recurrence.
  Re-radiation with intraoperative RT [image-guided radiation therapy (IGRT)] or brachytherapy may be considered in high-volume centers.
  Incidence of myelopathy increases after cumulative biological dose [biologically effective dose (BED)] of 120 Gy, but the risk is even more if Fraction size is >2.5 Gy/Fr.
  Re-radiation volumes should include a known disease only to minimize the volume of tissue receiving a very high dose in region of overlap. Prophylactic radiation of subclinical disease (like elective nodal RT) is not routinely indicated.
  Select your patients carefully for re-radiation with stereotactic body radiation therapy (SBRT). A good outcome is expected in smaller tumor and no skin involvement. Be careful if circumferential carotid involvement is there.
  Re-radiation dose: Postoperative 56–60 Gy at 1.8–2.0 Gy/Fr
  Definitive: 64–70 Gy at 1.8–2.0 Gy/Fr
  SBRT: 35–44 Gy in 5 Fr
- Any palliative RT regimen that might cause severe toxicities should be avoided. More hypofractionated regimens may be useful for patients with end-stage disease. For example, the QUAD SHOT regimen consists of a dose of 44.4 Gy, delivered in 12 fractions over three cycles, with each cycle being separated by 2–3 weeks. For IMRT, 54–63 Gy (1.6–1.8 Gy/Fr) is suggested. Delivery of 6 fractions/week is an acceptable accelerated schedule, if ChT is not prescribed concurrently. In general, postoperative RT is recommended for selected risk factors, including advanced T-stage, DOI, multiple positive nodes (without extranodal extension), or perineural/lymphatic/vascular invasion. Higher doses of postoperative RT alone (60–66 Gy), or with systemic therapy, are recommended for the high-risk features of extranodal extension and/or positive margins. The preferred interval is 6 weeks or less, between resection and commencement of postoperative

RT. Dosing schedules are the same regardless of whether or not systemic therapy is administered concurrently with postoperative RT.
- Hypofractionation may be considered for patients who are not good candidates for 6-7 weeks of RT due to comorbidities. The MARCH (Meta-analysis of Radiotherapy in Carcinomas of Head and neck) meta-analysis, including individual patient data from 15 randomized trials, analyzed the effect of hyperfractionated or accelerated RT on survival of patients with head and neck cancers. An absolute survival benefit for altered fractionation of 3.4% at 5 years was reported. This benefit, however, was limited to patients younger than 60 years of age. Hyperfractionation was associated with a benefit of 8% after 5 years. An update of the MARCH meta-analysis, including data from 33 trials, continued to show a survival benefit of hyperfractionation, compared to standard fractionation, in patients with locally advanced SCCHN.

IMRT dose painting refers to the method of assigning different dose levels to different structures within the same treatment fraction (e.g., 2.0 to gross tumor, 1.7 to microscopic tumor, <1.0 Gy to parotid gland) resulting in different total doses to different targets (e.g., 70, 56, <26 Gy). Although dose painting has been used to simplify radiation planning, hot spots associated with higher toxicity can occur.

Xerostomia is a common long-term side effect of RT, which can be reduced with the use of IMRT, drug therapy (e.g., pilocarpine, cevimeline), salivary substitutes, and other novel approaches (e.g., relocation of the submandibular gland). In patients with tumors that are periocular in location and/or invade the orbit, skull base, and/or cavernous sinus; in patients with tumors that extend intracranially or exhibit extensive perineural invasion; and in patients being treated with curative intent and/or have long life expectancies, achieving highly conformal dose distributions is crucial.

Brachytherapy is now being used less often because of improved local control and lower toxicities obtained with IMRT with or without systemic therapy. However, brachytherapy still has a role primarily for lip and oral cavity cancers.
- For patients whose cancer has been treated with RT, the recommended follow-up includes an assessment of thyroid function (6-12 months). Increased thyroid-stimulating hormone (TSH) levels have been detected in 20-25% of patients who have received neck irradiation.

MANAGEMENT OF RECURRENT/ METASTATIC ORAL CANCER

Management of recurrent/metastatic oral cancer is shown in **Figure 2**.

In selected patients with oligometastatic disease at diagnosis, local and/or regional treatment (with surgery or RT) can be considered for treatment with curative intent, especially after a response to upfront systemic treatment. On the other hand, in the presence of a high burden of distant metastases (e.g., more than two distant sites, mainly visceral involvement), starting systemic treatment is a priority and locoregional treatment should be carried out only if symptoms occur. Patients with locoregional recurrence not amenable to surgery and/or RT as well as those with metastatic disease are eligible for systemic treatment.

The standard of care (first-line therapy) for recurrent and/or metastatic disease has changed recently. The KEYNOTE-048 study showed that a combination of ChT [cisplatin

No platinum-based ChT during the last 6 months and PD-L1-positive tumor	No platinum-based ChT during the last 6 months and PD-L1 assessment not carried out	No platinum-based ChT during the last 6 months and PD-L1-negative tumor	Pretreated with platinum-based ChT within the last 6 months and immunotherapy-naïve	Pretreated with platinum-based ChT within the last 6 months and with prior immunotherapy
Standard: • Pembrolizumab monotherapy [I,A;MCBS4] • Pembrolizumab plus platinum/5-FU [I,A;MCBS4] *Options:* • Platinum/5-FU/ cetuximab if contraindication to immunotherapy and fit for platinum-based therapy [I,A;MCBS3] • Methotrexate or taxane or cetuximab and/or BSC if contraindication to immunotherapy and unfit for platinum-based therapy [III, C]	*Standard:* Pembrolizumab plus platinum/5-FU [I,A;MCBS4] *Options:* • Platinum/5-FU/ cetuximab if contraindication to immunotherapy and fit for platinum-based therapy [I,A;MCBS3] • Methotrexate or taxane or cetuximab and/or BSC if contraindication to platinum-based therapy [III, C]	*Standard:* Platinum/5-FU/ cetuximab [I,A;MCBS3] *Options:* • Pembrolizumab plus platinum/5-FU [I,A;MCBS4] • TPeX [II,B] • Methotrexate or taxane or cetuximab and/or BSC in case of contraindication to immunotherapy and unfit for platinum-based therapy [III, C]	*Standard:* Nivolumab [I,A;MCBS4] or pembrolizumab [I,A;MCBS4] *Option:* Taxane or methotrexate or cetuximab and/or BSC if contraindication to immunotherapy [III,C]	*Option:* Taxane or methotrexate or cetuximab and/or BSC [III,C]

Fig. 2: Management of recurrent and/or metastatic disease not amenable to curative RT or surgery (ESMO-2020). (5-FU: 5-fluorouracil; BSC: best supportive care; ChT: chemotherapy; CRT: chemoradiotherapy; M: metastasis; N: node; PD-L1: programmed death-ligand 1; RT: radiotherapy; T: tumor; TPeX: Cisplatin/Docetaxel/Cetuximab)

or carboplatin plus 5-fluorouracil (5-FU)] plus pembrolizumab, a monoclonal antibody targeting programmed cell death protein 1 (PD-1), significantly improved overall survival (OS) compared with the EXTREME regimen (cisplatin or carboplatin plus 5-FU plus cetuximab): median OS 13 versus 10.7 months. Objective response rate (ORR) and progression-free survival (PFS) were similar between the ChT plus cetuximab and ChT plus pembrolizumab arms [ORR 35.6% and 36.3%, PFS 4.9 and 5.1 months, grade 3–5 adverse events (AEs) 85.1% vs. 83.3%, respectively].

In the same trial, pembrolizumab monotherapy also improved median OS in patients with PD-L1-expressing SCCHN: 14.9 versus 10.7 months in the CPS ≥ 20 subgroup and 12.3 versus 10.3 months in the CPS ≥1 subgroup. As expected, pembrolizumab monotherapy was better tolerated than EXTREME (grade 3–5 AEs, 54.7% vs. 83.3%, respectively). Therefore, based on the KEYNOTE-048 results, two different approaches are validated for patients with locoregional relapse not amenable to locoregional salvage treatment and/or with distant metastases. A "chemo-free" approach with pembrolizumab monotherapy in patients with CPS >1 SCCHN should be considered, especially when a rapid tumor shrinkage is not needed. A second option, independent of the PD-L1 status, is the combination of pembrolizumab and ChT (cisplatin or carboplatin plus 5-FU), particularly in symptomatic patients or when a rapid tumor shrinkage is needed.

The Food and Drug Administration (FDA) recently approved pembrolizumab in combination with ChT as first-line treatment regardless of the PD-L1 expression and pembrolizumab alone for patients with PD-L1-expressing tumors (CPS > 1). In the first-line treatment of recurrent SCCHN, EXTREME is the standard of care for patients with contraindications to anti-PD-1 inhibitors and in patients with a tumor not expressing PD-L1. EXTREME can also be considered as second-line treatment after progression on an immune checkpoint inhibitor in fit patients considered eligible for platinum-based ChT. Similarly, TPeX can be considered as a treatment alternative to EXTREME for some patients (e.g., in case of dihydropyrimidine dehydrogenase deficiency (DPD)].

For patients who progress within 6 months of platinum therapy, given either as palliative treatment or as multimodal curative treatment, nivolumab has been shown to improve OS compared with single-agent systemic treatment (cetuximab, docetaxel, or methotrexate): 7.5 versus 5.1 months (CheckMate 141). Nivolumab is both FDA- and European Medicines Agency (EMA)- approved in this setting. Pembrolizumab is also approved by the FDA for the same indication and is approved by the EMA for patients whose tumors express PD-L1 with a TPS of ≤50%. After progression on platinum-based ChT and anti-PD-1 inhibitors, no standard of care exists. Cetuximab is approved by the FDA after platinum failure.

Taxanes with or without cetuximab and/or methotrexate are frequently used after platinum failure, although no randomized trials have demonstrated their benefit in this setting.

The risk of disease relapse is estimated at between 40 and 60% for patients with locally advanced disease, with most recurrences occurring within the first 2 years after the primary diagnosis. The incidence of second primaries is 2-4% per year and remains relatively constant over time. FDG-PET/CT is recommended 3 months after CRT for patients with node-positive disease to assess the necessity of neck dissection, otherwise imaging should be carried out if symptoms occur or in case of abnormalities found at clinical examination.

Pembrolizumab

Pembrolizumab is recommended as an option for untreated metastatic or unresectable recurrent HNSCC in adults whose tumors express PD-L1 with a CPS of 1 or more. This is only if:
- Pembrolizumab is given as a monotherapy
- Pembrolizumab is stopped at 2 years of uninterrupted treatment or earlier if the disease progresses.

Treatment of metastatic or unresectable recurrent HNSCC depends on where it starts. If it starts in the oral cavity (mouth), it is usually first treated with cetuximab combination therapy (cetuximab with platinum and 5-FU ChT). If it starts outside the oral cavity, it is treated with ChT (platinum and 5-FU) alone. If cancer starts in the oral cavity, pembrolizumab monotherapy works at least as well as cetuximab combination therapy and has lower overall costs. If the cancer starts outside the oral cavity, pembrolizumab monotherapy works better than ChT alone. Pembrolizumab monotherapy is therefore recommended for both types of HNSCC.

Combination therapy is usually offered to people with a high disease burden or whose disease is progressing rapidly or has relapsed after ChT. Monotherapy is offered to people with a low disease burden, with disease progressing at the expected rate, or to people who are not able to tolerate combination therapy.

Cetuximab combination therapy is a relevant comparator for cancer starting in the oral cavity, while ChT alone is relevant for cancer starting outside the oral cavity.

NUTRITION

- Prophylactic tube feeding [nasogastric tube (NG)/percutaneous endoscopic gastrostomy (PEG)] is considered in patients:
  - Severe weight loss prior to treatment → 5% weight loss in 1 month, >10% loss in 6 months
  - Ongoing dehydration or dysphagia, anorexia, pain interfering with the ability to drink or eat adequately
  - *Aspiration (severe)*: Even mild aspiration in elderly or with compromised cardiopulmonary function
  - Consider feeding tube placement if >2 criteria apply.
- Inadequate food intake (60% of estimated energy expenditure) anticipated for >10 days.
- Weight loss > 5% in 1 month
- Age > 60 years
- Severe mucositis, odynophagia, grade III dysphagia, aspiration

DENTAL MANAGEMENT

Radiotherapy for oral cancer causes xerostomia and salivary gland dysfunction which increase the risk of caries, dentoalveolar infection, and osteoradionecrosis. Radiation caries and dental hard tissue changes can appear within the first 3 months after RT:

- *Strategies for dry mouth—improve hydration*:
  - Avoid caffeinated products
  - Salivary substitutes
  - Alcohol-free mouth washes
  - Salivary stimulation—gustatory stimulants (chewing gum, lozenges), cholinergic agonists (pilocarpine)
- *Dental caries prevention*:
  - Diet counseling
  - Oral hygiene —brushing frequently, flossing, alcohol-free mouth wash
  - High-potency topical fluoride
  - Candidiasis—prevention and treatment
  - Frequent dental evaluation
- *Effect on bones/muscles*:
  - Pre RT evaluation—if extraction is required, do it 2 weeks before RT
  - Use custom-made mouth-opening devices
  - Treat active caries and periodontal disease before starting RT
  - Reevaluate 6–12 weeks after completion of RT

KEY POINTS

- Decisions are more important than incisions of surgery and precisions of RT.
- Choose investigations judiciously. Know what is expected from investigations.
- The objective of treatment is to achieve the highest possible cure rate with the lowest morbidity.
- The rapid development of molecular biology, identification of cancer genes, and signaling pathways show renewed promise for better outcomes.
- TSH test should be done every 6–12 months if neck is irradiated.
- SLN biopsy is an alternative to elective node dissection for identifying occult nodal metastasis in early oral cancer.
- Pembrolizumab is recommended as an option for untreated metastatic or unresectable recurrent SCCHN in adults whose tumors express PD-L1 with a CPS of 1 or more.
- PBT (proton beam therapy) is a viable option for patients with tumors in the periocular area, skull base + cavernous sinus who may still be treated with curative intent. PBT is useful for recurrent tumors.
- PET may complement or replace other imaging modalities when staging recurrent/refractory disease to detect distant metastases or second primaries that may impact the choice of further therapy.
- Follow-up recommendations are based on risk of relapse, second primary, treatment sequelae, and toxicities.

Index

Page numbers followed by *b* refer to box, *f* refer to figure, *fc* refer to flowchart, and *t* refer to table.

A

Abbe flap 133, 133*f*, 135*f*
Abducens nerve 43
Abscess, periapical 266*f*
Acetaldehyde 18, 19
Acetyl-L-carnitine 284
Acrylic cones 76
Actinic keratosis 29
Adenoid cystic carcinoma 155*f*
Adenomatoid odontogenic tumor 80, 83, 83*f*
Adenosquamous carcinoma 29, 33, 39
Adjuvant radiotherapy
    doses 236, 236*t*
    indications for 161
Air embolism 195
Airway 221
    assessment 108, 109*t*
    obstruction 195
    patency, assess for 123
    plan 109
Alar crescent excision 133
Alcohol 18, 74
    dehydrogenase 18
    intake 15, 102, 296
    major metabolite of 18
    mechanism of action of 19*f*
Aldehyde dehydrogenase 19
Allen's test 218
Alpha-lipoic acid 284
Alveolar ridge 303
Alveolectomy, upper 156
Alveolus 179
    carcinoma of 117
    mandibular 55*f*
Ameloblastoma 79, 80, 81*f*
    malignant 80, 84
        excision for 225
        variants of 84
    maxillary 81
    peripheral 79, 82
    solid 79

American Joint Committee on Cancer 254*f*, 315
Amifostine 284
Aminolevulinic acid 69
Amitriptyline 284
Analgesia
    postoperative 111
    topical 287
Andy gump deformity 174, 175, 175*f*
Anesthesia, general 77
Anisocytosis 30
Anisonucleosis 29
Ankyloglossia 41, 296, 298
    complete 41
    mild 41
    moderate 41
Anorexia 249
Anterolateral thigh
    flap 174, 222, 224, 227*f*
    types of 227
Anthropometry 102
Antibiotics
    perioperative 210
    prophylactic 221
Antioxidant 25
Anxiety 289
Apolipoprotein 27
Arrhythmias, cardiac 196
Arterial thrombosis, pale flap after 196*f*
Artery 213
    maxillary 193
Articulation 280
    therapy 281
Ascorbic acid 23, 68
Aspergillus niger 298
Aspiration 107, 249
    pneumonia 125
Axial flaps 204

B

Barium swallow procedure, modified 275

Bartholin's duct 164
Basaloid squamous cell carcinoma 29, 33, 39
B-cell lymphoma 97
Bence-Jones protein 97
Bernard's burrow 133
Bernard's flap 138*f*
Beta-carotene 68
Bidi 18
Biochemistry 103
Biopsy 41
    image-guided 260, 263
    incisional 42, 67
Bite excision 6
Black hairy tongue 298
Bleeding 64, 193, 195, 289
Bleomycin 68
Blood
    soaked sponge 91
    thinners 221
    type 119
Body
    image alteration 289
    mandibular 99*f*
    mass index 108
    weight 109
Bone 80, 98, 225, 324
    cyst, aneurysmal 80, 90, 90*f*
    exposure 152
    fibrosarcoma of 80, 95, 96*f*
    invasion 36
    management of 6, 144
    postradiation sarcoma of 80, 99
Bony
    exposure 157, 158
    mandible 53*f*
    metastasis 64
    resection 158, 159
Botulinum toxin, injection of 75
Brachytherapy 240, 242
    advantages of 242
    adverse effects of 243
    boost 240, 242

Index

doses 242
implant 241*f*
intraoperative 241, 242*f*
selection criteria for 242
types of 241
Brain 247
  metastasis 64
  specific angiogenesis inhibitor 27
Brainstem 247
Breast 13
  cancer 99*f*
Bronchopneumonia 198
Brush
  biopsy 67
  sensitivity of 67
Buccal fat pad flap 213, 214*f*
Buccal mucosa 15, 140, 179, 201, 213, 225, 247, 303
  anatomy of 140*f*
  arterial supply of 3*f*
  carcinoma of 117, 241*f*
  defects 224
  innervation of 4*f*
  management of 140
  maxillary 55*f*
Buccal myomucosal flap 131, 132*f*, 133*f*
Buccinator muscle 5
Buccinator myomucosal flap 9, 174
Bulky nodal disease 60
Burkitt lymphoma 80, 97

C

Cancer
  buccal mucosal 142
  genome atlas
    data 314
    network 38
  multiple 24
  pain management 112*f*
  prevention of 23
  recurrent 256, 256*t*
  registry development 14
  resection, principles of 128
  secondary prevention of 23
  stage of 141
  subsite of 58
  therapy, functional assessment of 291
  unresectable 142
Candidiasis 29, 267, 287

Capecitabine 258, 259
Carboplatin 252, 258
  chemotherapy 284
Carcinoembryonic antigen 34
Carcinoma
  ameloblastic 84
  buccal mucosa 243*f*, 244*f*
  cuniculatum 29
  in-situ 30
  lymphoepithelial 29
  odontogenic 80, 83, 85
  of alveolus, management of 157*fc*
  of hard palate, management of 157*fc*
  sarcomatoid 34, 34*f*
  ulcerated 142*f*
Carious tooth 266*f*
Carotenoids 20
Carotid artery
  common 318
  external 260
  internal 318
Carotid sinus syndrome 194
Catheters, size of 123
Cavernous sinus invasion 43, 62
Celecoxib 259
Celsus method 135*f*
Cementoblastoma 80, 85
Central giant cell granuloma 80, 89, 90*f*
Cephalic vein 218
Cerebrospinal fluid 287
Cerebrovascular accident 297
Cervical
  esophagus 177
  nodes 62
  plexus block 113
  spine movement 108
Cervix uteri 13
Cetuximab 64, 252, 322
  combination therapy 323
Cheek 213, 299, 300
  mucosa 2
  skin flap, necrosis of 197
Chemiluminescent light 67
Chemoprevention 24
  model of 24*f*
Chemoradiation 251, 253
  adjuvant 251, 252
  postoperative 252
  primary 251, 252
Chemoradiotherapy 60, 169, 322

concurrent 157, 161
postoperative 162
Chemotherapy 44, 95, 102, 106, 284, 322
  adjuvant 235
  combination 64
  concurrent 230, 235, 320
  dental management during 270
  dose of 61
  high-dose 98
  induction 169, 253
  neoadjuvant 149, 157, 317
  role of 146, 161
  single-agent 64
  systemic 64
  transarterial 261, 263
Cherubism 80, 90, 90*f*
Chest
  imaging 62
  infection 277
  pain 64
  X-ray 42, 58
Chimeric flaps 209
Chin skin, necrosis of 197*f*
Chondroma 80, 93
Chondrosarcoma 80, 95
  mesenchymal 80, 95
Chronic obstructive pulmonary disease 297
Chuttaa 18
Chyle leak 197
Cigarettes, smokers of 18
Circulation flaps 204
Cisplatin 252, 322
  high-dose 252
Clear-cell odontogenic carcinoma 80, 85
Cochlea 247
Colorectum 13
Combined positive score 253, 259, 314
Comorbidity 315
Compensatory technique 282
Complete blood count 119
Complex odontome 87*f*
Composite flaps 207
Computed tomography
  angiography 261
Computer-adaptive tests 291
Condyloma acuminatum 29
Conservative physical therapy 76
Constrictor muscles 246

Contaminated traumatic wounds 208
Contrast-enhanced computed tomography 42
Corkscrew device 76, 77f
Coronoidectomy 77
Coupling devices 211
Cranial nerve 11f
Cranial neuralgia 285
Cross vermilion flap 131f
Cryotherapy 71
Cuff pressure 123
Cupid's bow 131
Cutaneous flaps, axial perforator-based 207
Cyclooxygenase inhibitors 25
Cystic ameloblastomas 79, 81
Cytokeratin 34

D

Death
 causes of 302
 cancer-related 12
Deep femoral artery 218
Deep inferior epigastric artery perforator 222
Deep soft-tissue infiltration 142
Deep vein thrombosis 195
Defects needing bone 225
Dehydration 277
Deltopectoral flap 226
Dental
 alveoli 150
 assessment, pre-radiotherapy 264
 caries prevention 324
 examination 40
 factors 20
 implants 268, 271, 271f
 issues 288
 management 270, 324
  pre-radiotherapy 265
 prosthetic evaluation 156
 rehabilitation 221, 270
 status 108
 ulcer 302
Dentin, amorphous mass of 87f
Deoxyribonucleic acid 107
Depression 289
Dermatitis 249
Diabetes mellitus 297
Diarrhea, treatment of 125
Digastric tendon 193f

Dimethyl sulfoxide 68
Direct cutaneous flaps 204
Discoid lupus erythematosus 29, 66
Distant flaps 223
Distant metastasis 32, 48, 316
 classification 48
Docetaxel 258, 322
Doxepin 287
Drain care 125
Dry mouth, strategies for 324
Dynamic bite openers 76
Dynasplint trismus system 77, 77f
Dysguesia 249
Dyskeratosis 29
Dysphagia 170, 249, 274, 296
 causes of 274b
Dysplasia 29, 30, 67
 mild 30
 moderate 30
 moderate-to-high-grade 240

E

Eastern cooperative oncology group 64, 255
Elective lymph node dissection 318
Elective neck dissection 161
Elective nodal irradiation 180
El-Ganzouri's index 109, 109t
Enamel, amorphous mass of 87f
Endotracheal tube 108
End-tidal carbon dioxide 115
Epidermal growth factor receptor 25, 64, 148, 258
 inhibitors 28
Epidermolysis bullosa 66
Epigallocatechin gallate 24
Episode 297
Epithelial precursor lesions 29
Epithelial tumors 80
 classification of 29b
Epithelium, squamous 50
Epstein-Barr virus 97
Erlotinib 259
Erythematous gingival lesion 96f
Erythroleukoplakia 29, 31, 296
 hard palate 154f
Erythroplakia 29, 31, 69
Esophagus 13
Estlander flap 135, 136f
European Medicines Agency 323

European Organization for Research and Treatment of Cancer 252, 319
European Society for Medical Oncology 315f
Ewing's sarcoma 80, 95, 96
Excessive salivation 296
Exfoliative cytology 42
Extended radical neck dissection 178
External beam radiotherapy 240, 243
 adverse effects of 249t
 techniques of 243
Extracapsular extension 161
Extractions 265, 268
Extranodal extension 32, 36, 46, 48, 60, 141, 234, 240, 251
Extratumoral perineural invasion 36f
Extrinsic muscle invasion 41
Eyes 247

F

Face, muscles of 2f
Facial artery 193, 193f
 myomucosal flap 215, 215f
Facial nerve 128
Fascia, superficial 1
Fasciocutaneous flaps 204
Fear 289
Feeding
 intolerance, management of 125
 position 125
 tube
  placement 124
  selection 124
  types of 104, 105f
Femoral artery 218
Fetor oris 296
Fiberoptic
 bronchoscopy 109
 examination 162
Fibroblast growth factor receptor 37
Fibroma
 ameloblastic 80, 88
 cementifying 80, 86
 cemento-ossifying 88
 desmoplastic 80, 93
 juvenile ossifying 80, 88
 odontogenic 80, 85

Index

Fibro-odontoma, ameloblastic 80, 88
Fibro-osseous tumors 80, 88
Fibrosarcoma, ameloblastic 80, 86
Fibrosis 274
  subcutaneous 249
  submucous 40, 59
Fine-needle aspiration cytology 42, 54*f*, 317
Finger stretching 76
Flap
  after venous thrombosis 196*f*
  classification of 204
  design 209
  elevation 185
  failure 197
  loss 170
  necrosis 116
  reconstruction 174
  unwanted hairs in 198
  vascular compromise of 196
Flexor carpi radialis muscle 218
Fluid intake 102
Fluorodeoxyglucose-positron emission tomography 314
Fluorouracil 149, 258
Food and Drug Administration 322
Forehead flap 216, 217*f*
Fracture 64, 199
Free anterolateral thigh flap 218, 227
Free fibula
  flap 174, 220, 220*f*
  osseous 228
Free fibular osteocutaneous flap 224
Free microvascular flap 138
Free radial artery forearm flap 217, 226
Frenulum 164
Fries flap 138*f*
Fugimori type unilateral nasolabial flap 136*f*
Fujimori gate flap, bilateral 137, 138*f*
Functional oral intake scale 275*b*

G

Gardner syndrome 92
Gastric reflux 108

Gastrostomy
  percutaneous
    endoscopic 106, 324
    radiological 260, 262, 263
  tube 104
Giant cell
  lesions-containing multinucleated 80, 89
  tumor 80, 89
Gillies fan flap 133, 134*f*, 137*f*
  unilateral 136
Gingival mucosa 2
Gingivobuccal complex 2, 213
Gingivobuccal sulcus 17, 144
Gland
  sublingual 164
  submandibular 164, 246
Glass ionomer cement 265
Glioma 91
Globocan 2018 13*f*
Glossectomy 172
  partial 172, 174
  subtotal 172
  total 173
  types of 172
Glossopharyngeal nerve 165, 286
  block 113, 287*f*
Glutamine 284
Glutathione 284
Grafts, full-thickness 203, 203*f*
Granuloma, eosinophilic 89
Greater auricular nerve 189, 194, 195*f*
Greater palatine nerve 57*f*
Grimm flap 138*f*
Gums 213, 299, 300
Gutka 16, 17

H

Hand-Schüller-Christian disease 89
Hard palate 56, 155*f*, 179, 224, 303, 274
  bony landmarks of 153*f*
  malignant melanoma of 155*f*
Head and neck
  cancer 28, 29, 58, 73, 107, 183*t*, 231, 258, 264
    inventory 291
    treatment of 180
  cast fabrication 236
  endoscopy 314
  malignancies of 119

  radiation therapy 265
  squamous cell carcinoma 23, 37, 64, 180, 230, 257, 314
Health utilities index 291
Hemangiopericytoma 95
Hemiglossectomy 172
  compartmental 172
Hemimandibulectomy 7
Hemorrhage 260
  uncontrolled 260
Herpes simplex virus 287
Heterozygosity, loss of 38
High molecular weight keratin 34
Histiocytoma, malignant fibrous 80, 96
Human papillomavirus 19, 314
  infection 29
Humby knife 203*f*
Humidification 123
Hydroxyurea 252
Hyperbaric oxygen 75, 269
Hyperchromasia 30
Hyperparathyroidism 80, 89
Hyperplasia
  multifocal epithelial 29
  pseudoepitheliomatous 34, 35*f*
Hypertension 297
Hypertrophic scar 199, 199*f*
Hypofractionation 249, 321
Hypopharynx 177, 183
Hypothermia 195

I

Immunohistochemistry 34
Immunotherapy 64
Induction sequential systemic therapy 311
Infection 287, 289
Infranotch tumor 147*f*
Infratemporal fossa 3, 4, 6, 141, 145, 149, 154
  boundaries of 5*f*
  contents of 146*f*
Intensity-modulated radiotherapy 77, 236, 238*f*, 244, 248*f*, 320
  advantages of 249
Intensive care unit 122, 221, 262
Interferon-gamma 70
Intermuscular septum 220
International Classification of Diseases 283

International Society of Oral Oncology 266
Interstitial implant brachytherapy 241, 241f
Interventional Gasserian Ganglion Block 286
Interventional therapy 113
Intraoperative nursing care 120
Intravenous patient-controlled analgesia 112
Invasion, depth of 35, 44, 48, 55, 231
Island platysma 216
Itching 289

J

Jaw 85, 88
   bisphosphonate-related osteonecrosis of 270
   deviation of 198
   malignant nonodontogenic tumors of 93
   mobilization 276
   opening devices 77f
   protrusion 108, 109
   tumors 79
      classification of 80t
Jejunostomy tube 104
Johanson's step ladder advancement 136
   flap 137f
Jugular vein, internal 193
Jugular venous pressure 297

K

Kaposi's sarcoma 155
Karapandzic flap 136
   bilateral 135f, 136
   reverse 134
   unilateral 137f
Khaini 16, 17
Kharra 16
Kotlow's assessment 41
Kotlow's classification 41t

L

Lamina dura 3
Langerhans cell disease 80, 89
Large multilocular solid ameloblastoma 80f
Laryngoscopy, indirect 40
Larynx 177, 183, 246
   glottic 177
   subglottic 177
L-ascorbic acid 68
Laser
   ablation 68
   surgery 114
Lateral circumflex femoral artery 218
Latyshevsky, Apron flap incision of 185
Left external carotid artery angiogram 261f
Left greater palatine foramen 57f
Lens 247
Letterer-Siwe disease 89
Leukoplakia 30, 66, 69, 301
   speckled 31
   types of 67b
Lichen planus 29, 66, 69-71
Lidocaine 287
Ligature slip 193
Limberg flap 207f
Lingual artery 193, 215
Lingual nerve 165
Lingual swellings 1
Lips 1, 127, 128, 177, 251, 298, 299
   cancers of 12, 251
   carcinoma 315f
   defects 128, 135
      central 133f
      full-thickness 128fc, 129
      lateral 133f
      reconstructive strategies for 129
   functions of 127
   landmarks 127f
   oral cavity 13
   primary repair of 130f
   reconstruction 129
      goals of 128
   sparing 143f
   split, lateral 143f
   vascular anatomy of 128f
Liver function test 119
Liverpool oral rehabilitation 291
Local flaps 206, 213, 223
Low molecular weight keratin 34
Lower alveolus 150
   carcinoma of 150
Lower lip 128
   defects 135, 136f
   split incisions 143f
   vermilion flap 130
Lung 13
   collapse 198
   metastases, treatment of 257
Lycopene 25, 68
   mechanism of action of 27fc
Lymph node 48, 60, 176
   ablation 260, 263
   metastasis 36
      incidence of 232f
   multiple 60
   pathological 46, 54t
   regional 32, 46, 178, 316
   supraclavicular 318
Lymphatic 2, 141
   dissemination 53
   drainage 3, 128
   interventions 260, 262
   spread 151
Lymphoscintigraphy 191
Lymphovascular invasion 35, 60, 161, 162, 233

M

Macroglossia 301
Magnetic resonance
   angiography 222
   imaging 42, 51, 142, 151, 156, 166, 256
Malignancy, mimickers of 34
Malignant diseases 23
Mallampati grade 109
Mallampati score, modified 108
Malnutrition
   associated morbidity 102
   impact of 102
   screening tool 102
Malocclusion 198
Mandible 5, 8, 246, 269f
   bony landmarks of 150f
   carcinoma of 117
   fracture of 199
   lower border of 4
   segmental resection of 151
Mandibular
   alveolar ridge, anterior 177
   guiding prosthesis 270
      placement of 271f
   nerve 4, 11f, 52f, 193f
   reconstruction 228
   resections, types of 151f
Mandibulectomy 173
   segmental 53f, 151, 151f, 225
   types of 151

Marginal mandibulectomy 6, 53*f*, 144, 145*f*, 151*f*
   contraindications for 152
Masseteric flap 215
Mastication, muscles of 4
Masticator space 4, 4*f*, 55*f*
   involvement of 141
Mathes and Nahai classification 205*f*
Mawa 16
Maxilla
   anterior right 96*f*
   carcinoma of 117
   posterior 81*f*
   posterolateral wall of 5
Maxillary artery, internal 4
Maxillary defects 270
Maxillary reconstruction 228
Maxillectomy 225
   infrastructural 158, 159*f*
   partial 157*f*
McGregor flap 136, 137*f*
Meckel's cave 286*f*
Medial pterygoid muscle 4, 5
Medial sural artery perforator flap 219, 219*f*
Meningioma 91
Metastasis 322
   pulmonary 64
Metastatic cancers 240
   chemotherapy for 253
Metastatic carcinoma 80, 99
   management of 99
   prognosis of 100
Metastatic disease 64, 149
   management of 322*f*
Methotrexate 258, 259
Metronomic therapy 64, 259
Microvascular free flap 134
Mid-face, structure of 177
Midline lip split 143*f*, 171
Minimally invasive neck dissection 191
Minor salivary glands, malignant tumors of 46
Mobile tongue 29*b*
Monoclonal light chain 97
Monotherapy 240, 242
Mouth 241*f*, 296
   cancer of floor of 163
   floor of 1, 7, 51, 55*f*, 56, 163, 164*f*, 165*f*, 167, 169, 177, 179, 224, 225, 232*f*, 240, 247, 299, 300, 303

opening 75, 108, 109
swelling in 295
Mucosal defects 60
Mucosal melanoma 46, 155, 311
Mucosectomy 172
Mucositis 170, 249, 266, 274
   grades of 287*t*
Multidetector computed tomography 57
Multifocal leukoerythroplakia syndrome 154
Multilocular radiolucency 86*f*, 90*f*
Multiple-eyed catheters 123
Murphy's law 193
Muscles 4*f*, 127, 324
   changes of 274
   flaps 205*f*
   forming 165*f*
Muscular diaphragm 165
Myeloma, multiple 80, 97
Myocutaneous flap 225
Myomucosal advancement 130, 130*f*
Myxoma, odontogenic 80, 85, 86*f*

N

Nakajima flap 136
Nasal cavity 177
Nasogastric tube 104, 324
Nasolabial flap 136, 160, 174, 215
   bilateral 138*f*
Nasopharynx 61, 177
Nasotracheal tube 114
Nausea 249, 289
   postoperative 111
N-butyl cyanoacrylate 261
Near-total glossectomy 172
Neck 257
   disease, direct extension of 318
   dissection 144, 145, 173, 178, 183, 190, 191, 318, 319
      bilateral selective 189
      complications of 181
      history of 183
      lateral 178
      modified 117, 185
      posterolateral 178
      superselective 179
      terminology 184
      types of 184*t*
   examination of 40, 300, 301*f*
   hematoma 196*f*

incisions 184
   types of 185*b*, 186*f*
management of 167, 170, 176
movement 109
nodes 179
   clinical staging of 178
   levels of 176
   seven levels of 176
   staging 247*t*
   ultrasound 42
Negative pressure wound therapy 202
Neoplastic spindle cells 34*f*
Nerve
   injury 193
      peripheral 9
   sheath 91
Neural integration 280
Neuralgia, glossopharyngeal 286
Neurofibroma 80, 91, 92
Neurofibromatosis 91
   types of 91*t*
Neurofibrosarcoma 98
Neuromuscular electrical stimulation 276
Neuropathy 274, 285
   painful trigeminal 285
Neurotropism 35
Nicotiana rustica 17
Nitric oxide 284
Nivolumab 64
Nodal disease, primary 60
Nodal gross tumor volumes 236
Non-Hodgkin's lymphoma 97
Non-human papilloma virus 45
Nonsteroidal anti-inflammatory drugs 112, 112
Nuclear pleomorphism 29
Numerical rating scale 285
Nurses, responsibilities of 120
Nutrition 324
   postoperative 106
   support 104
      methods of 104
Nutritional assessment parameters 102
Nutritional screening 102

O

Obstructive sleep apnea 108
Odontoma 80, 87
Odontome, compound 87*f*
Oligometastasis 64

Index

Omohyoid tendon 188
Oncology, interventional 260
Operation theater 122
   preoperative care in 120
Opioid therapy 285*fc*
Optic
   chiasma 247
   nerves 247
Oral cancer 18, 40, 61, 176, 183, 200, 213, 273, 280, 281, 284*t*, 290, 292, 310, 312, 314, 318
   advanced 306-309
   chemotherapy for 251
   development of 20
   early stage 230, 239
   etiology of 12
   immobilization for 245*f*
   locally advanced
      resectable 239
      unresectable 240
   management of 59*fc*, 260
   metastatic 63, 321
   nutrition in 101
   primary treatment of 304
   radiotherapy for 239, 240
   recurrent 149*b*, 253, 258
   reirradiation for 249
   speech therapy in 280
   staging of 40, 51
   surgery 108
      anesthesia in 108
      emergency in 116
   treatment
      guidelines for 239
      principles of 58
Oral cavity 1, 29, 29*b*, 38, 50, 177, 183, 251, 256, 284
   anatomy of 201
   bony defects of 222
   boundaries of 1, 2*f*
   cancer 12, 23, 50, 230, 251, 253, 260, 283, 285, 303
      management of 315*f*
   carcinoma of 50, 58
   defects, typical 201
   lateral part of 54
   mucosa of 20
   proper 50, 50*f*, 55
   reconstruction 201
   routes of spread of 51
   squamous cell carcinoma 57
      management of 162*fc*
   structures of 201*f*
   surgical anatomy of 1
Oral cytology 67
Oral defects, reconstruction of 200, 224
Oral epithelial dysplasia 29
Oral health examination 265
Oral hygiene 125
Oral leukoplakia 66, 67
Oral lichen planus 31
   subtypes of 71
Oral mucosal
   defects, reconstructions of 213
   melanoma 315
Oral mucositis 287
Oral potentially malignant
      disorders 29
Oral premalignant lesions,
      management of 66
Oral rehabilitation 264
Oral squamous cell carcinoma,
      advanced 251
Oral submucosal fibrosis 17, 29, 66, 69, 70, 298
Oral tongue 9, 50*f*, 55, 167, 169, 179
Oral transit phase 273
Orbicularis oris muscle 1
Orbital fissure, inferior 5
Orbital invasion 43, 62
Orocutaneous fistula 152, 170, 197
Orofacial pain 285
   causes of 283
Oropharynx 177, 183, 256
Orthopantomogram 42, 142
Orthopantomography 271*f*
Ossifying fibroma 80, 88, 88*f*
Osteoblastoma 80, 92
Osteocutaneous flap 228
Osteoid
   osteoma 80, 92
   production of 94*f*
Osteoma 80, 92
   endosteal 92
   periosteal 92
Osteoradionecrosis 198, 199*f*, 249, 264, 268, 269, 269*f*, 269*t*, 288
   treatment of 268
Osteosarcoma 80, 93, 94, 94*f*, 95
   peripheral 80
Otalgia 11*f*
Ovary 13
Oxaliplatin 258

P

Paan 15, 17
   consumption, effects of 17*f*
Paclitaxel 252, 258, 284
Pain 64, 249, 283, 285, 289, 296
   assessment of 285
   causes of 284*t*
   management 260, 263
   mechanism of 283
Palatal defects 224
Palate 299, 300
Palliative care 283
   team 44
Palpation 299
Papillomas 29
Paradoxical maturation 29
Paramandibular disease 142
Parapharyngeal space 61
Parathyroid hormone 89
Parietal calvarium 4
Parotid
   bed tumor 242*f*
   gland 177, 246
Partial flap necrosis 197
Partial thickness lip defects 129
Passive jaw movement exercises 76
Pectoralis major
   flap 174
   muscle 225
Pembrolizumab 64, 259, 323
Pentoxifylline 70, 75
Perforator flaps 208
Perialar excision advancement
      flap 134*f*
Perineural extension 53*f*
Perineural invasion 35, 43, 60, 161, 162, 231, 318
Perineural spread 43, 62
Perinodal extension 60
Peripheral nervous system 61
Peronea magna 228
Peroxisome activator receptor
      gamma agonists 25
Phonation 280
Photodynamic therapy 69, 71
Physiotherapy 221
Pindborg tumor 82
Plasmacytoma, solitary 80, 98
Plate exposure 198, 199*f*

Platelet 119
  rich plasma 269
Platysma flap 138, 139f
Plica fimbriata 7
Polynuclear aromatic
      hydrocarbons 18
Polyphenol 25
Polyvinyl chloride 114, 117
Postchemotherapy 113
  dental management 270
Post-mandibular resection 271f
Post-oncosurgery 113
Postoperative adjuvant
    therapy 230
  treatment, basis of 319
Postoperative nursing care 122
Post-systemic therapy 313
Potassium 20
Power-Driven dermatome 204f
Precancerous lesions 66, 66t
Pre-chemotherapy dental
      assessment 269
Precursor lesions 29
Preoperative nursing care 119
Pre-radiation treatment 265
Primary systemic therapy 252, 311
Profunda artery perforator flap 220
Proliferative verrucous
      leukoplakia 29, 31, 66, 71
Proton beam therapy 320
Provitamin A 23
Pseudoaneurysm 260
Pterygoid plate 4, 81f
Pterygomaxillary fissure 5
Pterygopalatine fossa 55f
Punch biopsy 42
Pyriform sinus, apex of 177

Q

Quality assurance 238
Quality of life 58, 290, 291, 315
  poor 102
  radiation therapy instrument 291
Quality-adjusted life-years 291

R

Radial artery forearm flap 135f, 218f, 224, 226f

Radiation
  caries 267f
  therapy 73, 95, 101, 166, 169, 170, 264
    oncology group 75, 252
    postoperative 60, 161, 162, 168, 230, 234
    primary 161
    role of 161
Radical ablative surgery 95
Radical neck dissection 178, 184, 190
  development of 183
  limits of 190f
  modified 184
Radical radiation therapy 60, 239
Radiology, interventional 317
Radiotherapy 73, 106, 144, 230, 274, 284, 288, 315, 320, 322
  dental management during 266
  doses 248
  image-guided 245
  role of 146
Random pattern flap 204, 204f
Randomized controlled trials 239
Range of motion exercises 276, 277t
Reconstruction
  options for 60
  principles of 209
Reconstructive
  ladder 200f
  paradigm 200
  surgery 113, 170
  techniques 223
Recurrent head and neck cancer 255, 255b
  prognosis of 255
Red-glazed tongue 298, 301
Refeeding syndrome 103, 104, 105fc
Regional flaps 215, 223
Rehabilitation 61, 161, 210
  team 44
Reirradiation, role of 258
Re-radiation 63, 309, 320
  dose 320
Resection, principles of 59
Residual cancer 256t
  diagnosis of 256
Respiration 280, 281

Retinoid 20, 25
  signaling pathways 26f
Retinol 20
Retromolar extension 145
Retromolar trigone 1, 3, 51, 55, 140, 179, 213, 303
  cancer 140
  spread of 55f
Retropharyngeal node 54f
Rhomboid flap 207f
Robotic neck dissection 115, 191, 192f
Rotation flap 207f
Ryles tube care 124

S

Saliva, drooling of 198
Salivary gland 61, 287
  cancers 155
  damage 287
Salvage neck dissection 179
Salvage surgery 63, 255, 256b
  principles of 255
Sarcoma
  neurogenic 92
  osteogenic 155
Sarcomatous stroma 94f
Schwann cells 91
Schwannoma 80, 91
  malignant 98
Seizures 297
Selective neck dissection 157, 177, 178, 184, 189
Selenium 20, 23
Sensory 213
Sentinel lymph node 319
  biopsy 180
Seroma 197
Serum thyroid-stimulating hormone 162
Sialocele 198
Sialometaplasia, necrotizing 34, 35f
Simple linear wounds 208
Skin 1
  defects 60
  fibrosis 249
  grafts 129, 223
    full-thickness 203
    split-thickness 202
  involvement 318
  metastases 168
  reaction 170

Skull, base of 226
Small-volume bone 226
Smoking 102
Soft palate 224, 226
Soft tissue 177, 225, 274
   coverage 60
   defects of face 226
   dissection 157, 158
   loss 60
   reconstruction of 222
Speckled opaque foci 83*f*
Speech
   components of 280
   difficulty in 296
   impact 293
   poor 198
   therapy 273, 280, 281
      interventions 281
Sphenoid bone 4
   greater wing of 5
Spinal accessory nerve 184, 194, 194*f*
Spinal cord 246
Spindle cell carcinoma 29, 39
Split skin graft 174
Squamous cell 35
   carcinoma 12, 22, 29, 31, 31*f*, 35*f*, 36*f*, 44, 50, 66, 141, 151, 154, 179, 251
   conventional 39
   oral 28, 29, 37, 181*t*, 295
   oropharyngeal 20
   papillary 29, 33, 39
   staging of oral 49*t*, 52*b*
   subtypes of 29, 33
   types of 56*f*
   variants 39
   papilloma 29
Squamous dysplasia
   mild 30*f*
   moderate 30*f*
   severe 30*f*
Stacked wooden tongue depressors 76
Stellate ganglion block 287
Stensen's duct 2
Sternocleidomastoid muscle 183, 187, 194
Steroid 71
Stoma care 123
Stomach 13
Stomatitis, chemotherapy-induced 274

Submandibular dissection 187*f*
Submandibular nodes 176
Submandibular triangle clearance 186
Submental artery island flap 174
Submental flap 216
Submental nodes 176
Submental triangle clearance 186
Submitting neck dissection 191
Supraclavicular flap 174
Supraglottic swallow 276*f*
Supranotch tumor 147*f*
Supraomohyoid neck dissection 178, 189*f*, 192*f*
Surface mold brachytherapy 241, 242*f*
Surgery 169, 230, 284, 317
   role of 64, 144
Surgical
   anatomy 140, 153, 164, 213
   bed 248
   complications 170
   margins 46
   objectives 171
   principles 5, 8, 10
   reconstruction, principles of 200
   safety 121
      checklist 121
   steps 186
   technique 156, 171
   therapies 68
   tools 210
   treatment 77
Swallowing 273
   difficulty in 198
   exercise procedure 277, 279
   fiberoptic endoscopic evaluation of 275
   function, normal 273
   impact 293
   interventions 275
   maneuvers 276
   phases of 273*f*
   rehabilitation, goals of 275
Systemic therapy 258, 309, 311
   principles of 310

T

Tacrolimus 71
Tactile stimulation 277
Taste, loss of 170

Temporal bone
   squamous part of 5
   tympanic part of 5
Temporalis muscle 4
   flap 160, 216
Temporary prosthesis 270
Temporomandibular joint 11*f*, 246, 299
TheraBite jaw 277*f*
   motion rehabilitation system 76
TheraBite protocol 77
Thiazolidinediones 26
Thoracic duct injury 194
Thoracodorsal artery
   perforator flap 219
   scapular tip 160
Thoracoscopic surgery, video-assisted 197
Thyroid
   gland 177
   stimulating hormone 312
Thyromental distance 108, 109
Tissue
   autofluorescence 67
   expansion 208
Titanium
   plate, extrusion of 152
   reconstruction plate 174
TNM staging
   classification 45*t*, 48*t*
   nodal status in 47*t*
Tobacco 15
   chewing 15
   smoking 15
Tocopherol 23
Tongue 15, 164, 224, 232*f*, 247, 298, 300
   base of 9, 50*f*, 55*f*
   blood supply of 8*f*
   cancer of 163
   carcinoma 117, 241, 260, 301, 302
      spread of 302
   depressors 76
   deviation of tip of 296
   extrinsic muscle of 55
   flap 131, 132*f*, 215
   intrinsic muscles of 55
   isometric exercises 276
   management of 163
   mobilization 276
   movement of 41
   muscles of 10*f*

squamous cell carcinoma of 164
strengthening exercises 276
ulcers of 301
Tonsil 55f
Tracheostomy 7, 117
  complications after 274
  need for 171
  percutaneous 260, 262
  tube, care of 123
Transarterial embolization 260, 263
Transoral robotic surgery 114
Transverse myomucosal advancement 131f
Transverse vermilion advancement 130
Trigeminal nerve 128
  block 113
Trismus 73, 74, 78, 198, 249, 296, 298
  classification of 74, 75
  exercises for 76
  extra-articular causes of 74
  grades of 75
  intra-articular causes of 74
  prevention of 77
  problems with 74
  treatment of 75
Tube
  blockage, signs of 123
  dislodgement 124
  displacement 124
    signs of 124
  feeding, prophylactic 324
  obstruction 124
Tumors 3, 101, 173, 254, 322
  advanced 147
  bed margins 37
  benign
    epithelial odontogenic 79
    mesenchymal odontogenic 85
    nonodontogenic 88
  calcifying epithelial odontogenic 80, 82, 82f, 83
  category 45
  cells 34f
  deep infiltrative type of 60
  high grade of 60
  locoregionally advanced 168

malignant
  epithelial odontogenic 84
  mesenchymal odontogenic 86
  odontogenic 84
  peripheral nerve sheath 80, 98
  surface epithelial 29
mandibular 95
mesenchymal 80
mixed epithelial 80
  and mesenchymal odontogenic 87
necrosis factor 101
neurogenic 80, 91
nonodontogenic 80
odontogenic 79, 80
primary 32, 52, 230, 236, 247
proportion score 314
resection 173
second primary 23, 38
size 45
squamous odontogenic 80, 84
thickness 168, 232f

U

Ulcer 295
  aphthous 301
  carcinomatous 302
  chronic nonspecific 302
  dyspeptic 301
Ulcerative lesion 164f
Ultraviolet radiation 295
Union for international cancer control 166, 254
Unresectable tumors, chemoembolization of 260, 261
Upper alveolus
  and palate 153
  cancers of 154
Upper gingival-buccal cancers 154
Upper jugular nodes 176
Upper left canine 83f
Upper lip 128, 134f
  defects 131

V

Veins 213
  pterygoid plexus of 193

Venous drainage 3, 10, 141
Vermilion defect 130, 130f, 131, 132f
Verruca vulgaris 29
Verrucous carcinoma 29, 33, 39, 155
Vestibule 213
Videofluorography 275
Vincent's stomatitis 299
Viral markers 119
Visor flap 171
Visual analog scale 285
Vitamin
  A 20, 68
  C 20, 23, 68
  E 20, 23, 284
  water-soluble 68
Voice 293
Vomiting 249
  postoperative 111
von Recklinghausen's disease 91
Vortex approach 116
V-Y advancement flap 207f

W

Weaning criteria 124
Wedge biopsy 67
Weight loss 107, 249, 277
Wharton's duct 164
Workhorse flaps 225
Wound
  breakdown 170
  care 288
  closure 202
  malignant 288f, 289t
  necrotic 208

X

Xerostomia 170, 249, 264, 267, 274, 280, 287
X-ray mandible 42

Y

Yankauer's suction catheter 109

Z

Zarda 16, 17
Zygomaticus major muscle 5

EU GSPR Authorised Reprsentative
Logos Europe, 9 rue Nicolas Poussin
1700, La Rochelle, France
Phone: +33 (0) 6 67 93 73 78
E-mail: contact@logoseurope.eu

www.ingramcontent.com/pod-product-compliance
Ingram Content Group UK Ltd.
Pitfield, Milton Keynes, MK11 3LW, UK
UKHW050456150426
5217IPUK00025B/1713